Health Disparities in Contemporary Korean Society

Korean Communities across the World

Series Editor: Joong-Hwan Oh, Hunter College, CUNY

Korean Communities across the World publishes works that address aspects of (a) the Korean American community, (b) Korean society, (c) the Korean communities in other foreign lands, or (d) transnational Korean communities. In the field of (a) the Korean American community, this series welcomes contributions involving concepts such as Americanization, pluralism, social mobility, migration/immigration, social networks, social institutions, social capital, racism/discrimination, settlement, identity, or politics, as well as a specific topic related to family/marriage, gender roles, generations, work, education, culture, citizenship, health, ethnic community, housing, ethnic identity, racial relations, social justice, social policy, and political views, among others. In the field of (b) Korean society, this series embraces scholarship on current issues such as gender roles, age/aging, low fertility, immigration, urbanization, gentrification, economic inequality, high youth unemployment, sexuality, democracy, political power, social injustice, the nation's educational problems, social welfare, capitalism, consumerism, labor, health, housing, crime, environmental degradation, and the social life in the digital age and its impacts, among others. Contributors in the field of (c) Korean communities in other foreign lands are encouraged to submit works that expand our understanding about the formation, vicissitudes, and major issues of an ethnic Korean community outside of South Korea and the Unites States, such as cultural or linguistic retention, ethnic identity, assimilation, settlement patterns, citizenship, economic activities, family relations, social mobility, and racism/discrimination. Lastly, contributions relating to (d) transnational Korean communities may touch upon transnational connectivity in family, economy/finance, politics, culture, technology, social institutions, and people.

Newcomers and Global Migration in Contemporary South Korea: Across National Boundaries, edited by Sung-Choon Park and Joong-Hwan Oh

Health Disparities in Contemporary Korean Society: Issues and Subpopulations, edited by Sou Hyun Jang and Joong-Hwan Oh

Koreatowns: Exploring the Economics, Politics, and Identities of Korean Spatial Formation, by Jinwon Kim, Soo Mee Kim, and Stephen Suh

Korean International Students and the Making of Racialized Transnational Elites, by Sung-Choon Park

Transnational Mobility and Identity in and out of Korea, edited by Yonson Ahn

Korean Diaspora across the World: Homeland in History, Memory, Imagination, Media and Reality, edited by Eun-Jeong Han, Min Wha Han, and JongHwa Lee

Mediatized Transient Migrants: Korean Visa-Status Migrants' Transnational Everyday Lives and Media Use, by Claire Shinhea Lee

LA Rising: Korean Relations with Blacks and Latinos after Civil Unrest, by Kyeyoung Park

Medical Transnationalism: Korean Immigrants' Medical Tourism to Home Country, by Sou Hyun Jang

Transnational Return Migration of 1.5 Generation Korean New Zealanders: A Quest for Home, by Jane Yeonjae Lee

Transnational Communities in the Smartphone Age: The Korean Community in the Nation's Capital, edited by Dae Young Kim

Health Disparities in Contemporary Korean Society

Issues and Subpopulations

Edited by
Sou Hyun Jang and Joong-Hwan Oh

LEXINGTON BOOKS
Lanham • Boulder • New York • London

Published by Lexington Books
An imprint of The Rowman & Littlefield Publishing Group, Inc.
4501 Forbes Boulevard, Suite 200, Lanham, Maryland 20706
www.rowman.com

6 Tinworth Street, London SE11 5AL, United Kingdom

British Library Cataloguing in Publication Information Available

Library of Congress Cataloging-in-Publication Data

Names: Jang, Sou Hyun, editor. | Oh, Joong-Hwan, editor.
Title: Health disparities in contemporary Korean society : issues and subpopulations / edited by Sou Hyun Jang and Joong-Hwan Oh.
Description: Lanham : Lexington Books, [2020] | Series: Korean communities across the world | Includes bibliographical references and index. |
Identifiers: LCCN 2020031579 (print) | LCCN 2020031580 (ebook) | ISBN 9781793632104 (cloth) | ISBN 9781793632111 (epub)
Subjects: LCSH: Social medicine—Korea (South) | Health services Accessibility—Korea (South) | Public health—Korea (South) | Population—Health aspects.
Classification: LCC RA418.3.K6 H43 2020 (print) | LCC RA418.3.K6 (ebook) | DDC 362.1095195—dc23
LC record available at https://lccn.loc.gov/2020031579
LC ebook record available at https://lccn.loc.gov/2020031580

Contents

Acknowledgments

The purpose of this edited volume is to introduce central themes and issues around health disparities in contemporary Korean society. This work is intended for international readers who are less familiar with the development of this research field in Korean academia. We would like to thank Julie E. Kirsch, senior vice president and publisher at Rowman & Littlefield Publishing Group, Inc.; and Courtney Morales, editor at Lexington Books for their support in this project. We also acknowledge the support and assistance from staff members at Lexington Books who helped us with the publication process.

This edited volume informs the reader about factors associated with health disparities, such as socioeconomic status, social networks, and health insurance. It also highlights health disparities among various subgroups, such as employees, the elderly, children and adolescents, and female immigrant women and multiethnic youths. We would like to give special thanks to each author who permitted us to include his or her scholarly work in this edited volume, and who thoroughly examined the content around health disparities, suggesting some insightful policies aimed at tackling health disparities in contemporary Korean society. Finally, we would like to express our deepest gratitude to the Korea-based publishers who generously allowed us to include their published works. Without their support, this edited volume would not have been able to be shared with the world.

Introduction

South Korea (hereafter referred to as Korea) has experienced rapid economic and social changes since the late 1990s. Its financial crisis erupted in 1997, after which Korea received a financial aid package from the International Monetary Fund (IMF) until 2001. Since then, Korean society has been burdened with economic inequality (Im 2011). For example, the Gini coefficient, which measures the degree of income inequality in a country, has increased. Furthermore, since the so-called IMF era, Korean society has suffered from both high layoff and unemployment rates, decreased wages and household income, and an increased number of nonpermanent or temporary workers in the labor market (Im 2011; Kim 2005). Since 1997, households with lower incomes have experienced a quicker decrease in their annual incomes than households with higher incomes (Kim 2005). For example, households in the lowest income quintile experienced a 17.2 percent decrease in income between 1997 and 1998, while those in the highest quintile experienced only a 0.3 percent decrease during the same time period. Although it has been more than twenty years since the financial crisis of 1997, Korea is still in a state of shock due to economic inequality between its lower- and higher-income households (KOSIS 2016).

In addition, Korean society has encountered a great shift in its population composition in two ways. First, Korea is one of the world's fastest aging countries in terms of population distribution at the national level. Indeed, Korea obtained the status of an aging society in 2000. A nation is considered to be an aging society if the elderly population is above 10 percent (OECD 2007; Bae and Park 2009). A so-called aging society by 2018 (Ministry of the Interior and Safety 2017), Korea will enter a super-aged society by 2026 (Hyun et al. 2016). The proportion of the elderly population aged sixty-five years or older increased from 6.3 percent in 1997 to 15.7 percent in 2020

(Korean Statistical Information Service 2020) and is projected to be near 41.0 percent in 2060 (Statistics Korea 2018). Second, contemporary Korean society is no longer an ethnically homogeneous country, as it has recently experienced a steady rise in cultural and ethnic diversity with a growing number of immigrant women (most from other Asian countries such as China, Vietnam, Japan, and the Philippines) who married Korean men and their children. The number of such marriages almost doubled from about 94,000 in 2006 to 160,000 in 2018 (Statistics Korea 2019). Another consequence of the overall increase in intermarriages is that the number of multiethnic youths has also increased from slightly less than 5,000 in 2012 to more than 122,000 in 2018 (Statistics Korea and the Ministry of Gender Equality and Family 2019). Successfully combating racial and ethnic discrimination and social exclusion is an important task for Korean society in this new phase of population diversity (Lee et al. 2019).

Many books have examined the consequences and policy implications of economic inequality and social changes since the financial crisis of Korea. However, there are only a few books that address the influences of economic inequality and social changes on health disparities in Korea. These Korean-language books, which were not accessible to English-speaking readers, showed little interest in exploring the sources, characters, and consequences of health disparities within and across Korea's subpopulations or immigrants/minorities. Furthermore, most books on health disparities published in Korean academia rely only on the Korean translation of some English books on these issues, which identify approaches that would not necessarily apply to Korea.

Hence, this book aims to show the health disparities and health issues among subpopulations in contemporary Korean society and to introduce them to non-Korean-speaking readers worldwide. Its interdisciplinary approach covers a wide variety of themes and perspectives in health disparities in contemporary Korean society. This book is focused on answering the following central questions: What are the observed characteristics associated with disparities in health and health-care utilization in contemporary Korean society? What are the associated factors that cause these health disparities? Are socioeconomic factors associated with health disparities? If so, to what extent? Is economic inequality one of the important determining factors? Are there subpopulations (e.g., employees, elderly, children, and immigrants) at greater risk of worsening health status or difficulties in accessing health care? Are there particularly important health-related issues across different subpopulations? What are some policy implications for diminishing health disparities for each of these population groups?

To answer these questions, this book compiles relevant journal articles published between 2010 and 2019 in English via Korea-based publishers. The book is significant for the following reasons: first, it provides an opportunity for readers outside of Korea to understand the trends, essence, and different views of health disparities in Korean society, and why its economic inequality and other social forces are closely linked to the subject of health disparities. Second, the majority of books on health disparities in Korea arose from public health disciplines. This is why there needs to be a comprehensive volume that uses the lens of social science to address health disparities influenced by diverse socioeconomic factors. Finally, this book will expand the scope of health disparities among not only Koreans but also different subpopulations, including immigrants who recently settled in Korea.

THE FOCUS AND CONTENT OF CHAPTERS

This book has an introductory chapter, followed by two parts with fifteen chapters. Part I, "Disparities in Health and Health-care Utilization," examines the relationship between health disparities and socioeconomic factors (chapters 1 and 2). Part I also includes disparities in health insurance and health-care utilization, such as how catastrophic payments and poverty influence health care over the years (chapter 3), and the factors associated with health-care utilization among medical aid beneficiaries (chapter 4).

Chapter 1 finds that socioeconomic status is related to self-rated health status among Koreans; those who have higher educational attainment and higher income report better health. As indicated earlier, the labor market structure has changed since 1997, with an increased number of nonpermanent workers. Regarding employment status, a frequently used measure for socioeconomic status (along with educational attainment and income), chapter 1 also finds that nonpermanent employees, who are likely to be female, less educated, and with lower job satisfaction and job stability, tend to have worse self-reported health compared to their permanent employee counterparts. By contrast, chapter 2 finds that socioeconomic status (e.g., educational attainment, household income, employment status, and homeownership) is not significantly associated with self-rated health status among Koreans in Seoul. Rather, it focuses on the impact of social capital on health, finding that the cognitive dimension of social capital (e.g., a higher level of trust) is positively associated with health and well-being, whereas the structural dimension (e.g., organizational membership and political participation) did not have any effect on health and well-being among Koreans.

National health insurance in Korea, which was enacted in 1963, enforced since 1977, and achieved universal coverage in 1989, is a single-payer program (Jeong 2011). Despite the universal coverage of national health insurance, chapter 3 shows how catastrophic payments are more likely to occur among poorer households who tend to utilize drugs and outpatient care, while richer households tend to utilize inpatient and dental care. Chapter 4 examines individual- and group-level factors associated with health-care service utilization among Koreans who receive medical aid, which was introduced in 1977 to help poor Koreans receive needed health care. Unlike previous studies that focused on individual-level factors, chapter 4 suggests that group-level approaches should be considered because the social deprivation index, the number of beneficiaries, and case managers within the region were found to be associated with health-care service utilization among medical aid beneficiaries.

Part II, "Health Disparities among Different Population Groups," examines the sources of health disparities within and among different subpopulations, including employees (chapters 5–9), the elderly (chapters 10, 11), children and adolescents (chapters 12, 13), and female marriage immigrants and multiethnic youths (chapters 14, 15). Since the financial crisis, many Korean companies have switched from employing permanent workers to hiring non-permanent or temporary workers. Employees often encounter worse working conditions once they fill those roles (Kim 2003). Chapters 5–7 investigate how employees' declining working conditions influence health disparities. In particular, long working hours, night shifts, and working on-call are negatively related to employees' health. For example, employees who work more than sixty hours (chapter 5), who work night shifts (chapter 6), and work on-call (chapter 7) are more likely to have worse health status than employees who work less than forty hours and do not take on night shifts or on-call hours.

Chapters 8 and 9 focus on issues related to older employees' health. The increased number of older employees and factors related to their employment and working conditions are other challenges that face contemporary Korean society. Korea already has a high proportion of older employees (45 percent) compared to other countries (25 percent of Organization for Economic Co-operation and Development (OECD) average), but the proportion of older employees is expected to increase in the coming years (OECD 2018). Most companies in Korea set a mandatory age of retirement at sixty. However, the average age of retirement from one's core career is 49.1 years, and full retirement age is sixty-eight (National Assembly Research Service 2018). After retiring from their core careers, older employees tend to seek and maintain poor-quality jobs with low-job security; thus, temporary jobs are concentrated among the elderly (OECD 2018). In this vein, chapter 8 finds that an individual's socioeconomic and health characteristics as well as the type of occupation, employment status, and working hours are related to older employees' health-related quality of life. Chapter 9 shows that older employees in elementary and skilled manual occupations are at higher risk of being exposed to job-specific hazards, work-related musculoskeletal disorders, and general fatigue.

As mentioned earlier, the proportion of the elderly has rapidly increased in Korea's population. According to a report by Statistics Korea (2018), more elderly self-reported poor health status (39.7 percent) than good (37.0 percent) and fair (23.3 percent). Environmental satisfaction, including the level of safety, natural environment, and traffic conditions, is positively associated with subjective health-related quality among community elders in Korea (chapter 10). Chapter 11 explains the relationship between elderly Koreans' health status and their sexual satisfaction, which was mediated by limitations in independent living and how relationships vary by gender.

According to the OECD (2007), the female employment rate in Korea (52.5 percent) is lower than the OECD average (56.1 percent), but more female workers (77 percent) overwork (more than forty hours a week) than the average female workers among OECD countries (49 percent). Employees' long working hours influence not only their own health status, as described in chapter 5, but also the health of their family members. Chapter 12 finds that a mother's working hours are related to Korean children's health status, especially their obesity, but in opposite directions according to gender. Considering the context of contemporary Korean society, discussion involves possible explanations of why boys with overworking mothers are at a lower risk of being obese than girls with overworking mothers. In addition to the mother's working conditions, subjective socioeconomic status (e.g., subjective family economic status) is found to have a greater effect on the health of adolescents than objective socioeconomic status (e.g., parents' educational attainment and family affluence scale) (chapter 13).

Finally, this book discusses health-related factors among female marriage immigrants and multiethnic youth, whose numbers have increased in contemporary Korean society. Chapter 14 compares health status and health risks among female marriage immigrants from their origin countries, including Vietnam, China, the Philippines, Japan, and Cambodia. In general, female marriage immigrants from Vietnam report a lower prevalence of diseases than other female marriage immigrant ethnic groups. As the number of female marriage immigrants increased, the number of multiethnic youth has also increased. Most were born in Korea with a Korean-born parent and a foreign spouse (often from China or Southeast Asian Countries), but they are at higher risk of having mental illnesses such as depression, social anxiety, and suicide attempts. By systematically reviewing fifty-four articles on mental health among multiethnic youth, chapter 15 emphasizes the importance of sociodemographic factors, familial factors, social relationships, and cultural adjustment, and indicates the need for future interventions.

IMPLICATIONS AND SUGGESTIONS FOR FUTURE STUDIES

This book examines various factors related to health disparities among diverse groups of people in contemporary Korean society. To reduce health disparities in contemporary Korean society, we offer suggestions for future studies as well as policy implications. From a macroperspective, it seems critical that tackling differences in key demographic and socioeconomic statuses such as education, employment status, working conditions, income, age, gender, race and ethnicity, nativity, and social support should accompany the enactment of related social policies to mitigate the severity of health disparities. It would be difficult to reduce health disparities without any changes in a larger social structure because an individual's health is not only solely influenced by his or her biological factors but also shaped by various social factors. Thus, policies to reduce health disparities will not be effective unless efforts are made to reduce socioeconomic disparities.

From a microperspective, intervention studies are needed to practically reduce health disparities in Korea. Interventions to change individuals' perceptions and health behaviors are common in the field of public health, but not in social sciences. Since most chapters in this book are in the social sciences field, effective intervention for health disparities is less of a focus. However, most chapters deal with the need and the significance of intervention studies as ways to reduce health disparities, especially for populations at greater risk of being sick or underutilizing health care. We believe that even social scientists should pay more attention to intervention studies associating various social factors with health issues ultimately to enhance their broad understanding of both health inequality and equity in contemporary Korean society. In particular, health promotion programs at different places targeting different vulnerable groups could be a good strategy. For example, workplace-based health promotion programs at small workplaces that offer lower salaries, limited welfare, and worse working conditions (Bae 2005) would be helpful for employees at high risk of experiencing job-specific hazards and work-related disorders. Moreover, developing and disseminating linguistic and culturally tailored health promotion programs would be beneficial for immigrants and minority groups who have not been assimilated into Korean society.

We hope this book will provide a strong foundation for the development of future policies and interventions to reduce health disparities for disadvantaged and marginalized groups in contemporary Korean society.

Part I

DISPARITIES IN HEALTH AND HEALTH-CARE UTILIZATION

Chapter 1

Association between Employment Status and Self-Rated Health

Korean Working Conditions Survey

Kimin Kwon, Jae Bum Park,
Kyung-Jong Lee, and Yoon-Sik Cho

BACKGROUND

With[1] the global emergence of policies emphasizing labor flexibility, such as globalization and neoliberalism, which started several decades ago, the number of nonpermanent workers has increased [1]. In Korea, following the 1997 economic crisis, the labor structure changed with greater flexibility in the labor market, and this effect continues to this day. In this regard, employment status in the labor market shows diverse patterns. In particular, nonpermanent positions are increasing, and so too is the ratio of nonpermanent workers to permanent workers, which means that nonpermanent positions have come to play an important role in the labor market [2]. According to a report by Statistics Korea, the percentage of nonpermanent workers among all paid employees was 35.5 percent as of the third quarter of 2014. The reported conversion rate of nonpermanent workers to permanent workers was 22.4 percent, and the hourly wage of nonpermanent workers was just 64 percent of that of permanent workers, which is markedly lower than other Organization for Economic Co-operation and Development member countries [3]. An increase in the number of nonpermanent workers causes a variety of problems, and research on this topic is being actively conducted.

One study on several occupational groups reported that unstable employment negatively affects perceived health status [4]. Nonpermanent work is accompanied by job insecurity, income inequality, and the sense of loss in job stability, and the associated anxiety negatively affects health. Unstable employment plays a role in reducing social safety and stability, and causes problems related to time, standing within the workplace, welfare, and low wages.

However, according to epidemiological investigations published to date, the effects of unstable employment on health have not been consistent. The results of studies reporting harmful health effects of unstable employment show that transition from a permanent position to a nonpermanent position causes job insecurity and anxiety, which not only negatively affects an individual's marriage, work motivation, and psychological health, such as worries, depression, and stress but also has a large effect on family and group health [5–7]. Furthermore, compared to permanent positions, nonpermanent positions are associated with a harmful work environment, such as simple and repetitive tasks, and sociopsychologically disadvantageous work characteristics [8]. Most nonpermanent jobs have poorer work conditions, and long work hours and overtime work are known to be associated with deterioration in subjective health status and sociopsychological health [9]. Nonpermanent work decreases job satisfaction, increases health risks due to drinking or smoking, and affects mortality due to various cancers and causes. In a study conducted in Finland, the mortality rate of nonpermanent workers was 1.2–1.6 higher than that of permanent employees [2].

However, other cross-sectional studies did not report an association between nonpermanent employment and negative health effects [10–12].

Currently, the number of nonpermanent employees is increasing in Korea, and therefore it is necessary to investigate the actual difference in health status due to nonpermanent work. However, the majority of studies to date were conducted in Europe or North America and reports on unstable employment and accompanying health indicators in Korea are lacking. This is likely because there have not yet been many investigations on work environment and its effects on health, and there is no formalized questionnaire to determine health status.

We assessed self-rated health, reasoning that subjective health is determined by the environment and sociostatistical characteristics and that it could be considered a comprehensive health indicator by previous studies [13–17]. Therefore, based on the data from the third Korean Working Conditions Survey, measured using a structured questionnaire tool on workers nationwide, we aimed to understand the reason.

METHODS

Study Population

This study used data from the 2011 Korean Working Conditions Survey, the third survey of the Occupational Safety and Health Research Institute (previous surveys were conducted in 2006 and 2010). Data were collected on employees older than fifteen years of age living in sixteen cities or provinces (including Jeju Island) in the Republic of Korea. Trained interviewers collected data from each respondent. A total of 50,032 respondents met the criteria and were classified as employers, self-employed workers, paid workers, unpaid family workers, or others. We included data from 34,783 respondents, excluding employers, self-employed workers, unpaid family workers, others, and five respondents for whom there was incomplete data.

Subjects

Gender, age, educational level, monthly household income, alcohol, and smoking were chosen as the variables of the sociodemographic characteristics. Classification of employment status in this study was based on response to the question in the Korean Working Conditions Survey "What is your position at your workplace among the following?" Those who responded as "(1) Permanent worker" were defined as permanent employees, and those who responded as "(2) Temporary worker" or "(3) Daily worker" were defined as nonpermanent workers.

Subjective health status was assessed by self-rated health and was based on response to the question, "How is your health in general? Would you say it is . . . " Those who responded as "Very good" or "Good" were defined as having good subjective health status, and those who responded as "Fair" or "Bad" or "Very bad" were defined as having poor subjective health status.

Subjects were divided into nondrinkers, those who drank the moderate amount of one to two glasses of soju less than one to two times a week, and those who drink more than that. Subjects were divided into nonsmokers, those who smoked in the past but did not at the time of questioning, and current smokers.

Using the Korean Standard Classification of Occupations, occupations were classified as follows: white-collar jobs—professional technical jobs, senior management jobs, and office jobs; pink-collar jobs—sales jobs and service jobs; and blue-collar jobs—skilled jobs, semiskilled jobs, unskilled jobs, and agriculture and forestry jobs [15].

In terms of the work environment, we analyzed work hours, shift work, occupational group, tenure, job satisfaction, and job instability. Work hours were classified according to the Labor Standards Act, with fifty-two hours used as the standard, including forty legal working hours and twelve overtime work hours. Weekly work hours were divided into less than forty hours, more than forty but less than fifty-two hours, and more than fifty-two hours. Those who responded "Yes" to the question "I am a shift worker" were defined as shift workers, and those who answered "No" were defined as non-shift workers. Tenure was classified into less than one year, between one and ten years, and more than ten years. Job satisfaction was identified through the question "is satisfied in the working environment." Job instability was identified through the "I, within the next six months, would be to lose this job" question.

Work hazards were categorized as physical, ergonomic hazards. Respondents were asked how often they are exposed to physical, chemical, biological, and ergonomic factors while working. Exposures to ergonomic factors were collected from one of seven choices as follows: (1) throughout the entire work, (2) throughout nearly all of the work, (3) throughout three-fourths of the work, (4) throughout half of the work, (5) throughout one-fourth of the work, (6) hardly exposed, or (7) never exposed. The respondents who answered either answers one through five, as listed above, were regarded as being exposed to work hazards. Physical hazards were exposures to vibrations from hand tools or machinery, and to noises that cause people to communicate in a very loud voice. Ergonomic hazards were being exposed to a tiring or painful posture, having to lift or move people, having to lift or move heavy things, standing or walking for extended periods or performing repetitive hand or arm movements.

Data Analysis

We analyzed the difference in the sociodemographic characteristics and work environment between permanent and nonpermanent employees as well as the difference in the sociodemographic characteristics and work environment according to self-rated health. After an adjustment for sociodemographic characteristics, working conditions, and working environments, a logistic regression analysis was conducted to determine if any sociodemographic characteristics, working conditions, or working environments were associated with self-rated health. The survey weighting was carried out on the basis of the economically active population. All analyses were performed using SPSS for Windows version 19.0 (SPSS Inc., Chicago, IL, USA).

RESULTS

General Characteristics of the Study Participants

The employment status of the study subjects was divided into permanent and nonpermanent jobs. Out of the total paid workers, the number of permanent and nonpermanent employees was 27,564 (79.2 percent) and 7,219 (20.8 percent), respectively. The rate of nonpermanent employees in this study was lower than the 35.5 percent reported by Statistics Korea for the third quarter of

2014. The increase in nonpermanent employees observed in 2014 compared to in 2011 when the Korean Working Conditions Survey was conducted, can be explained, according to the analysis of Statistics Korea, by the effects of increased part-time employment of women with career discontinuity and the elderly population as the government implemented policies expanding flexible jobs. When we compared the difference in each factor according to employment status, more women than men, and more older individuals than younger individuals, had nonpermanent jobs. Distribution of nonpermanent jobs was significantly higher in subjects with a lower education level or a lower-income level (table 1.1).

In terms of work environment, distribution of nonpermanent jobs was significantly higher in subjects with shorter working hours, while in terms of occupational classification, it was highest in the blue-collar group. With shorter tenure, lower job satisfaction and the nonpermanent job distribution was higher. For physical hazard exposure, nonpermanent workers were more likely to be exposed to vibrations from hand tools or machinery and noise. For

Table 1.1 Comparison of the Sociodemographic Characteristics of Study Subjects According to Employment Status

		Employment Status		
Characteristics		*Permanent n=27,564*	*Nonpermanent n=7,219*	*P-value*
Sex	Male	16,919 (61.4)	3,612 (50.0)	<0.001
	Female	10,645 (38.6)	3,607 (50.0)	
Age (years)	≤29	5,652 (20.5)	1,735 (24.0)	<0.001
	30–39	8,837 (32.1)	1,042 (14.4)	
	40–49	7,740 (28.1)	1,521 (21.1)	
	50–59	4,228 (15.3)	1,674 (23.2)	
	≥60	1,108 (4.0)	1,247 (17.3)	
Education	≤Middle School	1,637 (5.9)	2,049 (28.4)	<0.001
	High School	9,207 (33.4)	3,556 (49.3)	
	≥Technical college	16,720 (60.7)	1,615 (22.4)	
Income (10,000 won/month)	<100	1,473 (5.3)	2,789 (38.6)	<0.001
	100–199	10,471 (38.0)	3,232 (44.8)	
	200–299	8,764 (31.8)	964 (13.4)	
	300–399	4,497 (16.3)	170 (2.4)	
	≥400	2,359 (8.6)	64 (0.9)	
Smoking	No	14,684 (53.3)	4,499 (62.3)	<0.001
	Past	3,020 (11.0)	661 (9.2)	
	Smoking	9,860 (35.8)	2,059 (28.5)	
Drinking	No	5,454 (19.8)	2,436 (33.7)	<0.001
	Optimal	3,543 (12.9)	852 (11.8)	
	Excessive	18,567 (67.4)	3,931 (54.5)	

Table 1.2 Comparison of the Working Environment of Study Subjects According to Employment Status

		Employment Status		
Characteristics		*Permanent n=27,564*	*Nonpermanent n=7,219*	P-*value*
Labor time per week (hours)	<40	10,764 (39.1)	3,664 (50.8)	<0.001
	40–52	9,482 (34.4)	1,576 (21.8)	
	>52	7,318 (26.5)	1,978 (27.4)	
Work type	White Collar	12,486 (45.3)	718 (9.9)	<0.001
	Pink Collar	6,970 (25.3)	2,674 (37.0)	
	Blue Collar	8,107 (29.4)	3,827 (53.0)	
Shift work	No	2,689 (90.2)	726 (89.9)	0.442
	Yes	24,875 (9.8)	6,492 (10.1)	
Tenure	<1	2,649 (9.6)	2,893 (40.1)	<0.001
	1–10	20,075 (72.8)	3,689 (51.1)	
	>10	4,840 (17.6)	638 (8.8)	
Job satisfaction	No	6,298 (22.8)	3,062 (42.4)	<0.001
	Yes	21,266 (77.2)	4,157 (57.6)	
Job instability	No	26,677 (96.8)	6,086 (84.3)	<0.001
	Yes	887 (3.2)	1,133 (15.7)	
Physical factors				
Noise	No	20,654 (74.9)	5,107 (70.7)	<0.001
	Yes	69,106 (25.1)	2,112 (29.3)	
Vibration	No	21,791 (79.1)	5,199 (72.0)	<0.001
	Yes	5,773 (20.9)	2,020 (28.0)	
Ergonomic factors				
Positions	No	14,695 (53.3)	2,661 (36.9)	<0.001
	Yes	12,868 (46.7)	4,558 (63.1)	
Moving people	No	25,160 (91.3)	6,353 (88.0)	<0.001
	Yes	2,403 (8.7)	866 (12.0)	
Moving heavy loads	No	19,219 (69.7)	3,523 (48.8)	<0.001
	Yes	8,345 (30.3)	3,696 (51.2)	
Standing	No	12,127 (44.0)	1,579 (21.9)	<0.001
	Yes	15,437 (56.0)	5,640 (78.1)	
Repetitive hand or arm	No	9,674 (35.1)	1,592 (22.1)	<0.001
	Yes	17,890 (64.9)	5,626 (77.9)	

ergonomic hazard exposure, nonpermanent workers tended to report a higher exposure to all of the surveyed items than permanent workers were (table 1.2).

The Relationship between Relevant Variables and Self-Rated Health

We investigated the characteristics of the subjects according to differences in self-rated heath. The number of subjects with good and poor self-rated health was 25,032 (72 percent) and 9,751 (28 percent), respectively. Among the general characteristics, a statistically significant difference in self-rated

Table 1.3 Comparison of Sociodemographic Characteristics of Study Subjects According to Self-rated Health

		Self-rated Health		
		Good n=25,032	Poor n=9,751	
Characteristics				P-*value*
Sex	Male	14,796 (59.1)	5,735 (58.8)	0.617
	Female	10,236 (40.9)	4,016 (41.2)	
Age (years)	≤29	6,078 (24.3)	1,309 (13.4)	<0.001
	30–39	7,537 (30.1)	2,342 (24.0)	
	40–49	6,590 (26.3)	2,670 (27.4)	
	50–59	3,642 (14.5)	2,260 (23.2)	
	≥60	1,185 (4.7)	1,170 (12.0)	
Education	≤Middle school	1,901 (7.6)	1,758 (18.3)	<0.001
	High school	9,016 (36.0)	3,747 (38.4)	
	≥Technical college	14,116 (56.4)	4,219 (43.3)	
Income (10,000 won/month)	<100	2,776 (11.1)	1,487 (15.2)	<0.001
	100–199	9,706 (38.8)	3,996 (41.0)	
	200–299	7,267 (29.0)	2,461 (25.2)	
	300–399	3,462 (13.8)	1,205 (12.4)	
	≥400	1,821 (7.3)	602 (6.2)	
Smoking	No	13,824 (55.2)	5,359 (55.0)	0.045
	Past	2,587 (10.3)	1,095 (11.2)	
	Smoking	8,622 (34.4)	3,297 (33.8)	
Drinking	No	5,512 (22.0)	2,379 (24.4)	<0.001
	Optimal	3,270 (13.1)	1,125 (11.5)	
	Excessive	16,250 (64.9)	6,247 (64.1)	

health was found for age, education level, income, smoking, and drinking. Health status was better when the subject was younger or the education level was higher (table 1.3).

In terms of work environment, a statistically significant difference in self-rated health was found in weekly work hours, occupational groups, shift work, and tenure. For weekly work hours, more subjects with a shorter work time rated their health status as good, and more subjects with a longer work time rated their health status as poor. For occupation groups, the ratio of subjects with a good self-rated health was highest in the white-collar group and lowest in the blue-collar group. Self-rated health was relatively higher in non-shift workers than in shift workers. Self-rated health was better with shorter tenure, satisfaction of job, stability of job. For physical hazard exposure, self-rated health was poor in both vibration and noise exposures. For ergonomic hazard exposure, self-rated health was poor in all of the surveyed item exposures (table 1.4).

In addition, the risk that the self-rated health of nonpermanent workers was poor was 1.67 times higher than for permanent workers if uncorrected, 1.3 times higher if sociodemographic factors were corrected for, and 1.2

Table 1.4 Comparison of Working Environment of Study Subjects According to Self-rated Health

Characteristics		*Self-rated Health* *Good* *n=25,032*	*Poor* *n=9,751*	*P-value*
Labor time per week (hours)	<40	10,920 (43.6)	3,508 (36.0)	<0.001
	40–52	7,857 (31.4)	3,201 (32.8)	
	>52	6,255 (25.0)	3,042 (31.2)	
Work type	White collar	10,223 (40.8)	2,981 (30.6)	<0.001
	Pink collar	7,050 (28.2)	2,595 (26.6)	
	Blue collar	7,759 (31.0)	4,175 (42.8)	
Shift work	No	2,367 (9.5)	1,049 (10.8)	<0.001
	Yes	22,666 (90.5)	8,702 (89.2)	
Tenure	<1	4,071 (16.3)	1,470 (15.1)	<0.001
	1–10	17,164 (68.6)	6,599 (67.7)	
	>10	3,796 (15.2)	1,682 (17.2)	
Employment status	Permanent	20,464 (81.8)	7,100 (72.8)	
	Precarious	4,568 (18.2)	2,651 (27.2)	
Job satisfaction	No	5,400 (21.6)	3,960 (40.6)	<0.001
	Yes	19,632 (78.4)	5,790 (59.4)	
Job instability	No	23,747 (94.9)	9,016 (92.5)	<0.001
	Yes	1,285 (5.1)	735 (7.5)	
Physical factors				
Noise	No	19,792 (79.1)	7,198 (73.8)	<0.001
	Yes	5,240 (20.9)	2,553 (26.2)	
Vibration	No	18,953 (75.7)	6,808 (69.8)	<0.001
	Yes	6,079 (24.3)	2,943 (30.2)	
Ergonomic factors				
Positions	No	13,655 (54.6)	3,701 (38.0)	<0.001
	Yes	11,377 (45.4)	6,050 (62.0)	
Moving people	No	22,799 (91.1)	8,714 (89.4)	<0.001
	Yes	2,233 (8.9)	1,036 (10.6)	
Moving heavy loads	No	17,235 (68.9)	5,507 (56.5)	<0.001
	Yes	7,797 (31.1)	4,244 (43.5)	
Standing	No	10,320 (41.2)	3,386 (34.7)	<0.001
	Yes	14,712 (58.8)	6,365 (65.3)	
Repetitive hand or arm	No	8,501 (34.0)	2,766 (28.4)	<0.001
	Yes	16,531 (66.0)	6,985 (71.6)	

times higher if both sociodemographic factors, and work environments and work hazards were corrected for (table 1.5).

DISCUSSION

In this study, to determine the health effects of nonpermanent employment, we investigated the relationship between self-rated heath status and

Table 1.5 Odds Ratio of Poor Self-Rated Health on Employment Status from Logistic Regression Models

		Crude (95 percent CI)	*Model 1[a] (95 percent CI)*	*Model 2[b] (95 percent CI)*
Employment status	Permanent	1	1	1
	Nonpermanent	1.67 (1.58–1.77)	1.30 (1.22–1.39)	1.20 (1.12–1.29)

CI confidence interval.
[a]Adjusted for sex, age, education, income, smoking, drinking.
[b]Adjusted for sex, age, education, income, smoking, drinking, labor time per week, work type, shift work, tenure, work environment, and all variables estimating one's working condition and physical, ergonomic factors.

employment status. This research demonstrates a significant relationship between employment status and perceived health, which is in line with previous studies [18]. A statistically significant difference was observed in all characteristics of the subjects depending on employment status, except for shift work. A higher percentage of people was engaged in nonpermanent jobs if they were older, less educated, or earned less income and exposed to various work hazard which was similar to the results of a previous report in Korea [6]. Also, the proportion of precarious workers who perceived themselves as not healthy was significantly higher than that of permanent workers.

Although the positive relationship between employment status and perceived health has been well established through previous research, in this study, we have examined the differences and the reasons. Even after adjustment for covariates, the odds of self-rated health were worse among nonpermanent workers than that among permanent workers. Therefore, employment status may influence these differences. Moreover, significant differences were found for the working environments, job satisfaction, job instability, and ergonomic hazards between nonpermanent and permanent workers. Working environments, job satisfaction, job instability, and ergonomic hazards were poorer than permanent workers in nonpermanent workers.

These differences in self-rated health may be considered because of the difference in the factors according to the employment status. In the previous study, precarious workers were found to be in a lower socioeconomic position and to have worse health status. By further controlling for sociodemographic covariates, the odds ratios were attenuated but remained significant. Job satisfaction, especially as related to job insecurity, and monthly wage further attenuated the effects [19]. The literature finds that a favorable work environment and high job security lead to better health conditions. Being employed with appropriate working conditions plays a protective role on physical health and psychiatric disorders [20].

Another study explored the pathways and mechanisms of the relation between employment conditions and health inequalities. Pathways, linking employment to health inequalities, were closely connected to hazardous working conditions (material and social deprivation, lack of social protection, and job insecurity), excessive demands, and unattainable work effort, with little power and few rewards (in salaries, fringe benefits, or job stability) [21]. In this study, physical and ergonomic hazards were associated with self-rated health.

In particular, workers in lower classes, with lower educational and occupational status, were more likely to report poor self-rated health. And physical workloads and other typical blue-collar job characteristics were found to be much more common among the lower classes. Therefore, blue-collar job characteristics contributed substantially to the social gradient found in general and physical health outcomes [22]. And precarious employment was associated with a high prevalence of occupational injuries, higher mortality rate, and inferior degree of mental health [23].

Lack of job satisfaction and job insecurity can be considered reasons for these health effects [24]. In the workers characteristics in this study, more nonpermanent workers were found among the subjects with less education, lower income, or those who engaged in manual labor. In fact, these characteristics are thought to have influenced subjective health status and job-related symptoms. In a study conducted in Japan, there was a difference in occupational group, tenure, work hours, marriage, and firm size between permanent and nonpermanent employees, and the nonpermanent employee group showed a poorer self-rated health and complained of musculoskeletal symptoms at a higher rate [25]. In another study that investigated specific job-related symptoms, nonpermanent jobs were associated with fatigue, back pain, and muscle pain [11]. In particular, in a study that classified jobs into permanent, nonpermanent, full-time, and part-time employment before analysis, deterioration of health was highest in full-time nonpermanent workers [26].

The results of previous study showed that a corresponding positive outcome based on self-assessed health was greater for employees that changed from precarious to nonprecarious jobs and for male employees with precarious jobs [27].

There is a possibility that the recognition of the state is insufficient because of the time and economic reasons. Workers with precarious employment, most notably hourly and dispatched workers, had a lower rate of health check-ups compared with full-time workers in permanent positions [28].

Although in terms of the general characteristics of the subjects, more men than women held permanent jobs, there was no difference in self-rated health between them. In this study, in terms of age-dependent effects, self-rated health was better for younger workers, and distribution of permanent employees was highest for subjects in their thirties. In particular, in workers over sixty years old, self-rated health of permanent employees was markedly decreased, which was consistent with the results of another study [13] on age-specific self-rated health. This indicated that job security and work environment for the elderly are poor in Korea.

Due to the nature of this research as a cross-sectional study, it has limitations in demonstrating causality between employment status and self-rated health. In addition, a change in self-rated health in one year cannot be an additional predictor [15] and can be considered as a temporary health status indicator at the time of survey. As mentioned above, although self-rated health has been used in various studies in the past, it is difficult to compare different studies because there is no systematic measurement tool assessing health status, and responders answer subjectively. Another limitation is that a self-reported questionnaire is used instead of objective measurements such as blood and imaging tests. In addition, since marital status, which can affect subjective health status, was not included in the Working Condition Survey, it could not be included as a variable for correction, which is another limitation.

In terms of the strengths of this study, it included a large population targeted in the Working Condition Survey, and approximately 50,000 samples were surveyed nationwide, unlike other domestic studies on health issues of nonpermanent workers. Therefore, it can be a representative study. In addition, since trained surveyors used a structured questionnaire for the investigation, the error in arbitrary interpretation of the questionnaire was minimized.

In this study, the self-rated health of nonpermanent workers was poorer than that of permanent workers, which further reinforces the existing hypothesis [29] that more health problems occur in nonpermanent employees than in permanent employees. Recognizing that nonpermanent workers are exposed to physical, mental, and social problems, we should discuss various ways to improve treatment of nonpermanent workers and solve the imbalance in employment status. Furthermore, in future studies, a systematic method to measure health status should be established, and a more in-depth study should be conducted with objective measurements.

CONCLUSION

This study was conducted to investigate the association between self-rated health and employment status based on the third Korea Working Condition Survey conducted in 2011. Perceived health was found to be worse in the nonpermanent workers than permanent workers. The inequalities between permanent and nonpermanent workers will be reduced and improve the working environments of nonpermanent workers.

NOTE

1. This chapter was previously published as Kwon, Kimin, Jae Bum Park, Kyung-Jong Lee, and Yoon-Sik Cho. "Association between employment status and self-rated health: Korean working conditions survey." *Annals of Occupational and Environmental Medicine* 28, no. 1 (2016): 43.

REFERENCES

1. Olsen KM. "The role of nonstandard workers in client organizations." *Ind Relat.* 2006; 61: 93–117.
2. Kivimaki M, Vahtera J, Virtanen M, Elovainio M, Pentti J, Ferrie JE, et al. "Temporary employment and risk of overall and cause-specific mortality." *Am J Epidemiol.* 2003; 158 (7): 663–8.
3. Statistics Korea. *Employed Persons by Status of Worker*, 2015. http://www.kosis.kr. Accessed March 2, 2015.
4. Hadden WC, Muntaner C, Benach J, Gimeno D, Benavides FG. "A glossary for the social epidemiology of work organisation: part 3, terms from the sociology of labour markets." *J Epidemiol Commun Health.* 2007; 61 (1): 6–8.
5. Bartely M, Ferrie J. "Glossary: Unemployment, job insecurity, and health." *J Epidemiol Commun Health.* 2001; 55: 776–81.
6. Kim IH, Paek DM, Cho SI. "Does non-standard work affect health?" *J Prev Med Public Health.* 2005; 38 (3): 337–44.
7. Marmot MG. "Job insecurity in a broader social and health context; Labour market changes and job insecurity: A challenge for social welfare and health promotion." *WHO Reg Publ Eur Ser.* 1999; 81: 1–9.
8. O'Campo P, Eaton WW, Muntaner C. "Labor marker experience, work organization, gender inequalities and health status: results from a prospective analysis of US employed women." *Soc Sci Med.* 2004; 58 (3): 585–94.
9. Robone S, Jones A, Rice N. "Contractual conditions, working conditions and their impact on health and well-being." *Eur J Health Econ.* 2011; 12 (5): 429–44.
10. Benach J, Gimeno D, Benavides FG, Martínez JM, Torné MM. "Types of employment and health in the European Union: changes from 1995 to 2000." *Eur J Public Health.* 2004; 14 (3): 314–21.
11. Benavides F, Benach J, Diez-Roux A, Roman C. "How do types of employment relate to health indicators? Findings from the Second European Survey on Working Conditions." *J Epidemiol Commun Health.* 2000; 54 (7): 494–501.
12. Virtanen P, Vahtera J, Kivinmaki M, Pentti J, Ferrie J. "Employment security and health." *J Epidemiol Commun Health.* 2002; 56: 569–74.
13. Jung-Min L, Won-Joong K, Hae-Sook S, Jin-Ho C, Myeong-Jin L, Hyun-Suk P. "Influences on health behaviors execution and self rated health as socioeconomic class by the age bracket." *J Korea Cont Assoc.* 2012; 12: 317–27.
14. Ware Jr JE, Brook RH, Davies AR, Lohr KN. "Choosing measures of health status for individuals in general populations." *Am J Public Health.* 1981; 71 (6): 620–5.

15. Mossey JM, Shapiro E. "Self-rated health: A predictor of mortality among the elderly." *Am J Public Health.* 1982; 72: 800–8.
16. Song J, Lee G, Kwon J, Park J, Choi H, Lim S. "The association between long working hours and self-rated health." *Ann Occup Environ Med.* 2014; 26: 2.
17. Schwarze J, Andersen HH, Anger S. "Self-rated health and changes in show self-rated health as predictors of mortality: first evidence from German panel data." *Quantific Simul Econ Process.* 2002; 203: 64.
18. Kim IH, Khang YH, Muntaner C, Chun H, Cho SI. "Gender, precarious work, and chronic diseases in South Korea". *Am J Ind Med.* 2008; 51: 748–57.
19. Kim MH, Kim CY, Park JK, Kawachi I. "Is precarious employment damaging to self-rated health? Results of propensity score matching methods, using longitudinal data in South Korea." *Soc Sci Med.* 2008; 67 (12): 1982–94.
20. Barnay T. "Health, work and working conditions: a review of the European economic literature." *Eur J Health Econ.* 2016; 17 (6): 693–709.
21. Muntaner C, Solar O, Vanroelen C, Martínez JM, Vergara M, Santana V, Castedo A, Kim IH, Benach J. "Unemployment, informal work, precarious employment, child labor, slavery, and health inequalities: pathways and mechanisms." *Int J Health Serv.* 2010; 40 (2): 281–95.
22. Hämmig O, Bauer GF. "The social gradient in work and health: a cross-sectional study exploring the relationship between working conditions and health inequalities." *BMC Public Health.* 2013; 13: 1170.
23. Inoue M, Nishikitani M, Tsurugano S, Yano E. "The health of permanent workers and workers with precarious employment: a literature review." *Sangyo Eiseigaku Zasshi.* 2011; 53 (4): 117–39.
24. Benach J, Tarafa M, Molinero V. "Multidimensional measurement of precarious employment: social distribution and its association with health in Catalonia." *Gac Sanit.* 2015; 29 (5): 375–8.
25. Tsurugano S, Inoue M, Yano E. "Precarious employment and health: analysis of the Comprehensive National Survey in Japan." *Ind Health.* 2012; 50 (3): 223–35.
26. Keuskamp D, Ziersch AM, Baum FE, LaMontagne AD. "Precarious employment, psychosocial working conditions, and health: cross-sectional associations in a population-based sample of working Australians." *Am J Ind Med.* 2013; 56: 838–44.
27. Bahk J, Han YJ, Kim SS. "Health inequity among waged workers by employment status." *J Prev Med Public Health.* 2007; 40 (5): 388–96.
28. Inoue M, Tsurugano S, Nishikitani M, Yano E. "Full-time workers with precarious employment face lower protection for receiving annual health check-ups." *Am J Ind Med.* 2012; 55 (10): 884–92.
29. Ferrie JE, Shipley MJ, Newman K, Stansfeld SA, Marmot M. "Self-reported job insecurity and health in the Whitehall II study: potential explanations of the relationship." *Soc Sci Med.* 2005; 60 (7): 1593–602.

Chapter 2

Social Capital and Its Association with Health and Well-Being

An Individual-Level Analysis in Seoul, South Korea

Sehee Han, Heaseung Kim, and Hee-Sun Lee

The[1] term "social capital" (Bourdieu 1986; Coleman 1988; Kadushin 2004; Lin 1999; Portes 1998; Putnam 1993, 2000; Snijders 1999) has been used and has gained popularity in a variety of fields, since the consideration of social capital could enhance policies or recommend interventions for reducing a variety of social problems (Besser 2009; Beaulieu et al. 2001; Hurtado, Kawachi, and Sudarsky 2011; Paxton 2002; Rose 2000; Snelgrove, Pikhart, and Stafford 2009; Suh 2008). Much research has demonstrated that social capital increases educational achievements and impacts social behaviors, such as finding jobs or voter choices (Granovetter 1973; Beaulieu et al. 2001; Gidengil, Harell, and Erickson 2001). One subject that has increasingly attracted researchers is the effect of social capital on health and well-being. Of the many possible returns of social capital, human well-being is the most important in a person's life, as well-being is a person's ultimate life goal. Among the concepts that have emerged over the past decade to improve citizens' well-being, socioeconomic inequality was the main concern (Mansyur et al. 2008). However, since we have experienced failures of policy or indifferent results of policy that mainly focused on fulfilling citizens' material needs, scholars, practitioners, and policymakers have recognized that other conditions such as social capital are necessary to improve public health and well-being (Szreter and Woolcock 2004). Some explanations exemplify links between social capital and health/well-being. One example shows that individuals who participate in organizations know a variety of people or have confidence in others are less likely to experience health problems and more likely to be satisfied with their lives, since the individuals could share their problems with others in order to resolve them and obtain information. Additionally, social capital may affect the health/well-being of citizens through their collective action to claim better welfare systems (Schultz, O'Brien, and Tadesse 2008). Empirical research supports this idea (Helliwell and Putnam 2004; Veenstra 2005). Although there is a lack of agreement on the concept of social capital (Brunie 2009), causing the association between social capital and health/well-being to vary, researchers generally agree that social capital is a crucial predictor of health and well-being.

Since social capital is a concept with multiple meanings, the measures vary from research to research. Some researchers, including Navarro (2002), make the critique that social capital's effect has been exaggerated, since social capital and its association with health and well-being is not found in all situations. One explanation for this problem is that social capital is often measured through a limited set of indicators, since researchers used data that were not designed to measure social capital (Berry and Welsh 2010). Thus, social capital requires careful conceptualization and operationalization. Despite these discrepancies regarding social capital, scholars generally agree that social capital can be categorized into two dimensions: structural and cognitive (Fujisawa, Hamano, and Takegawa 2009; Harpham 2008; Yamaoka 2008; Yip et al. 2007). Structural social capital refers to participation and social networks which can be confirmed objectively. Cognitive social capital is defined by mental processes, such as trust and reciprocity, which can be verified subjectively (Uphoff 2000). Indeed, many empirical studies have adopted the structural and cognitive dimensions of social capital framework.

The concept of well-being itself also invites controversy (Shin and Johnson 1978), as the concept has multiple meanings. Broadly, well-being has two dimensions. Diener (2000) defines well-being as "people's evaluations of their lives—evaluations that are both affective and cognitive," with the affective component referring to happiness and the cognitive component referring to life satisfaction. According to Gundelach and Kreiner (2004), happiness and life satisfaction are related as the subdimensions of well-being, but empirically reflect different aspects of well-being. Hence, it is likely that the same independent variables have a different effect on happiness and life satisfaction, and/or different independent variables have an effect on happiness and life satisfaction, so the variables need to be examined separately. Thus, this study included both happiness and life satisfaction as outcome variables and conducted analysis separately. Additionally, empirical studies regarding social capital and its association with health and well-being are sparse in Asian countries, especially South Korea, compared to Western countries. Thus, more research needs to be conducted in non-Western countries to confirm whether similar associations between social capital and health/well-being could be found in a study done in an Asian country.

The primary purpose of this study is to fill the knowledge gap regarding the association between social capital and health/well-being in non-Western societies. The main study question was, "Is social capital associated with health and well-being in Seoul, South Korea, after adjustment for sociodemographic and economic characteristics?" Based on the findings, we could draw implications about whether the concept of social capital can be applied to South Korea and whether the concept can be used to suggest policy recommendations. To examine this research question, a survey was conducted from June 2009 to September 2009. Additionally, this study geographically focused on Seoul because major differences in sociodemographic and socioeconomic situations between Seoul and other regions necessitate separate analyses. Furthermore, as the capital city of South Korea, Seoul merits initial research on the impacts of social capital.

To the best of our knowledge, no previous study has included the social networks measure as a structural social capital dimension and distinguished the subdimensions of well-being as happiness and life satisfaction. For these reasons, this study includes the social network measure as a structural social capital measure and estimates the impact of social capital on happiness and life satisfaction separately.

SOCIAL CAPITAL AND HEALTH/WELL-BEING

Literature linking social capital to health, and more recently, to well-being has been increasing (Helliwell and Putnam 2004; Yamaoka 2008; Yip et al. 2007). Kawachi et al. (2004) reviewed articles which examined the association between social capital and health/well-being, finding that many studies have shown that social capital is related to health and well-being. Although there is an agreement that social capital is an important determinant of health and well-being, the results varied depending on the definition of the concept and measure of social capital, level of analysis, and researched areas.

Helliwell and Putnam (2004), using data from the World Values Survey from the U.S. Benchmark Survey and a comparable Canadian survey, found that civic engagement, social ties, and trust, which are positively associated with health, have an effect on life satisfaction and happiness. Schultz, O'Brien, and Tadesse (2008), using data from the 2006 Social Capital Community Survey in Duluth, Minnesota, and Superior, Wisconsin, of the United States, examined the relationship between social capital (attitudes on trust, formal group involvement, informal socializing, organized group interaction, social support, and volunteer activity) and health. They found that individual social capital variables are associated with health. Recent research by Berry and Welsh (2010) empirically examined the relationship between social capital and physical functioning, mental health, and general health, using data from Wave 6 of the Household, Income and Labour Dynamics in Australia Survey. They found that social capital is associated with three forms of health. However, such relationships have not been confirmed from all studies. Using data from East Asia (Japan, South Korea, Singapore, and five cities in mainland China and Taiwan) in 2002–2004, Yamaoka (2008) found that while cognitive social capital is positively associated with health and well-being, structural social capital is negatively related to health. Additionally, Baron-Epel et al. (2008), using data from an Israeli health interview survey, which included adult Jews and adult Arabs, examined the association between social capital and health (e.g., social trust, neighborhood safety, perceived helpfulness, trust in authorities, and social support). They found that among Jews, those reporting higher levels of social capital reported better health. On the other hand, among Arabs, only those reporting higher levels of social support reported higher health. Moreover, Harpham, Emma, and Rodriguez (2004), using cross-sectional data from Cali, Colombia, did not find any relationship between social capital and self-reported mental health.

The findings also varied depending on the level of analysis. Some ecological research has found a relationship between social capital and outcomes related to health (Poortinga 2006b). At the U.S. state level, Kawachi et al. (1997) found that social capital is associated with self-rated health. Additionally, Veenstra (2002) found that social capital is related to health status in Saskatchewan, Canada. Contrary to these findings, some research did not find the association between social capital and health at the collective level (Veenstra 2000). Some research was conducted using a multilevel analysis. For example, Poortinga (2006a), using data from the European Social Survey, found that although individual levels of social capital are related to self-rated health, the same aggregate measures are not associated at the national level. However, using data from the 2000 and 2002 Health Survey for England, Poortinga (2006b) found that the aggregate social trust's effect on self-rated health was beyond the effect of individual social capital. Yip et al. (2007), using survey data from rural counties of Shandong province in China, found that social capital is associated with health and well-being. Namely, cognitive social capital (i.e., trust) has an effect on psychological health, general health, and well-being, both at the individual and village level. However, organizational membership, which is structural social capital, does not affect health and well-being except for village-level membership in voluntary organizations. Veenstra (2005) conducted similar research by examining the relationship between social capital and three measures of health and well-being (e.g., long-term limiting illness, depressive symptoms, and self-rated health) using multilevel analysis. Results showed that only a measure of depressive symptoms was associated with community-level social capital. Among individual-level social capital measures, trust in politicians and government and trust in community members were associated with outcome measures, but not participation in voluntary associations. A recent study by Snelgrove et al. (2010), which used data from the British Household Panel Survey, found that area social trust is associated with self-rated health. However, they found no evidence that area civic participation is related to self-rated health.

Although research examining the effect of social capital on health has been growing, fewer studies have been conducted in Asian countries compared to the studies conducted in Western countries (Ichida et al. 2009). Additionally, the variables used to measure social capital are inconsistent in various studies, thus the effect of social capital on health and well-being is varied. Moreover, the study of social capital and well-being is only recently burgeoning (Yip et al. 2007); therefore, few studies have been conducted to examine their relationships and only a few studies have distinguished between life satisfaction and happiness as a subdimension of well-being.

In sum, there is empirical evidence that shows social capital is beneficial for people's health and well-being with a few exceptions. Thus, we hypothesize that both cognitive and structural social capital are positively associated with health and well-being. Specifically, cognitive social capital is positively associated with health and well-being because increased structural social capital might stimulate information related to health and well-being, or the adoption of healthy behavioral norms (Kawachi and Berkman 2000; Snelgrove et al. 2009). Structural social capital is positively related to health and well-being because it might encourage the diffusion of ideas that promote behaviors and norms amenable to better health and well-being (Mitchell and Bossert 2007).

Conceptualization of Social Capital

The concept of social capital has been developed over a long period of time through studies by a number of researchers (Van der Gaag and Snijders 2005). However, there is no consensus on the notion of social capital (Brunie 2009). The premise of the social capital definition is simple and straightforward: social capital embeds in and derives from networks of people (Bekkers et al. 2008). Scholars generally agree with this definition (Bourdieu 1986; Coleman 1988, 1990; Erickson 1996; Lin 1999, 2001a, b; Portes 1998; Putnam 1993, 2000). However, the differences of social capital concepts and measures have emerged as well because some scholars (Paxton 1999; Portes 1998; Putnam 2000) define social capital as the trust and reciprocity derived from social networks of participation (Carpiano 2006) or as the networks themselves (Bourdieu 1986; Burt 1992; Flap and Volker 2001; Lin 2001a, b).

One group of researchers (Coleman 1998, 1990; Paxton 1999; Putnam 1993, 2000) understands social capital to derive from participation. Participation includes a number of different tasks and activities (Berry and Welsh 2010). It contains civic engagement, including volunteering and organizational involvement (Putnam 1995; Van der Gaag 2005) and political participation (Lofors and Sundquist 2007; Rich 1999). Putnam, a political scientist, has influenced most[2] research that understands social capital as being derived from participation, which increases trust, reciprocity, and vice versa (Magee 2009). Putnam (2000), in his recent book, Bowling Alone, defines social capital as "connections among individual's social networks and the norms of reciprocity and trustworthiness that arise from them." He argues that high degrees of trust, dense social networks, and high degrees of participation in collective action, such as volunteering or associational membership, indicate the presence of social capital. Miyata, Ikeda, and Kobayashi (2008) pointed out that the crucial point of Putnam's argument is that civic engagement is derived from diverse networks because people who know a wide range of others are likely to participate in the civic field, since at least some of the people they know are interested in political issues. Moreover, people who connect with a variety of others tend to participate in civic life because this enhances their trust in others as well as their value of reciprocity.

Another group of scholars (Burt 1992; Erickson 1996; Lin 2001) see social capital as an additional pool of resources embedded in the social networks of individuals, which can be useful for accomplishing individual goals (Van der Gaag 2005). Thus, social capital could be defined as "the total expected value of the benefits that this individual can obtain from his ties to other individuals" (Snijders 1999). Lin (2001b), a prominent scholar in this perspective, defines social capital as "resources embedded in one's social networks, resources that can be accessed or mobilized (used) through ties in the networks." Thus, one can capture the embedded resources through one's social networks, which are useful for a certain purpose. In addition to these differences, the theoretical concept of social capital is divided into micro- and macrolevels (Yamaoka 2008).

What becomes clear from the research presented above is that the concept of social capital is a very wide concept with complex meanings. In this study, we understand that the discrepancies regarding social capital broadly derive from whether researchers see participation related to factors, such as civic engagement and political participation, and intercorrelated with trust as a source of social capital or personal networks as a source of social capital. And within the participation perspective, there is a discrepancy in whether scholars regard social capital as a collective or an individual asset, or both. To better understand and measure social capital, social capital needs to be categorized into structural and cognitive dimensions (Chuang and Chuang 2008; Mitchell and Bossert 2007).

Since the aim of this study is to examine the effects of social capital on health and well-being at the individual level, this study conceptualizes social capital at the individual level. At this level, social capital refers to social resources derived and captured from one's social networks, contrary to the macrolevel social capital, which refers to the social resource of a group of people. To reconcile discrepancies regarding the concepts of social capital and measure social capital concretely, this study adopts structural and cognitive distinctions of social capital. The structural dimension reflects behavioral manifestations of social capital, which are associated with various forms of participation and social networks. The cognitive dimension reflects subjective attitudes of social networks, such as trust and reciprocity (Uphoff 2000).

DATA AND ANALYSIS

Data

We conducted a telephone survey from June 2009 to September 2009 to collect the data for the present study. The target respondents consisted of Seoul citizens who are twenty years of age and over. In the main, a stratified sampling method was used. Seoul's twenty-five districts were divided into two strata. Twenty-five districts in Seoul were categorized into two artificial regions, the Gangnam region, which includes the Gang-nam-gu, Seocho-gu, and Songpa-gu districts, and all other regions. We stratified the population size by the two artificial regions based on official census data. The Gangnam region is relatively wealthier and more urbanized than the other regions. By conducting a stratified sampling method, this variation can be considered in further analysis. Within the two artificial regions, the households were randomly chosen using a telephone book. Then, the respondents were selected using the birthday rule, which selects a respondent whose birthday was closest to the interview date. If the respondent did not want to or could not participate in the survey by phone for any reason, the respondent was asked to answer the questionnaire via e-mail. Additionally, we used the quota sampling method to gather data from seniors because the age group of twenty to fifty was initially overrepresented. By doing this, the present study gathered 1,432 cases of individual data (response rate: 54.3 percent including the e-mail surveys). However, 671 cases had to be dropped because their answers were substantially incomplete. The full sample includes 811 respondents, aged from twenty to seventy-nine years, from all twenty-five districts in Seoul.

Table 2.1 Summary of Variables

Characteristics		*Variables*
Social capital	Cognitive	Trust
	Structural	Network diversity, organization membership, political participation, and volunteer work
Health		Self-rated health
Well-being		Self-rated life satisfaction and happiness
Socioeconomic status		Region, gender, age, education, marital status, religion, employment status, home ownership, and household income

Measures

All variables were self-reported. Dependent variables included subjective life satisfaction, subjective happiness, and subjective health. Independent variables included social capital variables (i.e., network diversity, organization membership, political participation, volunteer work, and trust) and other variables, such as socioeconomic and demographic variables that are possibly related to each dependent variable as control variables (Dolan, Peasgood, and White 2008; Harpham, Emma, and Elizabeth 2002; Helliwell and Putnam 2004). Table 2.1 presents the summary of variables that are used in the present study.

Social Capital Variables

Structural Dimension

Network diversity, the dimension of structural social capital, was measured by using the position generator (Lin and Dumin 1986). This method, used by Lin and Dumin (1986), has been widely employed by empirical studies (Erikson 1996; Gidengil et al. 2001; Flap and Boxman 2005) and has been proven to have adaptability and flexibility to specific substantive settings (Erickson 2004). The original questionnaire used Choi's occupational prestige scale (Choi 2001) including twenty-five occupations, which describes the context of Korean society. The included twenty-five occupations are as follows: doctor, assemblyman, professor, owner of a large company, lawyer, local governor, clergy, pharmacist, school teacher, producer, entertainer, journalist, small-business owner, officer (armed forces), police officer, employee of a large company, nurse, computer programmer, technician, shop owner, skilled worker, salesman, driver, farmer, and construction worker. Network diversity was measured by summing the number of occupations accessed through the respondents' social networks. Thus, the range of the network diversity was from zero to twenty-five.

Organization membership was measured as another measure of the dimension of structural social capital. Organization membership was measured by asking the respondents to indicate whether they are members of the listed organizations. The listed organizations are hobby clubs, sports clubs, environmental/animal protection organizations, social clubs, human rights organizations, business organizations, consumer protection groups, alumni associations, hometown organizations, and labor unions. Respondents were subdivided into two groups: people who do not have any organization membership (coded = 0) and people who have organization membership (coded = 1).

The level of political participation was measured by adding up the responses to three statements: "Do you have any political party which you advocate for?"; "Are you a member of any political party?"; and "Did you vote in the 2007 presidential election?" Items were measured on a binary scale (yes = 1, no = 0). This additive scale was then recoded to a dummy variable, with score 0 reflecting a low level (coded = 0), and scores from one to three reflecting a high level (coded = 1). Volunteer work was measured with one item, which is similar to previous studies (Hurtado et al. 2011; Schultz et al. 2008). The respondents were asked how many times they usually participate in volunteer work in a year. The original 5-point scale was recoded to a dummy variable in which no volunteer work (coded = 0) reflected score 1, and high volunteer work (coded=1) included scores 2 to 5.

Cognitive Dimension

Trust, a dimension of cognitive social capital, was measured by two items related to trust and reciprocity: "Most people are trustworthy," and "If I provide useful help and information to someone, somebody will help me when I need help." These items were measured on a scale of 1–10, where 1 represented "strongly disagree" and 10 represented "strongly agree." A combined mean variable was calculated for the two items and used for further analysis (interitem correlation = 0.42).

Sociodemographic and SES Variables

Variables analyzed included gender, age, education, marital status, religious faith, personal income, employment status, and home ownership, which proved to have an impact on subjective life satisfaction, subjective happiness, and subjective health in literature (Blanchflower and Oswald 2000, 2004; Dolan, Peasgood, and White 2008; Fu 2005; Helliwell and Putnam 2004; Layard 2003; Yamaoka 2008).

Gender was categorized as male (coded = 1) or female (coded = 0). Age was measured by asking the respondent's age and used as a continuous scale.

Education was measured as the highest grade completed on a three-point scale, including (1) high school or below, (2) college or university, and (3) graduate school, with the high school or below group used as the reference. Marital status was originally classified into four categories. This was recoded as a dichotomous variable (1 = being married, 0 = others).[3] Religious faith was used as a dummy variable (1 = belonging to any, 0 = none). Household income was used as a continuous scale. Employment status was used as a dummy variable (1 = full-time worker, 0 = part-time worker). Home ownership was categorized into four parts: (1) family's property, (2) deposit based, (3) monthly rent, and (4) others. This was recoded as a dichotomous variable (1 = family's property, 0 = others). Finally, the districts were designated as the Gangnam region (coded = 1) or the non-Gangnam region (coded = 0).

Dependent Variables

Subjective life satisfaction was measured by one item. The respondents were asked: "All things considered, how satisfied are you with your life as a whole?" The original 10-point scale was recoded, where "low" encompassed 1 to 5 (coded = 1), "average" encompassed 6–7 (coded=2), and "high" encompassed 8 to 10 (coded=3). Subjective happiness was measured by one item. "Considering everything, would you say that you are very happy?" The original item was measured on a scale of 1–10, with 1 representing strongly disagree and 10 representing strongly agree. The responses of 1–5 (coded = 1) were classified as "low," 6–7 (coded = 2) were classified as "average," and 8–10 (coded 3) were classified as "high." Subjective health was assessed by one question: "How is your health in general?" The original 10-point scale was recoded, where the responses of 1–5 (coded = 1) representing "low," 6–7 (coded = 2) representing "average," and 8–10 (coded = 3) reflecting "high."[4] This measure is a good predictor of physical and mental health (Idler and Benyamini 1997).

Statistical Analysis

The aim of this study is to examine whether social capital affects self-rated health and well-being. To achieve this goal, ordinal logistic regression analysis was performed for each dependent variable since each dependent variable is an ordinal level. By conducting ordered logistic analysis, the association between social capital and self-rated health/well-being, after controlling for other variables, was confirmed. We estimate the following ordinal logistic model:

$$\Pr\left(Y = j|x\right) = F\left(\alpha j - x\beta\right) - F\left(aj - 1 - x\beta\right) \qquad (1)^5$$

where

$$x\beta=\beta 1\text{gangnam}+\beta 2\text{male}+\beta 3\text{edu1}+\beta 4\text{edu2}+\beta 4\text{married}+\beta 5\text{religion}+\beta 6\text{income}+\beta 7\text{employment}+\beta 8\text{home}+\beta 9\text{network}+\beta 10\text{membership}+\beta 11\text{participation}+\beta 12\text{volunteer}+(\beta 13\text{health})$$

Note: edu1: college or university, edu2: graduate school

In equation (1), Y refers to relevant dependent variables and β's function as regression parameters. When we conduct ordinal logistic analyses for life satisfaction and happiness, health is included as an independent variable. The odds ratio (OR), 95 percent confidence interval (95% CI), and p values are presented. The OR reflected an increase in the odds of a higher number of self-reported health and well-being. All analyses were conducted using STATA v.10 statistical package. All tests were two-tailed, with a significant level at 5 percent. Descriptive statistics of responses are presented first.

RESULTS

Descriptive Statistics

Table 2.2 provides the descriptive statistics of responses. About 17.3 percent of the respondents reported living in the Gangnam district. The gender distribution of the sample shows that male (52.3 percent) and female (47.7 percent) are distributed approximately equally. The mean age was about 37.5.

Table 2.2 Descriptive Statistics of Responses

Variables	*N (Mean)*	*Percentage (%)*
Control variables		
Region (Gangnam)	141	17.3
Gender (male)	424	52.3
Age	(37.5)	–
Education		
High school or below	137	16.9
College or university	543	67.0
Graduate school	131	16.1
Marital status (married)	446	55
Religion (faith in religion)	442	52
Employment status (employed full-time)	674	83.1
Home ownership (family's property)	409	50.4
Household income (won)	(375.4)	–
Social capital variables		
Network diversity	(9.0)	–
Organization membership (belonging to)	669	82.2
Level of political participation (high)	622	77
Volunteer work (high)	437	54
Trust	(6.2)	–

The majority (83.9 percent) had attained the educational level of above high school. More than half of the respondents (55 percent) were married. About 55 percent of respondents had faith in a religion. High proportions (83.1 percent) of the respondents were full-time workers. Slightly more than half of respondents (50.4 percent) reported that they own a house as family property (including the respondent's own). The mean monthly household income was 3,754,000 (*won*).[6] The mean network diversity was about 9. Thus, the respondent knows approximately nine different people whose occupations are different from their own. About 82.2 percent of respondents had at least one organizational membership. More than half of the respondents (54 percent) reported that they participated in volunteer work in the last year at least one time. More than half of the respondents (54 percent) answered that they did at least one form of political participation in the last year. Finally, the degree of agreement regarding trust and reciprocity was about 6.2.

Social Capital and Health

Table 2.3 presents the results of the relationships between social capital and self-rated health after adjustments for the control variables. In the ordinal logistic regression model, network diversity, volunteer work, and trust are statistically related to health among social capital variables (OR=1.05, 95%

Table 2.3 Ordinal Logistic Regression of Social Capital on Self-Rated Health (N = 811)

Variables	*Odds ratio*	*95% CI*
Control variables		
Region (Gangnam)	1.34	0.94–1.91
Gender (male)	1.31	0.99–1.73
Age	0.98*	0.96–0.99
Education		
(college or university)	0.91	0.62–1.35
(graduate school)	0.96	0.59–1.57
Marital status (married)	0.72	0.52–10.01
Religion (faith in religion)	0.97	0.73–1.30
Household income	1.00	0.99–1.01
Employment (employed full-time)	1.08	0.72–1.60
Home ownership (family's property)	1.15	0.87–1.52
Social capital variables		
Network diversity	1.05**	1.02–1.08
Organization membership (belonging to)	0.98	0.67–1.42
Political participation (high)	1.02	0.74–1.42
Volunteer work (high)	1.37*	1.02–1.85
Trust	1.65***	1.49–1.84
Cut point 1[a]	1.81***	(0.48)
Cut point 2[a]	3.66***	(0.50)

Notes: (1) *$p < 0.05$; **$p < 0.01$, ***$p < 0.001$. (2) [a]: βcoefficient (standard error).

CI=1.02–1.08; OR=1.37, 95% CI=1.02–1.85, OR=1.65, 95% CI=1.49–1.84, respectively). Thus, more network diversity and higher trust are associated with an increased probability of higher self-rated health. Similarly, a person with a high level of volunteer work participation reported a higher self-rated health compared to a person who did not do volunteer work. Among control variables, being older is associated with a decreased probability of higher health (OR = 0.98, 95% CI = 0.96–0.99).

Social Capital and Well-Being

Since life satisfaction and happiness are different dimensions of well-being (Pavot and Diener 1993; Gundelach and Kreiner 2004), ordinal logistic regression analysis was conducted separately for life satisfaction and happiness. Additionally, self-rated health was included as a control variable.[7] Although the causality between health and well-being is controversial, the causal link of health affecting well-being is more plausible (Dolan, Peasgood, and White 2008). Adding self-rated health decreases the influence of network diversity and trust on life satisfaction and happiness as expected (result not shown). Among social capital variables, network diversity and trust are statistically associated with life satisfaction even after health was included (OR = 1.08, 95% CI = 1.05–1.11; OR = 1.49, 95% CI = 1.33–1.66, respectively). Thus, an additional increase in network diversity per individual increases the likelihood of individuals to report average or high life satisfaction. Additionally, a one unit increase in trust enhances the odds of reporting a higher life satisfaction. In terms of control variables, gender (OR = 0.68, 95% CI = 0.51–0.91), having a college or university degree (OR=1.51, 95% CI=1.00–2.29), household income (OR=1.00, 95% CI=1.00–1.80), and health (OR=1.49, 95% CI=1.36–1.64) are statistically related to life satisfaction. Hence, being male is associated with a decreased probability of higher life satisfaction. Respondents who have college or university degrees reported higher life satisfaction compared to those who were educated at the high school level or below. Household income increases the OR of higher life satisfaction. In terms of happiness, network diversity and trust are statistically significant (OR = 1.07, 95% CI = 1.04–1.10, OR = 1.43, 95% CI = 1.28–1.60, respectively) social capital variables. Thus, a one unit increase in network diversity enhances in the OR of higher happiness. Additionally, respondents with a high level of trust are more likely to report higher happiness. Among control variables, age (OR = 0.98, 95% CI = 0.96–0.99), marital status (OR = 1.50, 95% CI = 1.06–2.11), and health (OR=1.38, 95% CI=1.26–1.51) are associated with happiness. Accordingly, being older is associated with a decreased probability of higher happiness. Respondents who are being married are more likely to report higher happiness. Among independent variables, self-rated

Table 2.4 Ordinal Logistic Regression of Social Capital on Subjective Well-Being (n=811)

	Life Satisfaction		*Happiness*	
Variables	*Odds Ratio*	*95% CI*	*Odds Ratio*	*95% CI*
Control variables				
Region (Gangnam)	1.16	0.80–1.68	1.33	0.92–1.93
Gender (male)	0.68**	0.51–0.91	0.75	0.56–1.00
Age	0.99	0.98–1.01	0.98*	0.96–0.99
Education				
(college or university)	1.51*	1.00–2.29	1.25	0.83–1.86
(graduate school)	1.30	0.78–2.16	1.16	0.71–1.92
Marital status (married)	1.36	0.96–1.92	1.50*	1.06–2.11
Religion (faith in religion)	1.19	0.89–1.60	1.12	0.84–1.50
Household income	1.00*	1.00–1.00	1.00	0.99–1.00
Employment				
(employed full-time)	0.66	0.43–1.01	0.70	0.46–1.06
Home ownership (family's property)	1.32	0.99–1.77	1.28	0.96–1.70
Health	1.49***	1.36–1.64	1.38***	1.26–1.51
Social capital variables				
Network diversity	1.08***	1.05–1.11	1.07***	1.04–1.10
Organization membership (belonging to)	1.18	0.80–1.72	1.12	0.77–1.63
Political participation (high)	1.31	0.94–1.83	1.39	0.99–1.95
Volunteer work (high)	1.05	0.77–1.43	1.10	0.81–1.49
Trust	1.49***	1.33–1.66	1.43***	1.28–1.60
Cut point 1[a]	4.94***	(0.57)	3.40***	(0.55)
Cut point 2[a]	7.39***	(0.61)	5.52***	(0.57)

Notes: 1) *p<.05; **p<.01; ***p<.001.
2) [a]: β coefficient (standard error).

health has relatively the largest influence on life satisfaction and happiness (result not shown). Additionally, except for network diversity and trust, none of the social capital variables are associated with life satisfaction and happiness, irrespective of whether self-rated health is included. The results are shown in table 2.4.

DISCUSSION

There is evidence that age, gender, education level, income, employment status, marital status, religiosity, and place of residence are related to health and well-being (Bartley 1994; Helliwell and Putnam 2004; Mansyur et al. 2008). Although there are suggestions that economic and social conditions are important factors in one's health and well-being, by themselves they are insufficient (Phongsavan et al. 2006). Thus, a significant amount of research has recently been conducted, and increasingly more research is examining the relationship between social capital and health/well-being in order to fill the gap. However, many questions still remain unanswered, and there are a few studies conducted for non-Western countries. The aims of this study were to confirm social capital's associations with health and well-being in Seoul, South Korea. We were especially concerned with whether social capital originated and studied in mainly Western societies has the same effect on health and well-being in non-Western countries. To achieve this research goal, a survey was conducted and ordinal logistic regression analysis was performed in Seoul, South Korea.

Our analyses provide evidence supporting the fact that the cognitive dimension of social capital is positively associated with all three dependent variables. However, the results are varied in terms of the structural dimension of social capital. Specifically, organization membership and political participation did not have an effect on any dependent variables. This tendency was also found in several studies that reported that organization membership does not have strong effect on health and well-being (Yip et al. 2007) and even has a negative effect on health (Yamaoka 2008). Several explanations are possible to explain these results. One possible explanation is that since many studies only included organization membership as a structural social capital measure, previous studies did not capture the effect of the other structural social capital variables such as social networks, allowing for the possibility that the previous studies overestimated the organization membership's effect on health and well-being. Thus, previous studies might have failed to consider more sophisticated social capital measures. It is also possible that since the organization membership measurement was originally developed in Western society, it is suitable for only Western societies. Additionally, the cultural aspect of South Korea might cause this result. Since hierarchical culture is prominent in South Korea compared to Western societies, some organizations might apply stress to lower-level members, especially in organizations where admission and quitting is not the member's individual decision. Although we did not measure health behavior, it is possible that some organizations encourage health behaviors such as drinking alcohol, which possibly affects health and well-being in return, as some studies suggest (Chuang and Chuang 2008). Since we measured organization membership with a single item, it was not possible to distinguish the type of organizations and it might cause some bias. Finally, we assumed that political participation could positively affect one's health and well-being because people who have higher levels of political participation could claim, solve, or change well-being issues related to policies that favor them. However, it is also possible that they experienced policy failures related to governmental programs or even experienced policy decisions that operate against their wishes that could possibly negatively affect well-being in return. Thus, it is likely that respondents who have the same level of political participation have inconsistent experiences regarding their political participation.

In this study, there is strong evidence that higher levels of trust are related to higher levels of self-rated health. In terms of structural social capital, network diversity and volunteer work are positively related to self-rated health. However, none of the other social capital measures were related to health. With regard to control variables, this study yields results that were consistent with previous studies. Old age is related to a low self-reported health as expected.

In terms of well-being, this study estimates social capital's effect on life satisfaction and happiness separately. Several researchers assumed that the two dimensions of well-being are the same; thus, they used the two terms interchangeably. However, the results suggested that each dependent variable was influenced by different variables. Although network diversity and trust were the most important predictors of both life satisfaction and happiness as expected, the influences of the independent variables changed with the fluctuations of each dependent variable. Specifically, gender, education, and household income were only related to life satisfaction. On the other hand, age and marital status were associated with only happiness. According to Helliwell and Putnam (2004), happiness reflects short-term, situation-dependent expressions of mood, compared to life satisfaction, which reflects long-term expressions of mood. Thus, it is a rather tentative conclusion that life satisfaction and happiness are different. Further research is necessary to establish a concrete conclusion.

There are some possible explanations as to why social capital affects self-rated health and well-being. One explanation is that, like previous studies suggest, separation, lack of trust, and lack of social contact, which are all indicators of social capital, were negatively associated with health and well-being as well (Kawachi 1999; Dolan, Peasgood, and White 2008). Since affluent people have access to multiple types of social capital and could easily access social resources such as medical care, emotional support, and information that provide a variety of solutions to solve their problems, they are, thus, less likely to experience and feel sadness and frustration. Overall, the current study's results indicate that the linkage between social capital to health and well-being in Seoul, South Korea, are more associated with personal network and trust compared to organization and political participation. This result indicates rather tentative policy implications that, with regard to the types of social capital, policy should be focused on improving citizens' health and well-being in Seoul. Our study suggests that policies should be considered for enhancing and strengthening citizens' personal networks and trust since this is a precursor of improving one's health and well-being in Seoul. Given the fact that even the most affluent societies in the world are not exempt from economic inequality problems, policies which solely aim at solving material deprivations are insufficient to enhance population health and well-being. Thus, policymakers should consider balancing between material assistance and social capital.

All research has limitations, including the present study. In order to generalize the analysis, we must acknowledge several limitations of the study. First, while this study used the probability sampling method, quota sampling method was also used, which may have caused sampling bias. Additionally, this study was based on a telephone survey to collect data. The bias may have occurred because people with unlisted numbers were excluded from the survey. This study used an e-mail survey as well. Thus, it may be possible that people who are not familiar with using e-mail or cannot access the Internet were denied a chance to participate in the survey. Second, the data set for the current study are cross-sectional samples. An important weakness of cross-sectional studies is that one cannot draw conclusions about the direction of the confirmed relationships, so the causality tends to be tentative. Thus, the cross-sectional characteristic of the data prevented exploration into the causal relationships between social capital and health/well-being. Although it is generally assumed that social capital has an effect on health and well-being, a reverse relationship may also be possible. It seems possible that the respondents who reported measures of higher social capital did so because they perceived a higher level of health and well-being.

Third, it is generally agreed that social capital is not only an individual characteristic but also a group characteristic as well (Fujisawa, Hamano, and Takegawa 2009; Snelgrove, Hynek, and Mai 2009). However, this study lacks the data to examine the group characteristic of social capital's association with health and well-being. This prevents us from reaching a concrete decision on the relationships between social capital and health and well-being since an individual analysis is not able to confirm the contextual effects. A lot of research provides evidence that collective social capital has an effect on health and well-being. Thus, multilevel modeling, which enables the inclusion of different levels of variables and cross-level interaction, should be considered in the future study. Fourth, the results may not be generalizable to all of South Korea. Since the dataset was gathered only from Seoul, it does not provide sufficient evidence to generalize the results in South Korea. Future research needs to consider a nationally representative sample. Finally, the data was based on self-reporting. Thus, the data involves subjective appraisal by the respondents, which is more uncertain than objective measure (Poortinga 2006b).

There are also several limitations derived from the measures of interest variables. In terms of social capital measures, the present study does not distinguish expressive and instrumental memberships of voluntary organizations. Since different characteristics of voluntary organizations can affect subjective well-being and health differently, it is recommended to measure them separately in future studies. Additionally, in terms of the position generator, the current study only chose twenty-five occupations; thus, it is possible to overlook other occupations that may serve as a crucial factor in establishing social capital for some people. Although the present study tries to consider the dimensions of the variety of occupations as Erikson (2004) argues, it may be subject to bias. With regard to the health measure, this study only included self-rated health reportings. Thus, we are not able to compare this study to other studies that used other health measures. Further research needs to consider multiple health outcomes, such as mental health. Additionally, we also used a single measure for each happiness and life satisfaction variable. Thus, the study is vulnerable to measurement error, which is a possible reason to cause bias. Future studies should measure well-being with multiple items to guarantee better reliability and validity of the variable.

These limitations aside, this study has provided additional evidence of the relationship between social capital and health and well-being, and suggestions of which future work should be considered in South Korea.

NOTES

1. This chapter was previously published as Sehee Han, Heaseung Kim, and Hee-Sun Lee. "Social Capital and Its Association with Health and Well-Being: An Individual-Level Analysis in Seoul, South Korea." *Korea Journal* 51, no. 4 (2011).

2. Some researchers have categorized social capital into bonding, bridging, and linking. Bonding social capital refers to relations between individuals with similar identities. Bridging social capital refers to relationships between individuals who are not alike. And political participation can be understood as "linking social capital," which is defined as the "norms of respect and networks of trusting relationships between people who are interacting across explicit, formal or institutionalized power or authority gradients in society" (Szreter and Woolcock 2004). Thus, it embraces relationships which connect people across vertical power differentials (Lofors and Sundquist 2007). An example of linking social capital is political participation, such as voting participation and political action (Chuang and Chuang 2008).

3. Originally, marital status was measured as single, married, divorced and separated, and others. Only three respondents (0.3 percent) answered on divorced and separated and no one answered on others. Thus, we recoded it as a dummy variable.

4. Using the original 10-point scale, preliminary analysis was conducted to ensure that there was no violation of the assumption of the proportional odds assumption on each dependent variable. Both an approximate LR test (Wolfe and Gould 1998) and a Wald test by Brant (1990) suggested that each model rejected the null-hypothesis that the βs are equal across each regression (Long and Freese 2006). Thus, we recoded

each dependent variable. The median scores of self-rated health, life satisfaction, and happiness were 7, respectively.

5. For an m-alternative ordered model, we define yi=j if αj–1 ≤ xβi+εi <αj for j=1 to m where α0=–∞ and αm=∞. Then Pr(y=j | x)=Pr(aj–1 ≤ xβ+<aj | x) which leads to equation number 1. F is the cumulative distribution fuction (c.d.f.) of εi. The cut-points α1 through αm–1 are estimated. For the ordinal logit model, F is logistic with Var(ε)=π2/3. Stata excludes an intercept from the regressors (Cameron and Trivedi 2010).

6. 1,300 won is around US$1.

7. Both a likelihood-ratio test for life satisfaction (LR×2 = 9.35, df = 8, $p = 0.314$) and for happiness (LR×2 = 11.88, df = 8, $p = 0.157$) and a Wald test for life satisfaction (χ_2 = 10.07, df = 8, $p = 0.260$) and for happiness (χ_2 = 11.98, df = 8, $p = 0.151$) suggested that the categories of self-rated health are evenly spaced. Thus, self-rated health was treated as an interval variable (from 1 = poor to 10 = good).

REFERENCES

Baron-Epel, Orna, et al. 2008. "Individual-Level Analysis of Social Capital and Health: A Comparison of Arab and Jewish Israelis." *Social Science and Medicine* 66(4): 900–910.

Bartley, Mel. 1994. "Unemployment and Ill Health: Understanding the Relationship." *Journal of Epidemiology and Community Health* 48(4): 333–337.

Beaulieu, Lionel J., et al. 2001. "For Whom Does the School Bell Toll?: Multi-Contextual Presence of Social Capital and Student Educational Achievement." *Journal of Socio-Economics* 30(2): 121.

Bekkers, René, et al. 2008. "Social Networks of Participants in Voluntary Associations." In *Social Capital: An International Research Program*, edited by Nan Lin and Bonnie H. Erickson, 185–205. New York, NY: Oxford University Press.

Berry, Helen L., and Jennifer A. Welsh. 2010. "Social Capital and Health in Australia: An Overview from the Household, Income and Labour Dynamics in Australia Survey." *Social Science and Medicine* 70(4): 588–596.

Besser, Terry L. 2009. "Change in Small Town Social Capital and Civic Engagement." *Journal of Rural Studies* 25(2): 185–193.

Bourdieu, Paul. 1986. "The Forms of Capital." In *Handbook of Theory and Research for the Sociology of Education*, edited by John G. Richardson. Westport, CT: Greenwood Press.

Brant, Rollin. 1990. "Assessing Proportionality in the Proportional Odds Model for Ordinal Logistic Regression." *Biometrics* 46: 1171–1178.

Brunie, Aurélie. 2009. "Meaningful Distinctions within a Concept: Relational, Collective, and Generalized Social Capital." *Social Science Research* 38(2): 251–265.

Burt, Ronald S. 1992. *Structural Holes: The Social Structure of Competition*. Cambridge, MA: Harvard University Press.

Cameron, Adrian D., and Pravin K. Trivedi. 2010. *Microeconometrics Using Stata*. Rev. ed. College Station, TX: Stata Press.

Carpiano, Richard M. 2006. "Toward a Neighborhood Resource-Based Theory of Social Capital for Health: Can Bourdieu and Sociology Help?" *Social Science and Medicine* 62(1): 165–175.

Choi, Tae Ryong. 2001. "Jigeop wisin-ui byeonhwa" (Changes in Occupational Prestige). *Hanguk sahoehak bipyeong* (Review of Korean Sociology) 1.

Chuang, Ying-Chih, and Kun-Yang Chuang. 2008. "Gender Differences in Relationships between Social Capital and Individual Smoking and Drinking Behavior in Taiwan." *Social Science and Medicine* 67(8): 1321–1330.

Coleman, James S. 1988. "Social Capital in the Creation of Human Capital." *American Journal of Sociology* 94: S95–S120.

———. 1990. *Foundations of Social Theory*. Cambridge, MA: Belknap Press of Harvard University Press.

Diener, Ed. 2000. "Subjective Well-Being: The Science of Happiness, and a Proposal for a National Index." *American Psychologist* 55(1): 34.

Dolan, Paul, Tessa Peasgood, and Mathew White. 2008. "Do We Really Know What Makes Us Happy? A Review of the Economic Literature on the Factors Associated with Subjective Well-Being." *Journal of Economics Psychology* 29(1): 94–122.

Erickson, Bonnie H. 1996. "Culture, Class, and Connections." *American Journal of Sociology* 102: 217–251.

———. 2004. "The Distribution of Gendered Social Capital in Canada." In *Creation and Returns of Social Capital*, edited by Henk Flap and Beate Völker, 27–50. London: Routledge.

Flap, Henk, and Beate Völker. 2001. "Goal Specific Social Capital and Job Satisfaction: Effects of Different Types of Networks on Instrumental and Social Aspects of Work." *Social Networks* 23(4): 297–320.

Flap, Henk, and Ed Boxman. 2005. "Getting Started: The Influence of Social Capital on the Start of the Occupational Career." In *Social Capital: Theory and Research*, edited by Nan Lin, Karen Cook, and Ronald S. Burt. New Brunswick, NJ and London: Aldine Transactions.

Frey, Bruno, and Alois Stutzer. 1999. *Measuring Preferences by Subjective Well-Being*. Zürich: University of Zurich, Mimeo.

Fujisawa, Yoshikazu, Tsuyoshi Hamano, and Shogo Takegawa. 2009. "Social Capital and Perceived Health in Japan: An Ecological and Multilevel Analysis." *Social Science and Medicine* 69(4): 500–505.

Gidengil, Elisabeth, Allison Harell, and Bonnie Erickson. 2001. "Network Diversity and Vote Choice: Women's Social Ties and Left Voting in Canada." *Politics and Gender* 3(2): 151–177.

Granovetter, Mark. 1973. "The Strength of Weak Ties." *American Journal of Sociology* 78(6): 1360–1380.

Gundelach, Peter, and Svend Kreiner. 2004. "Happiness and Life Satisfaction in Advanced European Countries." *Cross-Cultural Research* 38(4): 359–386.

Harpham, Trudy. 2008. "The Measurement of Community Social Capital through Surveys." In *Social Capital and Health*, edited by Ichiro Kawachi, S. V. Subramanian, and Daniel Kim. New York, NY: Springer.

Harpham, Trudy, Grant Emma, and Thomas Elizabeth. 2002. "Measuring Social Capital within Health Surveys: Key Issues." *Health Policy and Planning* 17(1): 106–111.
Harpham, Trudy, Grant Emma, and Carlos Rodriguez. 2004. "Mental Health and Social Capital in Cali, Colombia." *Social Science and Medicine* 58(11): 2267–2277.
Helliwell, John F., and Robert D. Putnam. 2004. "The Social Context of Well-Being." *Philosophical Transactions of the Royal Society London* 359: 1435–1446.
Hurtado, David, Ichiro Kawachi, and John Sudarsky. 2011. "Social Capital and Self-Rated Health in Colombia: The Good, the Bad and the Ugly." *Social Science and Medicine* 72(4): 584–590.
Ichida, Yukinobu, et al. 2009. "Social Capital, Income Inequality and Self-Rated Health in Chita Peninsular, Japan: A Multilevel Analysis of Older People in 25 Communities." *Social Science and Medicine* 69(4): 489–499.
Idler, Ellen L., and Benyamini Yael. 1997. "Self-rated Health and Mortality: A Review of Twenty-Seven Community Studies." *Journal of Health and Social Behavior* 38: 21–37.
Kadushin, Charles. 2004. "Too Much Investment in Social Capital?" *Social Networks* 26: 75–90.
Kawachi, Ichiro, and Lisa F. Berkman. 2000. "Social Cohesion, Social Capital, and Health." In *Social Epidemiology*, edited by Lisa F. Berkman and Ichiro Kawachi. New York, NY: Oxford University Press.
Kawachi, Ichiro, Bruce P. Kennedy, Kimberly Lochner, and Deborah Prothrow-Stith. 1997. "Social Capital, Income Inequality, and Mortality." *American Journal of Public Health* 87(9): 1491–1498.
Kawachi, Ichiro, et al. 2004. "Commentary: Reconciling the Three Accounts of Social Capital." *International Journal of Epidemiology* 33: 682–690.
Lin, Nan. 1999. "Building a Network Theory of Social Capital." *Connections* 22(1): 28–51.
———. 2001a. *Social Capital: A Theory of Social Structure and Action*. Cambridge: Cambridge University Press.
———. 2001b. "Building a Network Theory of Social Capital." In *Social Capital: Theory and Research*, edited by Nan Lin, Karen Cook, and Ronald S. Burt. New Brunswick, NJ and London: Aldine Transactions.
Lin, Nan, and Mary Dumin. 1986. "Access to Occupations through Social Ties." *Social Networks* 8(4): 365–385.
Lofors, Jonas, and Kristina Sundquist. 2007. "Low-linking Social Capital as a Predictor of Mental Disorders: A Cohort Study of 4.5 Million Swedes." *Social Science and Medicine* 64(1): 21–34.
Long, J. Scott, and Jeremy Freese. 2006. *Regression Models for Categorical Dependent Variables Using Stata*. College Station, TX: Stata Press.
Magee, Marc P. 2008. "Civic Participation and Social Capital: A Social Network Analysis in Two American Counties." In *Social Capital: An International Research Program*, edited by Nan Lin and Bonnie H. Erickson, 308–327. New York, NY: Oxford University Press.
Mansyur, Carol, et al. 2008. "Social Capital, Income Inequality, and Self-Rated Health in 45 Countries." *Social Science and Medicine* 66(1): 43–56.

Mitchell, Andrew D., and Thomas J. Bossert. 2007. "Measuring Dimensions of Social Capital: Evidence from Surveys in Poor Communities in Nicaragua." *Social Science and Medicine* 64(1): 50–63.

Miyata, Kakuko, Kenichi Ikeda, and Tetsuro Kobayashi. 2008. "The Internet, Social Capital, Civic Engagement, and Gender in Japan." In *Social Capital: An International Research Program*, edited by Nan Lin and Bonnie H. Erickson, 206–233. New York, NY: Oxford University Press.

Navarro, Vicente. 2002. "A Critique of Social Capital." *International Journal of Health Services* 32(3): 423–432.

Pavot, William, and Ed Diener. 1993. "Review of the Satisfaction with Life Scale." *Psychological Assessment* 5(2): 101–117.

Paxton, Pamela. 1999. "Is Social Capital Declining in the United States? A Multiple Indicator Assessment." *American Journal of Sociology* 105.1.

———. 2002. "Social Capital and Democracy: An Interdependent Relationship." *American Sociological Review* 67: 254–277.

Phongsavan, Philayrat, et al. 2006. "Social Capital, Socio-Economic Status and Psychological Distress among Australian Adults." *Social Science and Medicine* 63(10): 2546–2561.

Poortinga, Wouter. 2006a. "Social Capital: An Individual or Collective Resource for Health?" *Social Science and Medicine* 62(2): 292–302.

———. 2006b. "Social Relations or Social Capital? Individual and Community Health Effects of Bonding Social Capital." *Social Science and Medicine* 63(1): 255–270.

Portes, Alejandro. 1998. "Social Capital: Its Origins and Applications in Modern Sociology." *Annual Review of Sociology* 24(1): 1–24.

Putnam, Robert D. 1993. *Making Democracy Work: Civic Traditions in Modern Italy.* Princeton, NJ: Princeton University Press.

———. 1995. "Bowling Alone: America's Declining Social Capital." *Journal of Democracy* 6(1): 65–78.

———. 2000. *Bowling Alone: The Collapse and Revival of American Community.* London: Simon and Schuster.

Rich, Paul. 1999. "American Voluntarism, Social Capital, and Political Culture." *Annals of the American Academy of Political and Social Science* 565(1): 15–34.

Rose, Richard. 2000. "How Much Does Social Capital Add to Individual Health? A Survey Study of Russians." *Social Science and Medicine* 51(9): 1421–1435.

Schultz, Jennifer, A. Maureen O'Brien, and Bedassa Tadesse. 2008. "Social Capital and Self-Rated Health: Results from the US 2006 Social Capital Survey of One Community." *Social Science and Medicine* 67(4): 606–617.

Shin, D. C., and D. M. Johnson. 1978. "Avowed Happiness as an Overall Assessment of the Quality of Life." *Social Indicators Research* 5: 475–492.

Snelgrove, John W., Hynek Pikhart, and Mai Stafford. 2009. "A Multilevel Analysis of Social Capital and Self-Rated Health: Evidence from the British Household Panel Survey." *Social Science and Medicine* 68(11): 1993–2001.

Snijders, Tom A. B. 1999. "Prologue to the Measurement of Social Capital." *La Revue Tocqueville* 20(1): 27–44.

Szreter, Simon, and Michael Woolcock. 2004. "Health by Association? Social Capital, Social Theory, and the Political Economy of Public Health." *International Journal of Epidemiology* 33(4): 650–667.

Suh, Moon-Gi. 2008. "Social Capital and Development in Comparative Perspective." *Korean Journal of Sociology* 42(8): 105–123.

Uphoff, Norman. 2000. "Understanding Social Capital: Learning from the Analysis and Experience of Participation." In *Social Capital: A Multifaceted Perspective*, edited by Partha Dasgupta and Ismail Serageldin, 215–253. Washington, DC: World Bank.

Van der Gaag, Martin. 2005. *The Measurement of Individual Social Capital.* PhD diss., Groningen University.

Van der Gaag, Martin, and Tom A. B. Snijders. 2005. "The Resource Genera- tor: Social Capital Quantification with Concrete Items." *Social Networks* 27(1): 1–29.

Veenstra, Gerry. 2000. "Social Capital, SES and Health: An Individual-Level Analysis." *Social Science and Medicine* 50(5): 619–629.

———. 2002. "Social Capital and Health (Plus Wealth, Income Inequality and Regional Health Governance)." *Social Science and Medicine* 54(6): 849–868.

———. 2005. "Location, Location, Location: Contextual and Compositional Health Effects of Social Capital in British Columbia, Canada." *Social Science and Medicine* 60(9): 2059–2071.

Wolfe, Rory, and William Gould. 1998. "An Approximate Likelihood-Ratio Test for Ordinal Response Models." *Stata Technical Bulletin Reprints* 7(42).

Yamaoka, Kazue. 2008. "Social Capital and Health and Well-Being in East Asia: A Population-Based Study." *Social Science and Medicine* 66(4): 885–899.

Yip, Winnie, et al. 2007. "Does Social Capital Enhance Health and Well-Being? Evidence from Rural China." *Social Science and Medicine* 64(1): 35–49.

Chapter 3

Paying Out-of-Pocket for Health Care in Korea

Changes in Catastrophic and Poverty Impact over a Decade of 1996–2005

TaeJin Lee

It[1] has been almost forty years since social health insurance was initiated in Korea in 1977. The most noticeable achievement in the history of the social health insurance was the establishment of the national health insurance (NHI) system in 1989, which achieved universal coverage of the population in only twelve years after the initiation of the social health insurance. Another remarkable change was a full integration of insurance funds in 2000, which merged a total of 375 insurance funds and brought a single-payer insurance system into Korea. After recovering from a financial crisis that the new-born single-payer was destined to face, an insurer named National Health Insurance Corporation has made the extension of insurance coverage a priority among various health policy agendas.

In fact, the NHI has never been comprehensive in terms of insurance coverage despite its universality in terms of population coverage. Most outpatient services and high-probability inpatient services are covered, but many low-probability, high-cost services are excluded. High co-payments are also imposed on covered services. As a result, the insurer pays only about 70 percent of the expenditures on those services and items covered under the NHI, and patients have to pay out-of-pocket (OOP) for the remaining 30 percent and for the expenditures on the services not covered under the NHI as well.

OOP payments as a way of financing health care have consequences for the utilization of health care and subsequently for health [1–6]. If the share of OOP payments among health expenditures is too large, patients are forced to face a financial barrier to the utilization of health care. In the case of catastrophic illness, for example, some households would face a difficult choice between diverting a large fraction of household resources to cover the costs of treatment and forgoing treatment at the expense of health.

Moreover, the large proportion of OOP payments has differential consequences among households with varying incomes. A well-off household can perhaps finance medical expenses from savings. A less well-off household may be forced to cut back on necessities and consequently pushed into—or further into—poverty [7].

Several studies give evidence on the catastrophic and poverty impact of OOP payments derived from nationally representative expenditure data [8–12]. Two of those studies compared the catastrophic and poverty impact of OOP payments among Asian countries, respectively. One of the two studies included evidence on catastrophic payments in Korea based on the estimate of only one year and did not show the catastrophic impact of OOP payments during a longer period [12]. The other study on poverty impact did not even include Korea because of the incomparability of its poverty level with that of other Asian countries [11].

It would be interesting to look at changes in the catastrophic and poverty impact of OOP payments over a longer period. This is particularly the case with Korea whose health-care financing has relied heavily on OOP payments in spite of universal health insurance and which experienced an important change in the financing of health care in 2000. A separation policy, as described in the next section, lowered the proportion of OOP payments in the financing of health care. However, a closer look at its effect on OOP payments reveals that the benefits from lowering OOP payments were not equally distributed among different income groups and that the extent to which OOP payments were reduced differed by different types of health care such as outpatient and inpatient care. This, in turn, leads to a conjecture that there might be variations in the catastrophic impact of OOP payments among varying income groups and/or by different types of health care. A longitudinal analysis of those variations in the catastrophic and poverty impact of OOP payments would help better understand which segment of the population suffers most from large OOP payments. Using the data from a nationally representative household expenditure survey, this study aims to examine the trend in the catastrophic and impoverishing impact of OOP payments in Korea over the decade from 1996 to 2005. It also aims to investigate catastrophic impact by income quintiles and by type of service.

TREND IN HEALTH-CARE FINANCING IN KOREA

It is true that the NHI has contributed to reducing a financial barrier to the utilization of health services in Korea over the decade from 1996 to 2005.

However, the share of health-care funding through the NHI was lower than that of OOP payments until 2000 when the separation policy (SP) was implemented (table 3.1).

Before July 2000, physicians were allowed to both prescribe and dispense drugs, and pharmacists to dispense drugs without prescriptions from doctors. The expenditures on drugs dispensed directly by pharmacists were mostly paid OOP. Under the SP, physicians prescribe but do not dispense drugs at their practices, and pharmacists dispense drugs only with prescriptions from doctors. Thus, the NHI has taken over the expenditures on drugs otherwise previously paid OOP. That is probably the main reason that the share of the NHI funding started to exceed that of OOP payments from 2001. Table 3.1 shows that the share of the NHI funding increased by about 5 percentage points in 2001, while that of OOP payments decreased by a similar amount.

A more careful examination on the effect of the SP on OOP payments shows that its effect varies at two different levels. First and at the system level, the SP led to the reduction of the share of OOP payments in the financing of health care for the abovementioned reason. Second and at the patient level, however, the SP resulted in the increase in OOP payments that individual patients bore at the time of utilizing health services. This can be explained by the increase in both price and quantity of health services utilized. As an incentive for doctors to accept the SP, the government endorsed an over 30 percent increase in medical fees within one year in 2000. In addition, with the SP implemented, almost all patients utilizing outpatient care had to visit pharmacies with doctor's prescriptions, which led to an abrupt increase in patients' OOP payments.

On the other hand, the NHI had to experience a financial turmoil after the SP was implemented. For the same reason that the absolute amount of patients' OOP payments increased, the insurer's expenditures on health care went up rapidly. Facing with a large-scale deficit, the NHI chose to implement every single policy option to contain health expenditures as much as possible. For example, the government increased co-payments for outpatient visit to clinics as well as for drugs in 2001. This, in turn, led to additional increase in the OOP payments of households.

In Korea, poor households tend to spend a disproportionately large share of their resources on outpatient care and drugs, compared to their rich counterparts [13]. Thus, a substantive increase in OOP payments of households, resulting from the SP and the subsequent policy on co-payments, was likely to end up with the increase in catastrophic and poverty impact of OOP payments, in particular, on poor households.

After recovering from the deficit, the government tried to extend overall insurance coverage, but did not reverse the policy on co-payments for

Table 3.1 Trend in Health-Care Financing in Korea (Unit: %)

	1996	*1997*	*1998*	*1999*	*2000*	*2001*	*2002*	*2003*	*2004*	*2005*
Public	*38.9*	*41.4*	*46.6*	*46.9*	*46.8*	*53.0*	*51.7*	*51.9*	*52.5*	*53.0*
Government	7.9	8.5	9.3	10.7	10.1	10.5	10.8	10.6	10.9	11.9
Social security	31.0	32.9	37.3	36.2	36.7	42.5	40.9	41.3	41.6	41.1
Private	*61.1*	*58.5*	*54.1*	*53.1*	*53.2*	*47.0*	*48.4*	*48.1*	*47.4*	*47.0*
OOP	52.9	49.6	46.6	44.4	43.6	38.3	39.7	38.4	38.1	37.7
Private insurance	2.1	2.5	3.4	3	4.1	3.3	3.2	3.6	3.4	3.4
All other private	6.1	6.4	4.3	5.7	5.5	5.4	5.5	6.1	5.9	5.9
Total	100.0	100.0	100.0	100.0	100.0	100.0	100.0	100.0	100.0	100.0

Source: OECD Health Data 2007 [19].

Table 3.2 Benefit Extensions under the NHI (Selected lists)

Dates	*Coverage-extended items or changes in co-payments*
1996.1	CT
2000.7	Pre-natal care
2001.1	Home care
2004.1	Reduction of co-payment for outpatient care of patients with cancers or 62 kinds of rare diseases
2004.7	Introduction of upper limit of co-payments for medical expenditure
2005.1	MRI for selected diseases
	Exemption of co-payment for vaginal delivery
	Reduction of co-payment for outpatient care of mental diseases (30~50% → 20%)
2005.5	Extension of insurance-covered period for therapeutic agents for osteoporosis (90 → 180 days)
2005.8	Introduction of partial insurance coverage for 483 items including some materials for treatment
2005.9	Reduction of co-payment for catastrophic diseases including cancers (20% → 10%)
2006.1	Exemption of co-payment for inpatient care of children under 6
2006.6	Reimbursement of PET costs for patients with cancers, cardiac diseases or brain diseases
2006.11	Reimbursement of home oxygen therapy for COPD patients

Source: National Health Insurance Statistical Yearbook 2007.

outpatient care and drugs which was implemented at the time of financial crisis. Instead, the government chose to lower co-payments for specific diseases such as cancers, mental, and rare diseases. Table 3.2 shows that the insurer's efforts on coverage extension varied from including new technologies such as CT, MRI, and PET under the umbrella of the NHI to directly lowering the patients' co-payments for specific diseases at the time of utilizing health services [14]. It is noticeable that these efforts were made more frequently after 2004 when the NHI escaped its accumulated financial deficit. The benefits from extending insurance coverage were expected to be provided to all members of society regardless of their economic status, and extra attention was not paid to those most in financial need.

Of the health expenditure for those services and items covered by the NHI, only 65 percent was paid by the insurer in 1996; the remaining 35 percent was paid OOP by patients at the time of utilization (figure 3.1). Since then, health insurance coverage rate, defined as the proportion of health expenditures paid by the insurer out of total health expenditures for those services and items covered under the NHI, has increased to reach a peak of 72.5 percent in 2001, and has hung back afterwards, mainly due to the increase in the patients' co-payments. Overall, health insurance coverage rates display an upward trend over the years, except for the peak in 2001.

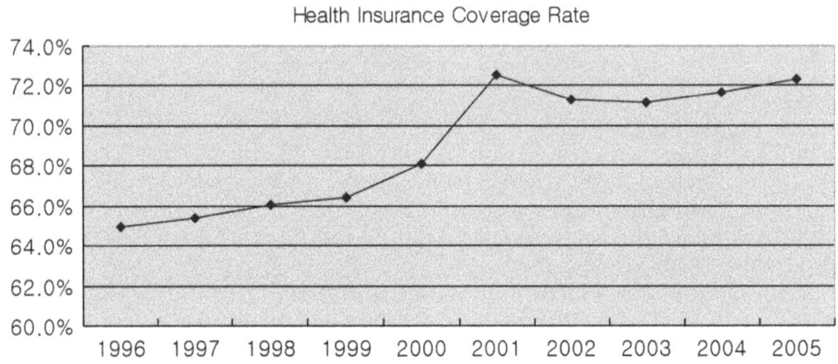

Figure 3.1 Trend in Health Insurance Coverage Rate in Korea. Figure created using data from the National Health Insurance Corporation. Note: Health insurance coverage rate is defined as "the actual health expenditure the NHI pays" divided by "total health expenditure for services included in the NHI's reimbursement list."

METHODS

The methodology used to measure the catastrophic and poverty impact of OOP payments is heavily based on that used in the Equity in Asia-Pacific Health System (EQUITAP) study [11, 12], which in turn draws on a seminal paper [9]. Thus, the explanation of the methodology here is maintained to a minimum.

Measuring the Catastrophic Effects of OOP Payments

Catastrophic payments are defined as OOP payments exceeding some threshold shares of household resources. Although the choice of the threshold share is subjective, 10 percent of total expenditure is used as a threshold in this study as in some previous studies [8, 9, 15]. The rationale is that at this threshold, households are forced to sacrifice other basic needs, sell productive assets, incur debt, or be impoverished [16].

The catastrophic payment headcount (H_C) represents the percentage of households incurring catastrophic payments and its measurement is described elsewhere [9, 12]. The concentration index (C_E) represents the correlation of catastrophic payments with household rank in the distribution of living standards. If households exceeding the threshold tend to be worse-off, CE will be negative, and vice versa.

Measuring the Impoverishing Effects of OOP Payments

High OOP payments can expose households to substantial financial risk, sometimes resulting in impoverishment. The impoverishing effect of OOP payments can be measured using the poverty headcount, which denotes the proportion of individuals who fall below a poverty line.

According to the recommendation that poverty be assessed after deduction of health-care payments since most of these payments cover essential needs [17], estimates of the poverty headcount are produced and compared before and after OOP payments for health care are deducted from household resources. In terms of a poverty threshold, two kinds of poverty lines are involved: pre-payment and post-payment poverty line. It is argued that the pre-payment poverty line should include an element for health spending, while the post-payment poverty line should not, and that it is necessary to deduct an amount from the poverty line corresponding to health spending to arrive at the post-payment poverty line [9]. As the pre-payment poverty threshold, the national poverty line (NPL) that the government announces every year is used in this study. To establish the post-payment poverty threshold, the average share of OOP payments among the third income quintile is subtracted from the NPL of each year.

How to estimate the poverty headcount before and after OOP payments for health care are deducted from household resources is described elsewhere [9]. The measures of the poverty impact of OOP payments are then simply defined as the difference between pre-payment and post-payment headcounts.

Data

To examine the trend in catastrophic and impoverishing impact of OOP payments in Korea over the decade between 1996 and 2005, the data from a nationally representative household expenditure survey was used. The household expenditure survey, administer by the National Statistical Office, is carried out nationwide every year for the purpose of helping the government with policymaking by providing basic information on household expenditures. The survey uses cluster sampling, and sampling weights were applied in the analysis to control for it. The average sample size was about 5,200 households during the period between 1996 and 2002, and increased to about 7,400 households during the period between 2003 and 2005. The response rate was, on average, around 80 percent each year. The survey uses one month recall period, and total expenditure for one month is reported and computed. Like in the EQUITAP study, OOP payments are defined here to include fees, co-payments, user charges for public care and purchases of medicines, appliances, diagnostic tests, and so on. Expenditures on Western and traditional care are included. The survey questions on OOP payments were consistent over the period of the study. Analyses were performed with STATA version 9.0.

RESULTS

The Catastrophic Impact of OOP Payments

Incidence of Catastrophic Payments

Table 3.3 provides the catastrophic payment headcount (H_C) and concentration index (C_E) over the decade of 1996–2005. The incidence of range of catastrophic payments over the decade amounts to a 10.2–11.8 percent of households at the threshold of 10 percent of total expenditures. The percentage of households with OOP payments in excess of this threshold was 11.8 percent in 1996, went down to 10.2 percent in 2001, and increased again to 11.8 percent in 2005. This statistically significant ($p < 0.05$) U-shaped incidence of catastrophic payments implies that OOP payments have increased rapidly relative to household budgets in recent years.

A negative concentration index means that the incidence of catastrophic payments decreases with household living standards. That is, the poorer households are more likely to spend large fractions of their total expenditures on health care. Over the decade, in particular since 2001, the strength of the negative correlation has increased, meaning that more of the poor households have experienced catastrophic payments.

Catastrophic Payments by Income Quintile

Incidence of catastrophic payments by income quintile is depicted in figure 3.2. At the threshold of 10 percent of total expenditures, incidence of catastrophic payments was similar among income quintile groups in 1996. While it did not change over time among the other quintiles, the incidence increased, particularly after 2001, among the poorest 20 percent group and the gap continued to be widened. It is evident that, although the NHI has tried to extend insurance coverage, the catastrophic impact of OOP payments for health care has been greatest among the poorest members of Korean society since 2001.

Catastrophic Payments by Type of Service

Incidence and intensity of catastrophic payments, segregated by type of service, are provided in table 3.4. In 2005, the percentages of households spending in excess of 10 percent of total expenditures on outpatient care, inpatient care, drug, and dental care are 2.5, 1.5, 3.0, and 1.6 percent, respectively. Compared to the catastrophic impact of total OOP payments, concentration indices of incidence of catastrophic payments of disaggregated OOP payments display a much clearer distinction between types of service, and the correlation of catastrophic payments with household rank in the distribution

Table 3.3 Incidence of Catastrophic Payments for Health Care

	1996	*1997*	*1998*	*1999*	*2000*	*2001*	*2002*	*2003*	*2004*	*2005*
OOP >10 percent of total expenditure										
Headcount (H_C)	11.80%	11.00%	10.43%	10.55%	10.36%	10.17%	10.44%	11.14%	11.01%	11.81%
	(0.13)	(0.13)	(0.12)	(0.12)	(0.12)	(0.12)	(0.12)	(0.11)	(0.11)	(0.11)
Concentration index (C_E)	0.0019	-0.0005	-0.0236	-0.0328	-0.0244	-0.0345	-0.0489	-0.0792	-0.0772	-0.0850

The figures in the parentheses are standard errors.
A least-squares regression of incidence of catastrophic payments on year in a quadratic functional form resulted in a coefficient for the quadratic term year^2 of 0.0007 ($p <$ 0.001) and for the term year of –2.883 ($p < 0.001$); adjusted $R^2 = 0.87$.

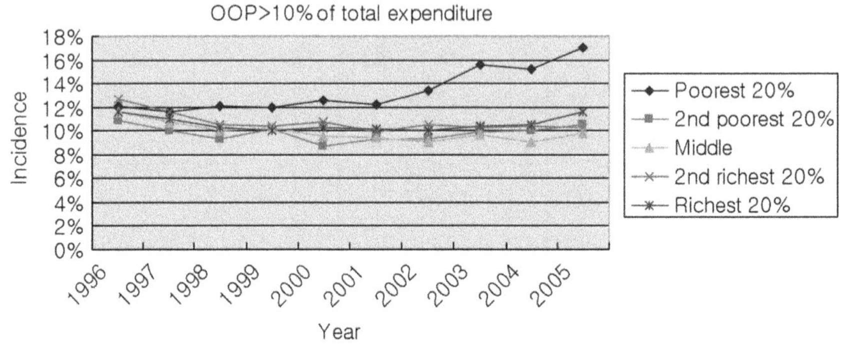

Figure 3.2 Incidence of Catastrophic Payments by Income Quintile.

Table 3.4 Catastrophic Payments by Type of Service (2005)

	OOP >10% Total Expenditure			
	Outpatient	*Inpatient*	*Drug*	*Dental*
Headcount measures				
Headcount (H_C)	2.45%	1.50%	2.98%	1.64%
Concentration index (C_E)	–0.1622	0.2451	–0.3518	0.351 3

of living standards is much stronger. For example, at the defined threshold of household expenditures, the poor are more likely to incur catastrophic payments on drug and outpatient care, while the better-off are more likely to spend in excess of the threshold on inpatient and dental care. This means that the poor may face a financial barrier to the utilization of inpatient and dental care, of which the insurance coverage is partial or very limited, so that they may be forced to substitute medication or outpatient care for inpatient care.

Table 3.5 shows the average OOP payments, by income quintile, of those households that experienced catastrophic payment and their breakdown by type of service. The average amount of OOP payments among those households experiencing catastrophic payment differs significantly by income quintile ($p < 0.005$). Out of the small amount of OOP payments, the poorest 20 percent households experiencing catastrophic payment spend a disproportionately large share on drug and outpatient care while, out of the large amount of OOP payments, the richest 20 percent households experiencing catastrophic payment spend a relatively even share on each service ($p < 0.005$).

The Poverty Impact of OOP Payments

The poverty headcounts based on household expenditures relative to the NPL are shown in table 3.6. The poverty headcounts, estimated before subtracting

Table 3.5 Breakdown of OOP Payments by Type of Service and by Income Quintile (2005)

Income quintile	*OOP payment (KW)*		*Percentage (%)*			
	Mean	*S.D.*	*Outpatient*	*Inpatient*	*Drug*	*Dental*
Poorest 20%	151,485	110,339	33.1	3.8	49.0	3.3
Second poorest 20%	299,716	183,328	33.1	7.4	36.7	9.7
Middle	435,847	290,013	27.8	14.5	31.9	13.8
Second richest 20%	645,655	436,932	25.6	14.7	25.3	22.1
Richest 20%	1,320,374	1,287,429	21.5	20.2	18.1	29.4
Total	537,250	742,275	28.7	11.3	33.8	14.5

KW denotes Korean Won.
The amount of OOP payment is the average OOP payments of those households that experienced catastrophic impact, and the percentage denotes the proportion of OOP payments spent on each type of service.

OOP payments from household expenditures, varied from 7.4 percent in 2004 to 16.8 percent in 1998. The highest poverty estimate in 1998, followed by that in 1999, has to do with an economic crisis in Korea that occurred at the end of 1997. As a consequence of the economic crisis, household expenditures shrank, and the number of households whose expenditures fell below the NPL increased steeply.

Subtraction of OOP payments from household expenditures did not change the general pattern of poverty headcounts by a great deal and increased the poverty headcounts by less than one percentage point each year. However, the differences between pre-payment and post-payment headcount were statistically significant ($p < 0.05$). In 2005, for example, the poverty headcount after subtracting OOP payments from household expenditures increased by 0.6 percentage points, equivalent to 292,550 people. Relative to the initial poverty headcount, adjustment for OOP payments increased the poverty estimate by 6.9 percent in 2005. Although the impoverishing effect of OOP payments appears to be moderate in Korea, there is a concern that, considering the number of individuals impoverished or the relative change in the poverty estimate, the impoverishing effect of OOP payments gradually tends to have become larger in recent years ($p < 0.01$).

DISCUSSION

Using the data from the nationally representative household expenditure survey, the trend in the catastrophic and impoverishing impact of OOP payments in Korea was examined during the period from 1996 to 2005. The main findings from the threshold analyses need further discussion.

Table 3.6 Poverty Headcounts

	1996	*1997*	*1998*	*1999*	*2000*	*2001*	*2002*	*2003*	*2004*	*2005*
Pre-payment	10.27	9.62	16.80	14.74	11.09	8.65	8.02	8.35	7.41	8.80
Headcount (%)	(0.12)	(0.12)	(0.15)	(0.14)	(0.13)	(0.11)	(0.11)	(0.09)	(0.09)	(0.10)
Postpayment	10.61	9.98	17.11	15.09	11.32	9.02	8.54	8.94	7.92	9.41
Headcount (%)	(0.12)	(0.12)	(0.15)	(0.14)	(0.13)	(0.12)	(0.11)	(0.10)	(0.09)	(0.10)
Change in poverty headcount										
Percentage point change (%)[1]	0.34	0.36	0.31	0.35	0.23	0.38	0.51	0.59	0.51	0.61
Number of individuals	154,666	165,355	144,743	165,032	108,340	179,053	243,916	284,107	245,597	292,550
Percentage change (%)[2]	3.31	3.74	1.86	2.40	2.08	4.37	6.38	7.11	6.90	6.90

The figures in the parentheses are standard errors.
[1]The differences between pre-payment and post-payment headcount were statistically significant ($p < 0.05$).
[2]A least-squares regression of percentage change in poverty headcount on year in a simple linear functional form resulted in a coefficient for the term year of 0.006 ($p = 0.004$); $R^2 = 0.66$.

First, although the proportion of health-care financing through the NHI has increased since 2001, the proportion of households spending in excess of the thresholds has not declined. Rather, the incidence of catastrophic payments produced the upward part of a U-shaped curve. The increasing trend of catastrophic payments can be explained by the fact that OOP payments for health-care increase faster than total household expenditures. During the period of 1996–2001, household expenditures increased annually by 4.7 percent, while OOP payments increased annually by 2.5 percent. After 2001, in contrast, the annual increase rate of OOP payments jumped up to 8.4 percent, while that of household expenditures remained at 4.2 percent, similar to previous years.

As mentioned above, the steep increase in OOP payments is attributable to the increase in both price and quantity of health services utilized after the implementation of the SP, as well as additional increase in co-payments for outpatient care and drugs. Despite the efforts to increase the overall insurance coverage rate, therefore, households' OOP payments went up from 2001, leading to a higher incidence of catastrophic payments and increased impoverishment as well.

Second, catastrophic payments occurred among the poor households more frequently compared to the better-off, and the negative concentration indices have been enlarged since 2001, which means more of the poor households have experienced catastrophic payments. The increasing and higher incidence of catastrophic payments among the poor households can be attributed to their limited household resources to cope with increased OOP payments for health care. As mentioned above, the annual increase rate of OOP payments more than tripled after 2001, compared to the period of 1996–2001. The increased OOP payments did not seem to affect consumption in the other income groups except the poorest 20 percent so that the incidence of catastrophic payments among each of these groups did not display great variations over the years. By contrast, the increased OOP payments disrupted severely the consumption of the poorest 20 percent group. Given that their household resources were limited, those with increased OOP payments ended up with reduced spending on other necessities rather than increasing overall household expenditures. Consequently, the incidence of catastrophic payments among the poorest 20 percent has been increasing since 2001 (figure 3.2). It is also noteworthy that the poor households are vulnerable to catastrophic payments even when they spend disproportionately large resources on drug and outpatient care, not on inpatient care.

Third, the incidence of catastrophic payments by type of service shows that the proportion of households spending in excess of the 10 percent threshold is higher for drug and outpatient care than for inpatient care. This may have to do with the demand for those services. By nature, health problems requiring outpatient care are more common compared to health problems requiring hospitalization. In the Korean context, however, the higher incidence of catastrophic payments in drug and outpatient care than in inpatient care has more to do with insurance coverage. Under the NHI, patients pay more for inpatient care than for outpatient care mainly because of many noncovered inpatient services. Thus, it is likely that patients substitute outpatient care and/or drugs for inpatient care, in particular, when they have limited resources.

In fact, it is observed that the poorest 20 percent of Korean households spend a disproportionately large share of their resources on drug and outpatient care, while the richest 20 percent spend an approximately equal share on different types of services. For example, among the poorest 20 percent of households, the budget share of OOP payments on drug is almost ten times as large as that on inpatient care. As shown in table 3.5, therefore, the poor households are more likely to experience catastrophic payments in drug and outpatient care while the better-off are in inpatient care. It is not easy to see with the data provided if the higher utilization of drug and outpatient care among the poor households helped them to meet their medical needs appropriately. However, a result from Korea National Health and Nutrition Examination Survey (KNHANES III) shows that the overall health status of the poor members of Korean society is worse than that of their nonpoor counterparts [18]. Considering the higher medical needs of the poor, there seems to be inequity in access to health services under the Korean NHI.

Fourth, just like the catastrophic impact, the poverty impact of OOP payments has been increasing in recent years. Further analysis shows that the average budget share of OOP payments among those households impoverished newly because of large OOP payments continued to increase in recent years, amounting to 33.9 percent in 2005, which was almost nine times higher than that of those households that remained nonimpoverished. In other words, spending about a third of household resources on OOP payments for health care ended up with 1.1 percent of the population, equivalent to 522,890 individuals, being newly impoverished in 2005.

On the other hand, the poverty impact was greatest among those households with household resources between 100 percent and 120 percent of the NPL. Adjusting for OOP payments increased the poverty estimate by 10.6 percentage points among those income groups. By contrast, among the households with household resources between 120 percent and 200 percent of the NPL, and over 200 percent of the NPL, the poverty headcount after adjusting for OOP payments increased by one percentage point and 0.3 percentage points, respectively. Therefore, it is evident that those households below 120 percent of the NPL are most vulnerable to OOP payments, and it is worthwhile to consider alleviating their financial burden at the time of utilizing health services in order to reduce the impoverishing effect of OOP payments.

This study has several limitations. First, though it estimated catastrophic impact of OOP payments over ten years, this study did not follow up each of those households that experienced catastrophic payments, and thus could not tell how long the catastrophic impact would last and how severe it would be. This has to do with the nature of the national household expenditure survey, which does not necessarily survey the same households each year. Second, this study identified only the households that incurred catastrophic payments and did not count those that forwent treatment due to lack of household resources. Taking account of unreported forgone treatment, large OOP payments would have a more detrimental effect on the welfare of patients. However, this study was at least successful in showing that the poor tend to seek relatively inexpensive services—drug and outpatient care—to meet their medical needs, irrespective of their medical appropriateness.

CONCLUSION

It was only a few years ago that the NHI was standing at the crossroads. In the light of its limited role of paying for health care, its proponents claimed that the NHI should extend its insurance coverage in order to cover up to 70 percent of total health expenditures, while others were looking for a gateway for relying further on private health insurance. At the crossroads, Korea has chosen a path for extending the insurance coverage of the NHI in order to relieve patients of the financial burden incurred by high OOP payments.

The findings of this study suggest that the NHI should pay attention to the increasing trend of the catastrophic and impoverishing impact of OOP payments since 2001, and in particular to the higher incidence of catastrophic payments among the poor, and to the financial barrier to the utilization of inpatient care. In conclusion, in order that the NHI may remain as a major way of financing health care in Korea, it is necessary not only to reduce overall OOP payments by extending insurance coverage particularly for inpatient care but also to ease the vulnerable households' financial burden by exempting them from some OOP payments.

NOTE

1. This chapter was previously published as Lee, TaeJin. "Paying out-of-pocket for health care in Korea: changes in catastrophic and poverty impact over a decade of 1996–2005." *The Korean Journal of Public Health* 54, no. 1 (2017): 31–41.

REFERENCES

1. Newhouse, J.P., Manning, W.G., Morris, C.N., Orr, L.L., Duan, N., Keeler, E.B., et al. (1981). "Some interim results from a controlled trial of cost sharing in health insurance." *New England Journal of Medicine*, 305(25), 1501–1507.
2. Leibowitz, A., Manning W.G., & Newhouse, J.P. (1985). "The demand for prescription drugs as a function of cost-sharing." *Social Science & Medicine*, 21(10), 1063–1069.
3. O'Brien, B. (1989). "The effect of patient charges on the utilisation of prescription medicines." *Journal of Health Economics*, 8(1), 109–132.
4. Ryan, M., & Birch, S. (1991). "Charging for health care: evidence on the utilisation of NHS prescribed drugs." *Social Science & Medicine*, 33(6), 681–687.
5. Brook, R.H., Ware, J.E.Jr., Rogers, W.H., Keeler, E.B., Davies, A.R., Donald, C.A., et al. (1983). "Does free care improve adults' health? Results from a randomized controlled trial." *New England Journal of Medicine*, 309(23), 1426–1434.
6. Keeler, E.B, Brook, R.H., Goldberg, G.A., Kamberg, C.J., & Newhouse, J.P. (1985). How free care reduced hypertension in the health insurance experiment. *Journal of American Medical Association*, 254(14), 1926–1931.
7. Van Doorslaer, E., O'Donnell, O., Rannan-Eliya, R., Somanathan, A., Adhikari, S.R., Akkazieva, B., et al. (2005). "Paying out-of-pocket for health care in Asia: catastrophic and poverty impact." *EQUITAP Project Working Paper # 2.*
8. Pradhan, M., & Prescott, N. (2002). "Social risk management options for medical care in Indonesia." *Health Economics*, 11(5), 431–446.
9. Wagstaff, A., & Van Doorslaer, E. (2003). "Catastrophe and impoverishment in paying for health care: with application to Vietnam 1993–98." *Health Economics*, 12(11), 921–934.
10. Xu, K., Evans, D.B., Kawabata, K., Zeramdini, R., Klavus, J., & Murray, C.J.L. (2003). "Household catastrophic health expenditure: a multicountry analysis." *Lancet*, 362(9378), 111–117.
11. Van Doorslaer, E., O'Donnell, O., Rannan-Eliya, R., Somanathan, A., Adhikari, S.R., Garg, C., et al. (2006). "Effect of health payments on poverty estimates in 11 countries in Asia: An analysis of household survey data." *Lancet*, 368(14), 1357–1364.
12. Van Doorslaer, E., O'Donnell, O., Rannan-Eliya, R., Somanathan, A., Adhikari, S.R., Garg, C., et al. (2007). "Catastrophic payments for health care in Asia." *Health Economics*, 16(11), 1159–1184.
13. Kim, H.R., Kang, Y.H., Yoon, K.J., & Kim, C.S. (2004). *Socioeconomic Health Inequalities and Counter Policies in Korea.* Seoul: Korea Institute of Health and Social Affairs.
14. Korea National Health Insurance Corporation. (2007). *National Health Insurance Statistical Yearbook.* Seoul: Korea National Health Insurance Corporation.
15. Ranson, M.K. (2002). "Reduction of catastrophic health care expenditures by a community-based health insurance scheme in Gujarat, India: current experiences and challenges." *Bulletin of the World Health Organization*, 80(8), 613–621.

16. Russell, S. (2004). "The economic burden of illness for households in developing countries: a review of studies focusing on malaria, tuberculosis, and human immunodeficiency virus/acquired immunodeficiency syndrome." *American Journal of Tropical Medicine and Hygiene*, 71(Suppl. 2), 147–155.
17. Short, K., & Garner, T. (2002). "Experimental poverty measures: accounting for medical expenditures." *Monthly Labor Review*, 125, 3–13.
18. Korea Institute of Health and Social Affairs. (2006). *The Third Korea National Health and Nutrition Examination Survey (KNHANES III)*. Seoul: Korea Institute of Health and Social Affairs.
19. OECD. (2007). *Health Data*. Paris: OECD.

Chapter 4

Multilevel Analysis of Health-Care Service Utilization among Medical Aid Beneficiaries in Korea

Yang Heui Ahn, Ok Kyung Ham, Soo Hyun Kim, and Chang Gi Park

As[1] one of Korea's social welfare programs, the medical aid program was introduced in 1977 as a public medical assistance program targeted at the poor. Due to an increase in the number of beneficiaries and expansion of services, as well as increased prevalence of chronic disease and an aging population, healthcare expenditure reimbursements for medical aid beneficiaries have continued to rise (Lee, Oh, & Choi, 2010). A previous study reported that the top 10 percent of beneficiaries who utilized a large amount of health-care services expended almost 60 percent of total medical aid expenditures; thus, these heavy users are regarded as targets of case management services to promote appropriate use of health-care services (Lee et al., 2010).

In Korea, a case management program for medical aid beneficiaries was initiated in 2003, in order to promote appropriate use, to ensure provision of quality health-care services and to safeguard health-care resources. Development of effective case management services requires elucidation of factors associated with use of health-care services. Few such studies have been conducted for identification of factors associated with health-care service utilization among medical aid beneficiaries in Korea (Ahn et al., 2011; Shin, Kim, Park, & Lee, 2010a; Shin et al., 2010b).

Ahn et al. (2011) sought to figure out factors associated with overuse and underuse of health-care services targeting medical aid beneficiaries, and others examined factors contributing overutilization of health-care services among medical aid beneficiaries; however, these studies considered only individual-level variables employing single-level model in the analysis of factors associated with health-care service utilization (Ahn et al., 2011; Shin et al., 2010a, b), while studies that examined community-level factors associated with health-care service utilization of medical aid beneficiaries have not been conducted in Korea. Single-level model only explains a limited portion of the variability in behavior (Ber-Ben, Dobbels, Engberg, Hill, & de Geest, 2012). The aim of this study was to identify individual- and group-level factors associated with overutilization of health-care services among medical aid beneficiaries in Korea by application of multilevel modeling to provide baseline data in the development of case management intervention programs for beneficiaries.

THEORETICAL FRAMEWORK

The theoretical model guiding this study was based on ecological model. Ecological models of health behavior emphasize the environmental and policy context of behavior, consider multiple-level influences in the development of interventions, and stimulate need for comprehensive population wide approaches to changing behaviors (Sallis, Owen, & Fisher, 2008). Ecological model posits that multiple-level factors can influence health behavior, including intrapersonal, interpersonal, organizational, community, and public policy levels (Sallis et al., 2008). Applying ecological model, Bae et al. (2008) analyzed factors associated with gastric cancer screening behavior of Koreans, and they found that intrapersonal (age), interpersonal (recommendation from family and family screening habits), and community (community health education, and social norm)-level factors were significantly associated with gastric cancer screening behavior.

World Health Organization (2002) argued that individual (biological and personal history factors), relationship (relationships with peers, intimate partners, and family members), community (community context in which social relationships are embedded), and societal (societal norms, policies, and cultural beliefs) factors interplay and influence behavior, thus ecological model provides key points for prevention and interventions. Therefore, utilizing ecological model, the current study sought to elucidate individual- and group (community)-level factors simultaneously that influence overutilization of health-care services among medical aid beneficiaries in Korea (figure 4.1).

METHODS

Sampling and Setting

Secondary data analysis was performed using data on health-care service reimbursement and medical aid case management progress from 16,370

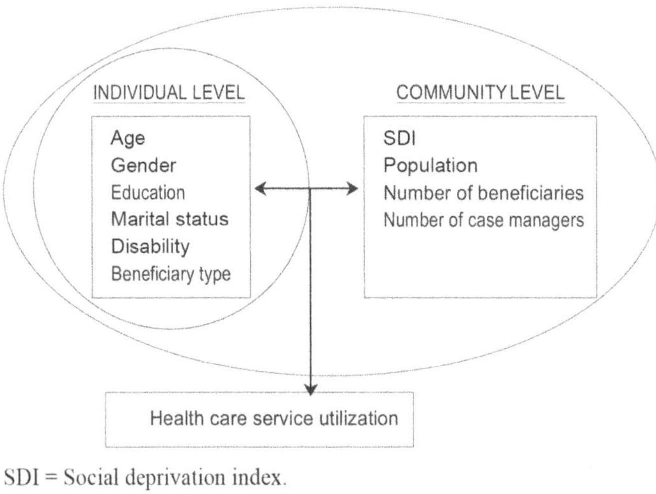

Figure 4.1 Theoretical Framework of the Study Based on Ecological Model. SDI = Social Deprivation Index.

beneficiaries who were heavy users of health-care services, and who obtained medical aid case management services from 232 local offices during the first half of 2009. After data cleaning and deletion of incomplete data, data on 15,948 (97.4 percent) beneficiaries from 229 local offices were used for analysis.

Heavy users were selected by case managers based on health-care service utilization data incurred during the previous year, thus for selection of 2009 case management target, data incurred during 2008 were assessed. Case managers received previous year's health-care service utilization data of all medical aid beneficiaries residing in their region from National Health Insurance Corporation (NHIC) for use with establishment of case management plan. Using the sorting menu of the Excel program, case managers ranked health-care service utilization data from highest to lowest. Variables included in the sorting were total health-care costs, length of health-care service utilization and hospitalization, overlapping days of medication (prescription of drugs with identical components exceeding 365 days within a year), and number of health-care organizations visited during the previous year.

Those ranked higher in most of the categories were assigned to the heavy user group, and case managers review individual medical record using integrated information support system, in order to assess whether or not beneficiaries utilized health-care services inappropriately considering their disease status, and whether or not they need case management services. Those ranked higher in most of the categories, but have multiple severe health conditions that need long-term and expensive health-care services, and appropriately utilized health-care services were not included as targets of case management services, and in turn excluded from the current study. The study was approved by the institutional review board of Yonsei University Wonju College of Medicine.

Dataset

Data on health-care service utilization incurred during the first half of 2009 were provided by the NHIC. Data related to sociodemographic and medical aid were provided by the Medical-Aid Case Management Center (MACMC), retrieved from center's database, which were collected by case managers during the case management services in 2009. Data of the 229 regions were retrieved from the Statistics Korea website (Statistics Korea, 2009) and government report (Shin et al., 2009). Data on health-care service utilization included total number of days of health-care service utilization during the first half of 2009, including clinic visits, hospitalization, and duration of drug prescription. Total number of days of health-care utilization was used as an outcome variable, because it is an important indicator in the management of beneficiary qualifications, and the beneficiaries should obtain approval from the local government if they need to use health-care services exceeds 365 days within a year (Korea Ministry of Health & Welfare, 2010).

Individual data included sociodemographic, medical aid beneficiary type, and existence of disability. Sociodemographic characteristics included age, gender, marital status, and education level. Medical aid beneficiary types include types 1 (those who have no copayments) and 2 (those who have upto 15 percent copayment rates), and those for persons of national merit, refugees, servicemen, and victims of natural disasters. Beneficiaries with disabilities were defined based on the physicians' diagnosis and disability registration record of local offices across Korea; disabilities included all types of impairment, including physical, sensory, and intellectual disabilities. Group data included social deprivation index (SDI), population size, and the number of medical aid beneficiaries and case managers within the region in 2009. The number of case managers was included as the group data because the number of case managers was associated with competencies of case managers (Song, 2011). The SDI for Korea was developed by Shin et al. (2009), considering low socioeconomic class, size of aged population, education level below high school, poor living environment, apartment houses, automobile ownership, single household family, and women as head of household. Mean z-scores of above indicators were used in the estimation of SDI with higher scores indicated more deprived regions. The Korean SDI was developed based on 2005 census data of Korea, and after review of SDI for England, Canada, New

Zealand, and Scotland. Verification of the construct and concurrent validity of the Korean SDI was provided by Shin et al.

Data Analysis

SPSS 19.0 was used for analysis. Descriptive statistical analysis was performed in order to illustrate individual-level and group-level data. Multilevel analysis was performed at two levels. In the analysis, individual beneficiaries were conceptualized as being nested within 229 regions. First, the null model without covariates was used to partition the total variance at the two levels. Second, analysis was performed for examination of associations between individual-level variables and health-care service utilization (Model 1). In model 2, group variables were added for simultaneous examination of the effects of individual- and group-level variables.

Null model

Level 1: $Y_{ij} = \beta_{0j} + e_{ij}$

Level 2: $\beta_{0j} = \alpha + u_j$

$Y_{ij} = \alpha + u_j + e_{ij}$

Y_{ij} denoted the value of the variable for health-care service utilization for *i*th beneficiaries within the *j*th region, α is the intercept, u_j is the level 2 random effect, and e_{ij} is the level 1 random error. Null model is the intercept only model, and only separates the variances of the dependent variable into two parts: the variance of groups (σ_u^2), and the variance of individuals (σ_e^2). The intraclass correlation (ICC) can be computed on the basis of these two variance components:

$$ICC = \sigma_u^2 / \left(\sigma_u^2 + \sigma_e^2\right)$$

The ICC refers to correlation among lower-level units (individual level) within higher-level units (group level). ICC measures the degree to which individuals share common characteristics due to closeness in space or time and is a proportion of variance in the outcome that is attributed to higher-level units (Lake, 2006).

Model 1

$$\begin{aligned} Yij = {} & \beta_{0j} + \beta_1 AGE_{ij} + \beta_2 GENDER_{ij} + \beta_3 EDUCATION_{ij} \\ & + \beta_4 MARRIAGE_{ij} + \beta_5 DISABILITY_{ij} \\ & + \beta_6 BENEFICIARYTYPE_{ij} + u_j + e_{ij} \end{aligned}$$

In model 1, β_{0j} is the intercept and could differ across groups, β is the effect of the covariate, and e_{ij} is the level 1 random error. Coefficients of model 1 (β_1, β_2, β_3, β_4, β_5, β_6) were modeled as fixed slopes.

Model 2

$$Y_{ij} = \beta_{0j} + \beta_{1j} \times AGE_{ij} + \beta_{2j} \times GENDER_{ij} + \beta_{3j} \times EDUCATION_{ij}$$
$$+ \beta_{4j} \times MARRIAGE_{ij} + \beta_{5j} \times DISABILITY_{ij}$$
$$+ \beta_{6j} \times BENEFICIARYTYPE_{ij} + \beta_7 SDI_j + \beta_8\, POPULATION_j$$
$$+ \beta_9\, BENEFICIARIES_j + \beta_{10}\, CASEMANAGERS_j + u_j + e_{ij}$$

In model 2, group-level variables were added. β_7, β_8, β_9, and β_{10} are the regression coefficients of the group-level variables, e_{ij} is the level 1 random error, and u_j is the level 2 random effect.

RESULTS

General Characteristics of the Participants

The mean age was 66.93 years (SD =12.51, range 11–100). Females constituted 64.5 percent (n = 10,281) of the beneficiaries, and 28 percent (n = 4,460) were married or cohabitating. Forty-two percent (n = 6,702) of participants had disabilities, and 35.5 percent (n = 5,660) had no school education. Seventy percent (n =11,255) were beneficiaries of the type 1 medical aid program, while 10.9 percent (n =1,737) were type 2 beneficiaries. The mean length of health-care service utilization in 2009 during the six-month period was 1,235.99 days (SD = 585.99) (table 4.1).

Attributes of Group-Level Characteristics

Group-level characteristics of 229 regions were illustrated. The mean SDI was –0.10 (SD = 0.83), and the mean number of the population was 292,585.34 (SD = 212,291.33) persons. The mean number of beneficiaries was 10,214.73 (SD = 6,034.24) persons, while the mean number of case managers for each regional office was 3.40 (SD = 2.78) persons (table 4.2).

Results of Multilevel Analysis

Null model

In the null model, statistical significance in the separate variances was observed at two levels ($p < 0.001$). ICC was estimated based on two variance

Table 4.1 General Characteristics of Medical Aid Beneficiaries (N = 15,948)

Individual Variable	*Distribution*	*n (%)*	*M± SD*	*Range*
Age (year)			66.93±12.51	11–100
Gender	Male	5,667 (35.5)		
	Female	10,281 (64.5)		
Marital status	Married/ cohabitating	4,460 (28.0)		
	Single	977 (6.1)		
	Widowed/ divorced/ separated	6,171 (38.7)		
	No response	4,340 (27.2)		
Education (*n* =19,946)	None	5,660 (35.5)		
	≤ 9 years	6,171 (38.7)		
	≥ 10 years	2,243 (14.1)		
	No response	1,874 (11.7)		
Disability	Yes	6,702 (42.0)		
	No	9,246 (58.0)		
Beneficiary type	Type 1	11,255 (70.6)		
	Type 2	1,737 (10.9)		
	Person of national merit	1,358 (8.5)		
	Other[a]	1,598 (10.0)		
Health-care service utilization (days/6 months)			1,235.99± 585.99	1–15,872

[a]Included refugees, servicemen, victims of natural disasters, and others.

Table 4.2 Attributes of Group-Level Characteristics According to the 229 Regions (N = 15,948)

Group Variables	*Range*	*M±SD*
SDI	– 1.42–1.69	–0.10± 0.83
Population	18,221–1,073,149	292,585.34± 212,291.33
Number of beneficiaries	468–27,773	10,214.73± 6,034.24
Number of case managers	1–10	3.40± 2.78

SDI=social deprivation index.

components, 69,267.68/ (313,859.17 + 69,267.68) = 0.181, indicating that variance at the group level accounted for 18.1 percent of the total variance of health-care service utilization. The results indicated that both individual and group variables could be considered in health-care service utilization.

Model 1

The results indicated a significant association of health-care service utilization with individual factors, including existence of disability and medical aid beneficiary type. The coefficient estimates of disability and beneficiary type were –35.98 and –97.17, respectively ($p < 0.05$), which implied decreased health-care service utilization by an average of 35.98 days by those with disabilities and average of 97.17 days for beneficiaries with other than type 1. Existence of statistically significant variance at the group level (74,194.58, $p < 0.001$) implied that the intercept could differ significantly across regions.

Model 2

The significant random intercept indicated that even after controlling for individual factors, health-care service utilization differs significantly across regions. Among group-level variables, SDI and number of case managers showed a negative association with health-care service utilization, while the number of beneficiaries showed a positive association with health-care service utilization ($p <.05$). Results of the chi-squared test for difference of variance between model 1 and model 2 indicated that model 2 showed a better fit ($\chi^2 = 40{,}813.04$, $p < 0.001$), which suggests that both individual- and group-level variables are good predictors for explaining variations in health-care service utilization among medical aid beneficiaries across regions (Cho, 2003) (table 4.3).

DISCUSSION

Using multilevel analysis, findings of the current study demonstrated an association of both individual- and group-level variables with health-care service utilization among medical aid beneficiaries in Korea. Using the null model, the estimated ICC was 0.181 (18.1 percent of the variance was explained with statistical significance by the group-level variables). ICC greater than 0.05 (5 percent) and 0.10 (10 percent) demonstrated meaningful and substantial differences across groups, respectively (Lee, 2009); thus, the ICC= 0.181 (18.1 percent) of the current study also indicated substantial differences in health-care service utilization across regions. Data collected from medical aid beneficiaries have a hierarchical structure and can be correlated with one another (Park & Lake, 2005). Using clustered data, estimated standard errors in a conventional regression are smaller than actual standard errors due to failure to account for the correlated structure of observations, which increase a type I error (Park & Lake). Thus, for the current study, application of multilevel analysis was appropriate. At the individual level, existence of disability and types of medical aid beneficiaries showed a significant association, while SDI, the number of beneficiaries, and case managers at the group level showed a significant association with health-care service utilization.

Table 4.3 Multilevel Analysis of Health-Care Service Utilization According to the 229 Regions (n = 15,948)

	Null Model		*Model 1*		*Model 2*	
Fixed Effect	*Estimates*	P	*Estimates*	p	*Estimates*	p
Individual level						
Intercept	1,209.39	<.001	1,325.70	<.001	1,254.37	<.001
Age			0.77	.121	0.61	.258
Gender			−1.73	.890	−11.42	.395
Education			−27.06	.099	−19.12	.287
Marital status			19.21	.114	15.62	.232
Disability			−28.67	.014	−35.98	.005
Beneficiary type			−111.49	<.001	−97.17	<.001
Group level						
SDI					−73.17	.044
Population					0.00	.678
Number of beneficiaries					0.02	.005
Number of case managers					−47.02	.007
Random Effect	*Variance Component*	*p*	*Variance Component*	*p*	*Variance Component*	*p*
Residual	313,859.17	<.001	320,318.59	<.001	285,288.65	<.001
Intercept (Variance)	69,267.68	<.001	74,194.58	<.001	62,038.82	<.001
Deviance	247,649.77		165,740.62		124,927.58	
X^2			81,909.15	<.001	40,813.04	<.001

SDI= social deprivation index.

Variables: Gender 1= male, 2= female; education 1= less than or equal to nine years, 2= more than nine years; marriage1= without spouse (single, divorces, widowed, or separated), 2= with spouse; disability 0= not disabled, 1= disabled; beneficiary type 1= type 1, 2= other (type 2, those for persons of national merit, refugees, servicemen, and victims of natural disasters).

The results indicated significant variation in health-care service utilization by region. These differences could be explained by group-level variables.

Findings from a previous study illustrated that beneficiaries with disability were more likely to be in poor health and to have more health-care service needs (Park et al., 2006). However, barriers to health-care service utilization, such as transportation, communication, financial problems, and lack of expert providers, prohibit them from utilization of needed health-care services (Eun et al., 2006), which is consistent with results of the current study. In the current study, due to barriers indicated above (transportation, communication etc.), beneficiaries with disabilities may have utilized health-care services less often than those without disabilities, even though their health-care service needs were greater. The beneficiaries included in the current study were heavy users of health-care services who were in the top 1 percent of 1.84 million beneficiaries (Korea Ministry of Health & Welfare, 2010); thus, they may have different attributes with regard to use of health-care services, compared with those not included in this category. However, negative association between disability and health-care service utilization may imply that case managers need to ensure that health-care needs of the beneficiaries with disabilities are met and/or that quality and continuity of health-care services are assured.

Findings of the current study also revealed an association of beneficiary type with health-care service utilization, and those who were type 1 medical aid beneficiaries (those who have no copayments) were more likely to overuse health-care services, regardless of health conditions; therefore, it is obvious that due to insensitivity to health-care costs, removal of financial barriers with type 1 medical aid may promote increased use of health-care services. Thus, for the sake of public interest, in education of medical aid beneficiaries, responsibility for use of common goods (free health-care services) should be fostered.

A previous study contended that those living in deprived regions were less likely to utilize preventive health-care services (Chang, 2012), which is consistent with the current study that SDI was negatively associated with health-care service utilization. SDI showed strong positive association with standardized mortality (Shin et al., 2009), and others argued for an association of deprivation with unhealthy lifestyles (Hanlon et al., 1998), thus beneficiaries living in deprived areas could be priority target of case management services to enhance health and quality of life and to promote optimal use of health-care services.

The ecological model posits that multiple-level factors such as intrapersonal, interpersonal, and community-level factors were associated with behavior (Sallis et al., 2008). Applying ecological model, Bae et al. (2008) demonstrated that intrapersonal (age) and community factors (community health education, and social norm) were associated with use of preventive health-care services in Korea, while Medlensky, Esplen, Gallinger, McLaughlin, and Goel (2003) investigated that individual (age, and perceived benefits and barriers), family (encourage from family), physician (advice from physician), and societal-level (screening advertisement) factors were associated with colorectal screening behavior in Canada. This could be applied to the results of the current study demonstrating that individual or intrapersonal level (existence of disabilities and type of medical aid), and group or community-level factors (SDI, and number of case managers and beneficiaries) may have had an influence on behaviors of individual beneficiaries in health-care service utilization. Influence of group-level factors outside beneficiaries in health-care service utilization may imply that education targeting beneficiaries is insufficient for promotion of appropriate health-care service utilization. Future interventions should include use of multilevel approaches applying ecological model (Sallis et al., 2008), such as enhancing awareness of health-care providers and communities, and/or change in public health policy.

Andersen's Behavioral Model, which is the most frequently used theoretical model for explaining use of health-care services could also be applied to the current study. The model consists of three determinant factors: predisposing, enabling, and need factors (Kim, Nam, Chae, & Lee, 2008). Findings of the current study revealed a significant association of enabling (beneficiary type and case managers) and need factors (existence of disability) with health-care service utilization, and indicated that community resources (case managers) may influence health-care service utilization by medical aid beneficiaries.

The significant negative association observed between the number of case managers and health-care service utilization may indicate effectiveness of case management programs in promotion of appropriate use of health-care services. A previous study reported on the effectiveness of administration of a case management program in decreasing health-care service utilization among medical aid beneficiaries with less severe conditions (Lim, 2010), which is consistent with results of the current study. On the part of beneficiaries, those with less severe conditions may have overused unnecessary health-care services with minimum or no co-payments. On the part of the providers, a fee-for-service payment system reimbursed by the government may result in increased frequency of use of nonessential health-care services. It is assumed that administration of case management programs could result in effective curtailment of unnecessary or nonessential use of health-care services that were previously overused by beneficiaries with less severe conditions. Kim (2012) investigated that case management services targeting medical aid beneficiaries were effective in promoting self-care abilities and quality of life of the beneficiaries, while decreasing health-care service utilization such as clinic visits, drug prescription duration, and health-care costs. The study results may indicate that strengthening of systematic medical aid case management services will help to meet the ever-increasing needs of the beneficiaries in line with increased elderly population and chronic diseases, while to safeguard health-care resources (Kim).

Policy implications of the current study may include in order to assure quality and continuity of health-care services, assignment of additional case managers in regions with an insufficient number of case managers are needed, since results of the current study revealed reverse relationship between the number of case managers and health-care service utilization, moreover, average 3.40 (SD = 2.78) case managers were assigned within the region, with an average of 10,215 (SD = 6,034) beneficiaries. In assigning case managers, level of deprivation and number of beneficiaries with disabilities within the region should be considered, rather than assigning case managers proportional to the number of beneficiaries.

Limitation of the current study includes due to difficulties in obtaining regional data, most of the regional data were restricted to those related to the case management services such as number of beneficiaries and number of case managers. The current study entered total number of days of health-care service utilization (combining clinic visits, hospitalization, and drug prescription days) into the equation as an outcome variable, instead of analyzing factors of these three services, separately. Total number of days of health-care service utilization is an important indicator in the management of beneficiary qualifications; however, future studies are recommended to separately examine factors of three different types of services (clinic visits, hospitalization, and drug prescription days) to verify whether factors of service utilization differ by the types of services. The current study only considered the existence of disability as a health-related variable in analysis of factors of health-care service utilization. Future studies are recommended to consider other health-related variables such as pain, depression, and disease characteristics in understanding factors of health-care service utilization. Another limitation is that 229 administrative districts were employed in the classification of regions, which might not have well represented true contextual effects in health-care service utilization of medical aid beneficiaries. Lastly, applying ecological model, the current study only considered individual- and community-level variables as predictors of health-care service utilization, while interpersonal and public policy-level variables were not included, thus future studies are recommended to include social network, social norm, and/or local public health policy in the analysis of factors of health-care service utilization.

CONCLUSION

By application of multilevel modeling, this study sought to identify individual- and group-level factors associated with health-care service utilization among Korean medical aid beneficiaries. At the individual level, existence of disability and types of medical aid beneficiaries showed a significant association, while at the group level, SDI, and number of beneficiaries and case managers within the region showed a significant association with health-care service utilization. Results of the current study illustrated that variance at the group level accounted for 18.1 percent of the total variance in health-care service utilization. Influence of group-level factors outside beneficiaries in health-care service utilization may imply a necessity for the use of group-level approaches. Thus, case management should include promotion of appropriate use of health-care services targeting beneficiaries, while assuring quality and continuity of health-care services on the part of case managers and health-care providers, as well as to include public health policy change and enhancing community awareness. Further investigations are needed in order to determine whether interpersonal and public policy-level factors (social network, social norm, and local public health policy, etc.) are associated with health-care service utilization.

NOTE

1. This chapter was previously published as Ahn, Yang Heui, Ok Kyung Ham, Soo Hyun Kim, and Chang Gi Park. "Multilevel analysis of health care service utilization among medical aid beneficiaries in Korea." *Journal of Korean Academy of Nursing* 42, no. 7 (2012): 928–935.

REFERENCES

Ahn, Y. H., Kim, E. S., Ham, O. K., Kim, S. H., Hwang, S. S., Chun, S. H., et al. (2011). Factors associated with the overuse or underuse of health care services among medical aid beneficiaries in Korea. *Journal of Community Health Nursing, 28*, 190–203. doi:10.1080/07370016.2011.614837.

Bae, S. S., Jo, H. S., Kim, D. H., Choi, Y. J., Lee, H. J., Lee, T. J., et al. (2008). Factors associated with gastric cancer screening of Koreans: Based on a socio-ecological model. *Journal of Preventive Medicine& Public Health, 41*(2), 100–106.

Berben, L., Dobbels, F., Engberg, S., Hill, M. N., & de Geest, S. (2012). An ecological perspective on medication adherence. *Western Journal of Nursing Research, 34*(5), 635–653. doi:10.1177/0193945911434518.

Chang, Y. (2012). *Determinants of Gastric Cancer Screening Attendance in Korea: A Multi-Level Analysis.* Unpublished Master's Thesis, Seoul National University, Seoul.

Cho, S. H. (2003). Using multilevel analysis in patient and organizational outcomes research. *Nursing Research, 52*(1), 61–65.

Eun, S. J., Hong, J. Y., Lee, J. Y., Lee, J. S., Kim, Y., Kim, Y. I., et al. (2006). Differences in medical care utilization rates of the disabled and the non-disabled with ambulatory care sensitive conditions. *Journal of Preventive Medicine and Public Health, 39*(5), 411–418.

Hanlon, P., Walsh, D., Whyte, B. W., Scott, S. N., Lightbody, P., & Gilhooly, M. L. M. (1998). Hospital use by an ageing cohort: An investigation into the association between biological, behavioural, and social risk markers and subsequent hospital utilization. *Journal of Public Health Medicine, 20*(4), 467–476.

Kim, E. Y., Nam, E. S., Chae, Y. R., & Lee, H. K. (2008). Factors affecting the elderly's preference for utilization of long-term care services based on Andersen's Behavioral Model. *Journal of the Korean Gerontological Society, 28*(3), 585–602.

Kim, S. A. (2012). *The Effect of Case Management Intervention by Medical Aid Case Manager: Centered on Medical Aid Recipients with Chronic Disease.* Unpublished Master's Thesis, Hanyang University, Seoul.

Korea Ministry of Health & Welfare. (2010). *2010 Medical Aid Program Guide.* Seoul: Author.

Lake, E. T. (2006). Multilevel models in health outcomes research part II: Statistical and analytic issues. *Applied Nursing Research, 19*(2), 113–115. doi:10.1016/j.apnr.2006.01.001.

Lee, H. J., Oh, J. J., & Choi, J. M. (2010). Comparison of case management between tele care regions and general care regions in Korean Medicaid. *Journal of Korean Academy of Nursing Administration, 16*(4), 381–388.

Lee, S. H. (2009). Multi-level analysis of factors related to quality of service in long-term care hospitals. *Journal of Korean Academy of Nursing, 39*(3), 409–421. doi:10.4040/jkan.2009.39.3.409.

Lim, S. J. (2010). Change in healthcare utilization by disease severity after case management for Medicaid. *Journal of Korean Academy of Community Health Nursing, 21*(3), 321–332.

Medlensky, L., Esplen, M. J., Gallinger, S., McLaughlin, J. R., & Goel, V. (2003). Relatives of colorectal cancer patients: Factors associated with screening behavior. *American Journal of Preventive Medicine, 25*(3), 187–194. doi:10.1016/S0749-3797(03)00202-2.

Park, J. H., Lee, J. S., Lee, J. Y., Hong, J. Y., Kim, S. Y., Kim, S. O., et al. (2006). Factors affecting national health insurance mass screening participation in the disabled. *Journal of Preventive Medicine and Public Health, 39*(6), 511–519.

Park, S., & Lake, E. T. (2005). Multilevel modeling of a clustered continuous outcome. *Nursing Research, 54*(6), 406–413. doi:10.1097/00006199-200511000-00007.

Sallis, J. F., Owen, N., & Fisher, E. B. (2008). Ecological models of health behavior. In K. Glanz, B. K. Rimer, & K. Viswanath (Eds.), *Health Behavior and Health Education: Theory, Research, and Practice* (4th ed.). San Fransisco, CA: Jossey-Bass.

Shin, S. M., Kim, E. S., Park, C. K., & Lee, H. W. (2010a). The medical use of the disabled among overusers of medical aid in Korea. *Journal of Preventive Medicine and Public Health, 43*(1), 35–41. doi:10.3961/jpmph.2010.43.1.35.

Shin, S. M., Kim, M. J., Kim, E. S., Lee, H. W., Park, C. G., & Kim, H. K. (2010b). Medical aid service overuse assessed by case managers in Korea. *Journal of Advanced Nursing, 66*(10), 2257–2265. doi:10.1111/j.1365-2648.2010.05364.x.

Shin, Y. J., Yoon, T. H., Kim, M. H., Cho, H. J., Kim, M. K., Yoo, W. S., et al. (2009). *Health Promotion Strategies and Programs Development for Health Inequalities Alleviation.* Seoul: Industry-University Cooperation Foundation Hanyang University·Korea Health Promotion Foundation.

Song, M. K. (2011). *Factors Related to Competencies of Medical Aid Case Managers.* Unpublished Master's Thesis, Hanyang University, Seoul.

Statistics Korea. (2009). *Database.* Retrieved December 15, 2011, from http:// kostat .go.kr/portal/korea/index.action.

World Health Organization. (2002). *World Report on Violence and Health.* Retrieved May 16, 2012, from http://www.emro.who.int/violence-inju-ries-disabilities/health-topics/.

Part II

HEALTH DISPARITIES AMONG DIFFERENT POPULATION GROUPS

Chapter 5

The Association between Long Working Hours and Self-Rated Health

Jun-Taek Song, Goeun Lee, Jongho Kwon, Jung-Woo Park, Hyunrim Choi, and Sinye Lim

The[1] relationship between working hours and health is an important issue in the field of occupational research. Many previous studies have shown that long working hours have negative impacts on workers' health. It has been reported that workers working long hours have a higher risk of myocardial infarction [1,2], noninsulin-dependent diabetes (NIDD) [3], and retiring due to disabilities [4]. Working long hours not only affects a worker's health but also has a negative effect on the worker's family [5,6]. Further, it has been reported to cause an increase in the number of accidents and errors in the workplace [7,8]. Caruso et al. presented a conceptual framework for the study of long working hours and stated that long working hours affect sleep and recovery, heighten job demands, increase the time of being exposed to dangerous factors in the workplace, and cause physiological changes, having adverse effects on the workers' health [5].

The International Labour Organisation (ILO) founded in 1919 presented "Controls on Working Hours as an Urgent Improvement Subject" in its constitution at the time of its founding [9]. Then, in November 1996, the European Community implemented regulations on working hours, including the rights of a laborer to refuse to work more than forty-eight hours a week [10]. According to the Fifth European Working Conditions Survey published in 2012, as a result of such efforts, the number of laborers working more than forty-eight hours per week has decreased steadily among wage workers in the European countries [11]. In Korea, the number of working hours in a week cannot exceed forty hours excluding the break time according to the Labor Standards Act, while overtime work hours are regulated to not exceed twelve hours per week [12]. However, despite such regulations, a recent annual report of the statistics of the Organization for Economic Co-operation and

Development (OECD) revealed Korea's average annual working hours to be 2,193 hours in 2010, ranking number one among OECD countries [13].

The self-rated health level is used widely as an indicator of the health condition of an individual, as it reflects the present state of an illness as well as the general health condition of an individual [14,15]. In a research conducted in the United States, it was reported that the odds ratio (OR) of workers working seventy hours or more per week who rated their general health condition and answered that their condition was poor or fair as compared to workers working thirty-five to forty hours per week with the same response was 1.94 (95% confidence interval (CI), 1.07 – 3.51) [16]. Despite the fact that Korea has the longest annual average working hours among the OECD countries, not many studies have been conducted on the relationship between working hours and their impact on workers' health. Some studies on working hours and mental health have been conducted, including studies on long working hours conducted using domestic data showing that workers working long hours have a higher risk of suicidal ideation [17] or show depressive symptomatology [18,19]. However, there have been few studies conducted on the effects of long working hours on general health or self-rated health. Therefore, this study has been conducted using the Korean Labor and Income Panel Study (KLIPS) data to analyze the working hours of full-time wage workers to determine the association between long working hours and self-rated health.

STUDY POPULATION AND METHODS

KLIPS was funded by Ministry of Employment and Labor and conducted with the approval of the Statistics Korea (approval number: 33601). KLIPS was a publicly opened dataset and did not contain any personal information; therefore, ethical approval for this study was waived.

Study Population

The research data of the eleventh KLIPS conducted in 2008 have been used in this study. KLIPS represents 10 percent of the sample survey population from the 1995 census on total population and housing, on the basis of a study on 5,000 households living in nonrural areas and panel sample members (all members of households living in the 5,000 households) representing household members. Further, KLIPS is a longitudinal study that includes follow-up surveys on panel sample members' economic activities, labor movement, income, expenditures, education, job training, and social activities, surveyed once a year starting from 1998 [20].

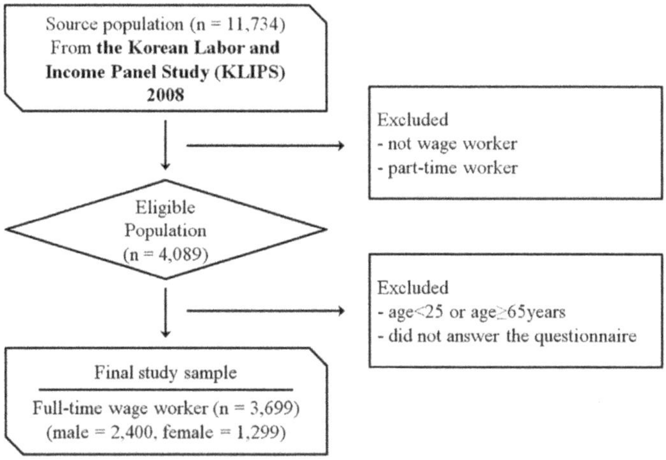

Figure 5.1 Flowchart of Study Population.

Among the 11,734 study subjects of the eleventh KLIPS conducted in 2008, the subjects of this study were 4,089 people who reported that they were full-time wage workers. The study subjects have been restricted to those between the age of twenty-five years or above and less than sixty-five years, considering the employment age of university graduates and the retirement age of workers so that, after excluding the missing data, the study participants finally included 3,699 people (figure 5.1).

Materials and Methods

Working Hours

Under Korea's Labor Standards Act, working hours are limited as follows: The first clause of Article 50 states that "working hours per week shall not exceed forty hours, excluding break times," while the first clause of Article 53 states that "if the parties concerned reach agreement, the working hours stipulated in Article 50 may be extended by up to 12 hours per week," allowing a total number of working hours of up to fifty-two hours under the law [12]. Moreover, in a study on the approval criteria of cardiovascular diseases caused by overwork, if the number of working hours per week right before an occurrence of a cardiovascular disease exceeds sixty hours, then the case is defined as short-term overwork [21].

In this study, the study subjects have been categorized into a less than forty hours group, more than forty hours, and up to fifty-two hours group, more than fifty-two hours and up to sixty hours group, and more than sixty hours group, on the basis of the Labor Standards Act and overwork standards. For cases with a fixed number of regular working hours, the number of working hours per week has been estimated by adding the answers of the questions "What are your current regular working hours per week excluding meal times?" and "In your current job, how many hours do you work overtime on average in a week?" For cases without a fixed number of regular working hours, the answer to the question, "In your current job, how many hours do you work on average in a week?" has been used.

Outcome Variable

The outcome variable of self-rated health has been surveyed on a scale of five levels including "very good," "good," "fair," "poor," and "very poor," on the basis of evaluation conducted by workers on their own at the time of the study. Among the five levels "very good" and "good" were defined as the "healthy group," while the remaining levels were defined as the "unhealthy group."

Measurement of Covariates

Other individual variables including the participants' sociodemographic characteristics, occupational characteristics, and items related to health-related behavior characteristics have been reconstructed by category. Gender, age, marital status, educational status, and monthly household income were chosen as the variables of the sociodemographic characteristics. The marital status variable had the values of "single," "married with a spouse," and others ("separated," "divorced," and "widow/widower"). The educational status was categorized into a below junior high school group, high school group, and above college group after answering the question, "What is your highest level of education? Or are you currently studying?" The monthly household income variable has six portions including earned income, financial income, real estate income, social insurance income, transfer income, and other income with the monthly income calculated by adding all portions of income divided by the square root of the number of family members.

Occupation, employment type, shift work status, and tenure have been chosen as the occupational variables. In the case of the occupation variable, "legislative officials," "senior officials and managers," "specialists," "engineers and associate experts," and "office workers" have been categorized as nonmanual workers, while the remaining occupations including "service workers" and "sales workers" have been categorized as manual workers. The employment type variable has been categorized into regular workers and irregular workers on the basis of the answers chosen by the workers, while the shift work variable was categorized into the shift work group for those who answered that they worked in shifts and the daytime work group for those who answered that they did not work in shifts. The tenure variable has been categorized into the below one year group, the more than one year up to ten years group, and the more than ten years group.

Smoking, alcohol consumption, and exercise have been chosen as the variables for health-related behavior characteristics. In the case of the smoking variable, subjects who answered "currently smoking" were categorized as the smoking group, while those who answered "smoked in the past but quit smoking" and "never smoked before" were categorized as the nonsmoking group. In the case of the alcohol consumption variable, subjects who answered "currently drinking" were categorized as the alcohol-consuming group, while those who answered "drank in the past but quit drinking," and "never drank before" were categorized as the nonalcohol-consuming group. In the case of the exercise variable, subjects who answered "yes, I exercise" were categorized as the exercise group, while those who answered "hardly exercise" were categorized as the nonexercise group.

Statistical Analysis

Frequency analysis and the chi-squared test were conducted in order to understand the relationship between the participants' working hours and each individual variable as well as the relationship between self-rated health and each individual variable. It has been predicted that gender and cumulative exposure time will be found to be important contributors in the relationship between the number of working hours and self-rated health. Female workers were expected to have different characteristics from male workers on the basis of a previous study showing that female workers earn lower wages or have less job control than male workers [22] and the cumulative exposure time is believed to have a great impact on self-rated health because the number of working hours closely affects the workers' lifestyle. On the basis of this fact, the following three types of models were formed and logistic regression analyses were carried out after controlling the relevant variables:

Model 1: Logistic regression analysis model of the study participants after controlling for the sociodemographic characteristics, occupational characteristics, and health-related behavior characteristics.

Model 2: Logistic regression analysis model of the study participants after controlling for the relevant variables after gender stratification.

Model 3: Logistic regression analysis model of the study participants after controlling for the relevant variables after tenure stratification.

SPSS statistics 20.0 (IBM Corp., Armonk, NY, USA) has been used for the statistical analysis, with a significance level of less than 5 percent.

RESULTS

General Characteristics of the Study Participants

Among the 3,699 study participants, there were 2,400 (64.9 percent) male participants and 1,299 (35.1 percent) female participants, with 29.7 percent of them in the group working less than forty hours per week, 39.7 percent in the group working more than forty hours and up to fifty-two hours per week, 19.7 percent in the group working more than fifty-two hours and up to sixty hours per week, and 10.9 percent in the group working more than sixty hours per week (table 5.1). The average working hours per week for all the study participants was 48.8 hours, with longer working hours per week for male workers, manual workers, regular workers, and shift workers than for female workers, nonmanual workers, irregular workers, and daytime workers.

In the cases of both male and female workers, there was no significant difference found between each working hour group with respect to age distribution and marital status (tables 5.2 and 5.3). With respect to educational status, the group having completed high school or beyond was the largest percentage in the group working more than forty hours and up to fifty-two hours per week for female workers. By contrast, in the case of male workers, the group with an educational status of below junior high school showed the largest percentage in the group working less than forty hours per week ($p < 0.001$) (tables 5.2 and 5.3). With respect to the monthly household income, both male and female workers showed the highest income level in the group working less than forty hours per week; in the case of male workers, the monthly household income tended to drop significantly as the number of working hours increased ($p < 0.001$), but the female group showed no statistically significant difference.

With respect to the occupational characteristics of both male and female study participants, manual workers were more common than nonmanual workers in the group working more than fifty-two hours per week ($p < 0.001$). With respect to the employment type, irregular male workers formed a higher proportion of the number of employees working less than forty hours per week and a lower proportion of those working more than forty hours and up to fifty-two hours per week than regular male workers ($p = 0.008$), while in the case of female workers, no significant difference between the groups by employment type was observed. Both male and female shift workers formed a higher proportion of the number of workers working more than fifty-two hours per week and a lower proportion of workers working less than fifty-two hours per week than daytime workers, although the difference was significant for just the males ($p = 0.011$). In

Table 5.1 Weekly Working Hours by Study Subjects' Characteristics

Variables		Total	Weekly Working Hours			
		Total *N Mean ± SD*[†]	*≤40* *%[*] Mean ± SD*[†]	*40 < x ≤ 52* *%[*] Mean ± SD*[†]	*52 < x ≤ 60* *%[*] Mean ± SD*[†]	*>60* *%[*] Mean ± SD*[†]
Total		3,699	29.7	39.7	19.7	10.9
		48.8 ± 12.5	36.8 ± 6.8	47.0 ± 2.8	57.1 ± 2.8	73.5 ± 11.0
Gender	Male	2,400	28.5	39.7	20.7	11.1
		49.2 ± 12.7	36.7 ± 6.8	47.0 ± 2.8	57.1 ± 2.8	74.1 ± 11.9
	Female	1,299	31.8	39.9	17.8	10.5
		48.2 ± 12.0	36.9 ± 6.9	46.9 ± 2.8	57.3 ± 2.8	72.3 ± 8.7
Age	25–34	1,248	30.0	41.2	18.7	10.1
		48.7 ± 12.0	37.5 ± 6.3	47.0 ± 2.8	57.2 ± 2.8	73.4 ± 11.6
	35–44	1,139	28.9	40.5	19.9	10.7
		49.1 ± 12.8	36.7 ± 7.1	47.1 ± 2.7	57.0 ± 2.8	74.9 ± 11.7
	45–54	897	29.9	37.1	20.8	12.2
		49.0 ± 12.7	36.3 ± 6.9	47.0 ± 2.8	57.1 ± 2.8	72.4 ± 10.3
	55–64	415	30.4	38.8	19.5	11.3
		48.4 ± 12.6	36.0 ± 7.2	46.4 ± 2.7	57.3 ± 2.8	72.9 ± 8.3
Occupation	Nonmanual	1,802	31.8	43.2	16.1	8.9
		47.8 ± 11.7	37.2 ± 6.6	46.7 ± 2.8	57.1 ± 2.8	73.6 ± 10.4
	Manual	1,897	27.6	36.5	23.0	12.9
		49.9 ± 13.1	36.3 ± 7.0	47.3 ± 2.7	57.2 ± 2.8	73.5 ± 11.4
Employment type	Regular worker	2,767	28.4	40.9	19.6	11.1
		49.1 ± 12.4	37.2 ± 6.6	46.9 ± 2.8	57.0 ± 2.8	73.9 ± 11.2
	Irregular worker	932	33.4	36.2	19.9	10.5
		48.0 ± 12.8	35.9 ± 7.3	47.0 ± 2.7	57.4 ± 2.8	72.5 ± 10.1
Shift work	No	3,330	30.3	40.0	19.3	10.4
		48.5 ± 12.4	36.7 ± 6.9	46.9 ± 2.8	57.1 ± 2.8	73.3 ± 11.0
	Yes	369	24.1	37.4	22.8	15.7

(Continued)

Table 5.1 Weekly Working Hours by Study Subjects' Characteristics *(Continued)*

			Weekly Working Hours			
		Total	*≤40*	*40 < x ≤ 52*	*52 < x ≤ 60*	*>60*
Variables		*N Mean ± SD*†	*%* Mean ± SD*†	*%* Mean ± SD*†	*%* Mean ± SD*†	*%* Mean ± SD*†
		51.6 ± 13.1	38.0 ± 5.1	47.2 ± 2.8	57.1 ± 2.7	74.8 ± 10.6
Tenure	≤1	988	28.9	41.0	18.8	11.3
(years)		49.0 ± 12.7	36.6 ± 6.7	47.1 ± 2.8	57.4 ± 2.8	74.0 ± 10.7
	1 < x ≤ 10	2,013	29.6	38.3	20.4	11.7
		49.1 ± 12.8	36.8 ± 7.1	47.0 ± 2.7	57.1 ± 2.7	73.5 ± 11.6
	>10	698	30.8	42.2	18.8	8.2
		47.8 ± 11.1	37.1 ± 6.2	46.8 ± 3.0	56.8 ± 2.8	72.6 ± 8.6

*: Row percentage, †SD: Standard deviation.

Table 5.2 General Characteristics of the Male Subjects

Variables		Total	Weekly Working Hours				
		n (%*)	≤40 %†	40 < x ≤ 52 %†	52 < x ≤ 60 %†	>60 %†	p-value
Age (years)	Mean ± SD‡	40.0 ± 10.0	41.5 ± 10.2	40.8 ± 9.9	40.8 ± 9.9	41.1 ± 9.9	0.479§
	25–34	759(31.6)	27.3	40.7	20.5	11.5	0.811‖
	35–44	786(32.8)	27.0	40.8	21.4	10.8	
	45–54	566(23.6)	31.5	36.7	20.5	11.3	
	55–64	289(12.0)	30.1	39.5	19.7	10.7	
Marital status	Never married	520(21.7)	28.3	41.9	20.0	9.8	0.196‖
	Married	1,766(73.6)	28.4	39.7	20.6	11.3	
	Others	114(4.7)	31.6	28.1	25.4	14.9	
Educational status	≤Junior high school	304(12.7)	34.2	29.6	22.7	13.5	<0.001‖
	High school	819(34.1)	25.8	37.6	23.8	12.8	
	≥College	1,277(53.2)	28.9	43.4	18.2	9.5	
Household income (KRW/month)¶	Mean ± SD‡	207.7 ± 260.5	224.6 ± 302.9	214.4 ± 273.7	190.1 ± 209.4	173.6 ± 155.4	<0.001**
Occupation	Nonmanual	1,097(45.7)	29.4	44.0	17.6	9.0	<0.001‖
	Manual	1,303(54.3)	27.8	36.0	23.3	12.9	
Employment type	Regular worker	1,879(78.3)	27.0	41.0	20.6	11.4	0.008‖
	Irregular worker	521(21.7)	34.0	34.7	21.3	10.0	
Shift work	No	2,110(87.9)	29.3	39.8	20.4	10.5	0.011‖
	Yes	290(12.1)	22.8	38.6	22.8	15.8	
Tenure (years)	Mean ± SD‡	7.06 ± 7.58	7.46 ± 7.77	7.40 ± 7.99	6.42 ± 6.96	6.00 ± 6.48	0.122**
	≤1	567(23.6)	27.3	40.4	21.2	11.1	0.015‖
	1 < x ≤ 10	1,288(53.7)	28.2	37.7	21.4	12.7	
	>10	545(22.7)	30.5	43.5	18.7	7.3	
Smoking	No	1,012(42.2)	30.1	41.7	19.0	9.2	0.008‖
	Yes	1,388(57.8)	27.3	38.2	22.0	12.5	
Alcohol consumption	No	370(15.4)	27.3	44.1	18.6	10.0	0.291‖
	Yes	2,030(84.6)	28.7	38.9	21.1	11.3	
Exercise	No	1,721(71.7)	27.6	37.6	22.3	12.5	<0.001‖
	Yes	679(28.3)	30.8	44.9	16.6	7.7	

*: Column percentage, †: Row percentage, ‡SD: Standard deviation, §: Tested by ANOVA, ‖: Tested by chi-squared test,
¶: KRW = 10,000 Korean won (approximately US$10), **: tested by Kruskal–Wallis test.

Table 5.3 General Characteristics of the Female Subjects

Variables		Total	Weekly Working Hours				p-value
		n(%*)	≤40 %†	40 < x ≤ 52 %†	52 < x ≤ 60 %†	>60 %†	
Age (years)	Mean ± SD‡	39.8 ± 10.2	39.0 ± 10.1	39.5 ± 10.3	41.0 ± 10.0	41.3 ± 10.4	0.022§
	25–34	489(37.6)	34.2	42.1	15.7	8.0	0.090‖
	35–44	353(27.2)	33.1	39.7	16.7	10.5	
	45–54	331(25.5)	27.2	37.8	21.4	13.6	
	55–64	126(9.7)	31.0	37.3	19.0	12.7	
Marital status	Never married	303(23.3)	34.0	39.9	16.2	9.9	0.252‖
	Married	858(66.1)	32.5	39.3	17.5	10.7	
	Others	138(10.6)	22.4	43.5	23.2	10.9	
Educational status	≤Junior high school	281(21.6)	27.1	34.5	24.9	13.5	<0.001‖
	High school	433(33.3)	27.5	42.5	19.4	10.6	
	≥College	585(45.1)	37.3	40.5	13.2	9.0	
Household income (KRW/month)¶	Mean ± SD‡	228.9 ± 333.6	241.7 ± 329.7	231.1 ± 362.8	209.2 ± 260.7	214.6 ± 340.9	0.640§
Occupation	Nonmanual	705(54.3)	35.6	41.8	13.9	8.7	<0.001‖
	Manual	594(45.7)	27.3	37.5	22.4	12.8	
Employment type	Regular worker	888(68.4)	31.4	40.8	17.6	10.2	0.803‖
	Irregular worker	411(31.6)	32.6	38.0	18.2	11.2	
Shift work	No	1,220(93.9)	32.0	40.3	17.5	10.2	0.249‖
	Yes	79(6.1)	29.1	32.9	22.8	15.2	
Tenure (years)	Mean ± SD‡	4.67 ± 5.57	4.71 ± 5.25	4.65 ± 5.82	4.62 ± 5.44	4.75 ± 5.78	0.995§
	≤1	421(32.4)	30.9	41.8	15.7	11.6	0.775‖
	1 < x ≤ 10	725(55.8)	32.3	39.2	18.7	9.8	
	>10	153(11.8)	32.0	37.9	19.0	11.1	
Smoking	No	1,281(98.6)	31.7	40.1	17.7	10.5	0.463‖
	Yes	18(1.4)	38.9	22.2	22.2	16.7	
Alcohol consumption	No	631(48.6)	31.1	41.2	16.6	11.1	0.573‖
	Yes	668(51.4)	32.5	38.6	18.9	10.0	
Exercise	No	1,083(83.4)	31.1	40.5	17.3	11.1	0.223‖
	Yes	216(16.6)	35.2	36.6	20.3	7.9	

*: Column percentage, †: Row percentage, ‡SD: Standard deviation, §: Tested by ANOVA, ‖: Tested by chi-squared test, ¶: KRW = 10,000 Korean won (approximately US$10).

the case of male workers, the percentage of participants working more than fifty-two hours per week was considerably lower for the group who had worked for more than ten years than for the group who had worked for less than ten years ($p = 0.015$). By contrast, in the case of female workers, the percentage of those working more than fifty-two hours per week was higher in the group who had worked for more than ten years, even though the difference was statistically nonsignificant. With respect to the health-related behavior characteristic variables of the study participants, the smoking group, alcohol-consuming group, and nonexercising group formed a higher proportion of the number of male and female workers working more than fifty-two hours per week (tables 5.2 and 5.3).

The Relationship between Relevant Variables and Prevalence of Poor Self-Rated Health

In the case of male workers, the prevalence of poor self-rated health with respect to the number of working hours per week was 27.9 percent for the group working less than forty hours per week, 26.2 percent for the group working more than forty hours and up to fifty-two hours per week, 27.8 percent for the group working more than fifty-two hours and up to sixty hours per week, and 31.5 percent for the group working more than sixty hours per week, showing a U-shaped form with no statistically significant differences (table 5.4). In the case of female workers, the prevalence of poor self-rated health was 32.7 percent for the group working less than forty hours per week, 36.7 percent for the group working more than forty hours and up to fifty-two hours per week, 40.3 percent for the group working more than fifty-two hours and up to sixty hours per week, and 51.8 percent for the group working more than sixty hours per week, showing a significantly higher rate in the unhealthy group for subjects working more hours per week with a dose-response pattern ($p < 0.001$). The self-rated health level with respect to the sociodemographic characteristics showed a significantly higher rate in the unhealthy group for older people and participants with lower educational status in the cases of both male and female workers ($p < 0.001$). With respect to the marital status variables, the people in the divorced, separated, or widow/widower group showed a higher unhealthy rate ($p < 0.001$). The self-rated health level with respect to occupational characteristics showed that manual workers had a higher unhealthy rate than nonmanual workers in the cases of both male and female workers. With respect to the employment type, irregular workers had a higher unhealthy rate than regular workers ($p < 0.001$). In the cases of both male and female workers, there was no significant difference in the self-rated health level with respect to shift work. The unhealthy rate with respect to the number of years of tenure showed no significant difference in the case

Table 5.4 Prevalence of Poor Self-Rated Health According to Sociodemographic Characteristics

Variables		*Total* Prevalence of Poor Self-Rated Health %*	*Total* p-value†	*Male* Prevalence of Poor Self-Rated Health %*	*Male* p-value†	*Female* Prevalence of Poor Self-Rated Health %*	*Female* p-value†
Weekly working hours	≤40	29.7	0.007	27.9	0.387	32.7	<0.001
	40 < x ≤ 52	29.9		26.2		36.7	
	52 < x ≤ 60	31.7		27.8		40.3	
	>60	38.4		31.5		51.8	
Age (years)	25–34	22.2	<0.001	20.8	<0.001	24.3	<0.001
	35–44	26.4		23.0		34.0	
	45–54	39.9		34.1		49.8	
	55–64	51.8		45.0		67.5	
Marital status	Never married	21.5	<0.001	19.8	<0.001	24.4	<0.001
	Married	31.7		28.3		38.8	
	Others	56.0		51.8		59.4	
Educational status	≤Junior high school	53.5	<0.001	46.7	<0.001	60.9	<0.001
	High school	31.2		28.8		35.8	
	≥College	24.0		22.2		27.9	
Occupation	Nonmanual	24.5	<0.001	22.7	<0.001	27.4	<0.001
	Manual	37.4		31.7		49.8	
Employment type	Regular worker	27.1	<0.001	24.5	<0.001	32.4	<0.001
	Irregular worker	43.1		38.6		48.9	
Shift work	No	31.1	0.796	28.6	0.673	37.3	0.307
	Yes	31.7		27.4		43.0	

Tenure	≤1	34.2	0.015	27.0	0.346	43.9	0.005
(years)	1 < × ≤ 10	30.8		28.7		34.5	
	>10	27.7		25.5		35.3	
Smoking	No	32.4	0.031	26.1	0.161	37.4	0.114
	Yes	29.0		28.7		55.6	
Alcohol consumption	No	37.9	<0.001	32.7	0.017	40.9	0.019
	Yes	28.6		26.7		34.6	
Exercise	No	37.4	<0.001	29.5	<0.001	37.9	0.722
	Yes	24.5		22.8		36.6	

*: Row percentage.
†: Tested by chi-squared test.

Table 5.5 OR and 95% CI for Poor Self-Rated Health

			Number of Workers		
		Weekly Working Hours	*Good Health*	*Poor Health*	*OR (95% CI)*
Model 1*		≤40	771	326	1.00
		40 < x ≤ 52	1,031	439	1.06 (0.89–1.27)
		52 < x ≤ 60	497	231	1.07 (0.86–1.33)
		>60	249	155	1.42 (1.10–1.83)
Model 2†	Male	≤40	493	191	1.00
		40 < x ≤ 52	703	249	1.00 (0.79–1.26)
		52 < x ≤ 60	359	138	0.98 (0.75–1.28)
		>60	183	84	1.14 (0.83–1.57)
	Female	≤40	278	135	1.00
		40 > x ≤ 52	328	190	1.17 (0.88–1.57)
		52 > x ≤ 60	138	93	1.22 (0.85–1.74)
		>60	66	71	1.97 (1.30–2.99)
Model 3‡	Tenure ≤1 year	≤40	180	105	1.00
		40 < x ≤ 52	277	128	0.88 (0.63–1.24)
		52 < x ≤ 60	122	64	0.93 (0.62–1.42)
		>60	71	41	0.95 (0.59–1.55)
	Tenure 1 < x ≤ 10 years	≤40	430	167	1.00
		40 < x ≤ 52	544	226	1.14 (0.89–1.46)
		52 < x ≤ 60	279	132	1.15 (0.86–1.55)
		>60	140	95	1.75 (1.25–2.45)
	Tenure >10 years	≤40	161	54	1.00
		40 < x ≤ 52	210	85	1.27 (0.84–1.93)
		52 < x ≤ 60	96	35	1.05 (0.62–1.76)
		>60	38	19	1.37 (0.71–2.65)

*: Model adjusted for gender, age, marital status, income, educational status, occupation, employment type, tenure, shift work, smoking, alcohol consumption, and exercise.
†: Model 1 after stratification by gender.
‡: Model 1 after stratification by tenure.

of male workers, but in the case of female workers, the group that had been working for less than one year showed a significantly higher unhealthy rate (p = 0.005). The self-rated health level with respect to the health-related behavior characteristics for male workers showed that the smoking group had a higher unhealthy rate but with no significant difference, while the non-alcohol-consuming group ($p = 0.017$) and the nonexercise group ($p < 0.001$) showed a significantly higher unhealthy rate. In the case of female workers, the smoking group and the nonexercise group showed a higher unhealthy rate, although statistically insignificant, while the nonalcohol-consuming group showed a significantly higher unhealthy rate ($p = 0.019$).

The Relationship between Weekly Working Hours and Self-Rated Health Level

The OR of the group with poor self-rated health level with respect to the weekly working hours was analyzed with the group working less than forty hours used as a reference (table 5.5). Model 1, after controlling for the variables of the study participants' sociodemographic characteristics, occupational characteristics, and health-related behavior characteristics, showed an OR of 1.06 (95% CI, 0.89–1.27) for the group working more than forty hours and up to fifty-two hours, 1.07 (95% CI, 0.86–1.33) for the group working more than fifty-two hours and up to sixty hours, and 1.42 (95% CI, 1.10–1.83) for the group working more than sixty hours.

Model 2 was constructed after gender stratification and then controlled for the relevant variables. In model 2, the female workers with a poor self-rated health level showed an OR of 1.17 (95% CI, 0.88–1.57) for the group working more than forty hours and up to fifty-two hours, 1.22 (95% CI, 0.85–1.74) for the group working more than fifty-two hours and up to sixty hours, and 1.97 (95% CI, 1.30–2.99) for the group working more than sixty hours, showing a higher OR of poor self-rated health level than the results of model 1. However, in the case of male workers, the OR of 1.14 (95% CI, 0.83–1.57) was higher than the reference group only in the group working more than sixty hours.

Model 3 was constructed after tenure stratification and then controlled for the relevant variables. The OR of poor self-rated health level for workers with more than one year up to ten years of tenure was 1.14 (95% CI, 0.89–1.46) for the group working more than forty hours and up to fifty-two hours, 1.15 (95% CI, 0.86–1.55) for the group working more than fifty-two hours and up to sixty hours, and 1.75 (95% CI, 1.25–2.45) for the group working more than sixty hours, showing a higher OR of poor self-rated health level than the results of model 1. However, the OR of workers with less than one year of tenure with a poor self-rated health level decreased and showed a U-shaped pattern. Further, in the case of workers with more than ten years of tenure, the OR of the group working more than forty hours and up to fifty-two hours was 1.27 (95% CI, 0.84–1.93), 1.05 (95% CI, 0.62–1.76) for the group working more than fifty-two hours and up to sixty hours, and 1.37 (95% CI, 0.71–2.65) for the group working more than sixty hours.

DISCUSSION

In this study, the results of the analysis on weekly working hours of full-time wage workers among the eleventh KLIPS study participants showed that the average number of weekly working hours was 48.8 hours, with the male workers showing a higher rate of working hours of more than fifty-two hours per week than female workers. It has been found that 30.6 percent of the participants of this study worked for more than fifty-two hours per week, which is the permitted standard of the Labor Standards Act. This is similar to the results of the fourth Korea National Health and Nutrition Examination Survey conducted on full-time wage workers, in which the weekly working hours were 48.3 hours and the rate of employees working more than fifty-two hours per week was 29.6 percent [19]. Considering both sources of data, around 30 percent of Korea's full-time wage workers are working for more than the number of hours permitted by the Labor Standards Act, and the reason for this is assumed to be the fact that Korea's Labor Standards Act does not have a separate regulation for working on Sundays and holidays. Moreover, the average number of working hours per week of the study participants, which was 48.8 hours, was 11.3 hours more than the average weekly working hours of European countries found in the Fifth European Working Conditions Survey, which was 37.5 hours [11]. Korea's actual conditions of long working hours can thus be seen not only through the OECD reports but also through this study.

The results of this study on the relationship between weekly working hours and the self-rated health level showed that the health level was getting worse in a dose-dependent manner as the number of working hours increased, and the group working more than sixty hours per week showed the worst health level. Such an effect was considerably more significant in the case of female workers and workers with more than one year of tenure. Thus far, studies using domestic Korean data on the health effects of long working hours have mostly been related to mental health. It has been reported that in a study conducted on public sector workers, the size of the group showing high-risk depressive symptoms increased with an increase in the number of weekly working hours and the OR of depressive symptoms in workers working more than ten hours daily more than seven times a month was 1.63 (95% CI, 1.10–2.43) [18]. The results of the fourth Korea National Health and Nutrition Examination Survey conducted on full-time wage workers revealed that the OR of depressive symptomatology for the group working more than sixty hours per week was 1.62 (95% CI, 1.20–2.18) as compared to the group working less than fifty-two hours per week [19]. Another study conducted on full-time wage workers of the fourth Korea National Health and Nutrition Examination Survey reported that the OR of suicidal ideation for the group working more than sixty hours per week was 1.38 ($p = 0.020$) as compared to the group working more than forty hours and up to fifty-one hours per week [17]. This study found that long working hours have negative impacts not only on workers' mental health but also on their self-rated health level, showing an increase in fair, poor, and very poor self-rated health with an increase in the number of working hours; further, this unhealthy rate was the highest when the number of working hours exceeded sixty hours per week, which is the standard of overwork.

In previous studies, the mechanism of the impact of long working hours on health was explained by dividing it into the direct pathway of a physiological recovery mechanism and the indirect pathway of a behavioral lifestyle mechanism [23–26]. The physiological recovery mechanism explained that insufficiency in recovery is caused by a lack of sleeping hours resulting from long working hours and that this has a negative impact on workers' health [27–31]. Further, it has been reported that insufficient recovery from labor can cause blood pressure elevation [32], sympathetic nerve activation [1,24], and an increase in the morbidity rate of cardiovascular diseases [33]. The behavioral lifestyle mechanism explains that changes in lifestyle such as an increase in the percentage of smoking and alcohol-consuming groups and decrease in the percentage of workers exercising regularly due to long working hours have a negative impact on the workers' health [34–36]. It also explains that there is an increase in the number of workers showing unhealthy eating habits including an increase in the intake of foods high in fat or calories and decrease in the consumption of foods beneficial to health such as vegetables and fruits [37,38]. Although the physiological recovery mechanism could not be verified through this study, the health impact of long working hours could be found to reach a certain level through the behavioral lifestyle mechanism. The results of this study showed that the percentage of the group working more than fifty-two hours was higher in the smoking, alcohol-consuming, and nonexercising groups than in the nonsmoking, nonalcohol-consuming, and nonexercising groups in the cases of both male and female workers (tables 5.2 and 5.3).

In this study, the behavioral lifestyle mechanism was identified through the fact that the smoking, alcohol-consuming, and nonexercising groups with unhealthy lifestyles had a higher percentage of workers working long hours and the self-rated health level in accordance with health-related behavior characteristics showed a higher percentage of unhealthy workers among the smoking, nonalcohol-consuming, and nonexercising groups in the cases of both male and female workers. The psychological impact of alcohol consumption, specifically stress reduction, may be explained for the high percentage of unhealthy workers in the nonalcohol-consuming group. In a social survey conducted in Korea in 2012, the results showed that proportion of respondents who answered that they were in good health in a self-health evaluation was 45.6 percent for the alcohol-consuming group and 34 percent for the nonalcohol-consuming group [39]. This finding may be explained by a psychological effect, in that the alcohol-consuming group may believe they are in better health than they are. The positive effects of mild-to-moderate alcohol consumption can also be considered. In a previous study on the risk of alcohol consumption and cardiovascular disorders, it was proven that irrespective of the type of alcohol, mild-to-moderate alcohol consumption may lower the risk of coronary artery disease [40]. Another study reported that a moderate intake of wine decreases oxidative stress and reduces atherosclerosis by enhancing cholesterol efflux from the vessel walls and inhibiting platelet adhesion [41].

In this study, the result of reanalysis after gender stratification showed a more noticeable tendency of having a poorer self-rated health level as the number of working hours increased in the case of female workers. This is mainly attributed to the burden of household chores for females. According to the Time Use Survey conducted in 2009 in Korea, the house-work time for weekdays was 27 min for husbands and 185 min for wives in a two-income household [42]. Therefore, female workers use most of the remaining time after work on household chores, leaving insufficient time for recovery and being more vulnerable to poor health due to long working hours. Korea's gender difference in the labor market should also be considered. Korea's labor market has a gender separation structure with male workers mostly taking up the higher level of occupational status with high wages and high job control and the female workers taking up the lower level with low wages and low job control; it has been reported that the U.S. labor market also shows a similar pattern [22]. This is mainly attributed to the fact that females, excluding some women with professional jobs, experience career discontinuity due to pregnancy and childbirth and show a tendency to take jobs unrelated to their past career during the reemployment process. With respect to the distribution of the age structure of this study, the percentage of the male subjects aged thirty-five to forty-four years was the highest, at 32.8 percent, but the percentage of female subjects aged twenty-five to thirty-four years was the highest, at 37.6 percent. According to the job strain model presented by Karasek et al., the group with high job control was classified as the active group, while the group with low job control was classified as the high job strain group, in the case of high work demands [43]. It has been identified that the group with a high job strain level will be affected with negative health impacts such as having a relatively higher risk of diabetes or cardiovascular diseases as compared to the other groups [44,45]. Thus, there is a possibility that female workers working long hours may show a relatively high job strain level due to career discontinuity, which leads to the belief that female workers are more vulnerable to poor health when working long hours. However, there is a need for additional studies in the future as this study does not cover psychosocial stress.

In this study, the self-rated health level was reanalyzed after tenure stratification. As a result of this, the OR of a poor self-rated health level increased with a dose-response pattern related to long working hours when the tenure exceeded one year and the effect was attenuated when the tenure exceeded ten years. Further, it was suggested that the cumulative exposure time until the working hours affect workers' health be estimated. This is because for the physiological recovery mechanism, a certain amount of cumulative exposure time is required in order for the insufficient recovery time resulting from working long hours to have a negative impact on the workers' health and for the behavioral lifestyle mechanism, a certain amount of exposure time is required for workers exposed to long working hours to make changes in lifestyle and for this to have a negative impact on the workers' health. The results of a systematic review analyzing the effect of the lifestyle changes on the metabolic syndrome showed that the group that changed to a healthy lifestyle showed a noticeable recovery rate from the metabolic syndrome that was two times higher than that of the comparison group after an average of one year had passed [46]. In another study, the group that maintained the changed lifestyle for more than one year was reported showing significant improvements in the risk factors of cardiovascular diseases such as obesity or blood lipid disorders as compared to the comparison group [47]. In this study, a significant difference in the self-rated health level was observed only in workers with a tenure of more than one year, which means that a cumulative exposure time of more than one year is expected in order for long working hours to have a negative impact on workers' health. Further, the health effects brought about by an improved lifestyle can be believed to be the reason why the OR of the poor self-rated health level caused by the high number of working hours decreased for the group with a tenure of exceeding ten years. The healthy worker effect is a bias observed commonly in the field of occupational epidemiology that arises because those with health problems tend to drop out of the working population, leaving the working population relatively healthier than the general population [48]. There is a possibility that only relatively healthy workers work in the same workplace for more than ten years because those with health disorders resulting from a negative health impact of long working hours would have stopped working in the middle of the career. Therefore, workers working for a long period of time of more than ten years would end up being relatively healthy people with a low percentage of selecting "unhealthy" in the self-rated health level; this implies, that the data collected on the impact of working hours on the self-rated health level may be distorted, hiding the true extent of the impact of long working hours.

This study has the following limitations: First, in this cross-sectional study, there is a limitation in explaining the relationship between the number of working hours and the self-rated health level by analyzing just the eleventh year (2008) data among the longitudinal KLIPS data. Second, there is a possibility of an information bias because the KLIPS data were collected using self-report through questionnaires. Third, the research results cannot be said to be fully adjusted because there is insufficient data to verify the study participants' alcohol consumption, past medical history, past work experience, and number of working hours. Despite these limitations, this study identified the relationship between the number of working hours and the self-rated health level by using the KLIPS data, which represent Korea's urban household members. The results of this study showed that after controlling for various relevant variables, the group working more than sixty hours per week exhibited a significantly increased risk of poor self-rated health as compared to the group working less than forty hours per week and that such an impact was much more significant in the case of the female workers and the workers with more than one year of tenure. Long-term follow-up studies may be needed to show the various health impacts of long working hours.

NOTE

1. This chapter was previously published as Song, Jun-Taek, Goeun Lee, Jongho Kwon, Jung-Woo Park, Hyunrim Choi, and Sinye Lim. "The association between long working hours and self-rated health." *Annals of Occupational and Environmental Medicine* 26, no. 1 (2014): 2.

REFERENCES

1. Sokejima S, Kagamimori S: "Working hours as a risk factor for acute myocardial infarction in Japan: case-control study." *BMJ* 1998, 317(7161):775–780.
2. Liu Y, Tanaka H, Fukuoka Heart Study Group: "Overtime work, insufficient sleep, and risk of non-fatal acute myocardial infarction in Japanese men." *Occup Environ Med* 2002, 59(7):447–451.
3. Kroenke CH, Spiegelman D, Manson J, Schernhammer ES, Colditz GA, Kawachi I: "Work characteristics and incidence of type 2 diabetes in women." *Am J Epidemiol* 2007, 165(2):175–183.
4. Krause N, Lynch J, Kaplan GA, Cohen RD, Goldberg DE, Salonen JT: "Predictors of disability retirement." *Scand J Work Environ Health* 1997, 23(6):403–413.
5. Caruso CC, Bushnell T, Eggerth D, Heitmann A, Kojola B, Newman K, Rosa RR, Sauter SL, Vila B: "Long working hours, safety, and health: toward a National Research Agenda." *Am J Ind Med* 2006, 49(11):930–942.
6. Caruso CC: "Possible broad impacts of long work hours." *Ind Health* 2006, 44(4):531–536.
7. Olds DM, Clarke SP: "The effect of work hours on adverse events and errors in health care." *J Safety Res* 2010, 41(2):153–162.

8. Dembe AE, Erickson JB, Delbos RG, Banks SM: The impact of overtime and long work hours on occupational injuries and illnesses: new evidence from the United States. *Occup Environ Med* 2005, 62(9):588–597.
9. International Labour Office Geneva: *Constitution of the International Labour Organisation and Selected Texts*. International Labour Organisation, 2010:5. Available: http://www.ilo.org/public/english/bureau/leg/download/constitution.pdf [cited March 25, 2013].
10. Spurgeon A, Harrington JM, Cooper CL: Health and safety problems associated with long working hours: a review of the current position. *Occup Environ Med* 1997, 54(6):367–375.
11. European Foundation for the Improvement of Living and Working Conditions: *Fifth European Working Conditions Survey*. Dublin, Ireland: Publications Office of the European Union, Luxembourg, 2012:33.
12. Ministry of Government Legislation: *Labor Standards Act. Laws on Green Growth, and Economic Investment in Korea*. Gil-Job-Ie Media, 2013:983–985. Available: http://world.moleg.go.kr/World/EastAsia/KR/law/14466 [cited on March 25, 2013].
13. OECD: *OECD Factbook 2011–2012 Economic, Environmental and Social Statistics*. Paris, France: OECD Publishing, 2011:164–165. doi:10.1787/factbook-2011-en [cited on March 30, 2013].
14. Ross CE, Bird CE: Sex stratification and health lifestyle: consequences for men's and women's perceived health. *J Health Soc Behav* 1994, 35(2):161–178.
15. Idler EL, Benyamini Y: Self-rated health and mortality: a review of twenty-seven community studies. *J Health Soc Behav* 1997, 38(1):21–37.
16. Grosch JW, Caruso CC, Rosa RR, Sauter SL: "Long hours of work in the U.S.: associations with demographic and organizational characteristics, psychosocial working conditions, and health." *Am J Ind Med* 2006, 49(11):943–952.
17. Kim KW, Park SG, Kim HC, Lim JH, Lee SJ, Jeon SH, Huh YS: "Association between long working hours and suicidal ideation." *Korean J Occup Environ Med* 2012, 24(4):339–346. Korean.
18. Heo HT, Kim DW, Lee JS, Jo HA, Jang SS, Kim SY, Kim IA: "An association between working schedules and depression in public sector employees." *Korean J Occup Environ Med* 2012, 24(4):347–355. Korean.
19. Kim I, Kim H, Lim S, Lee M, Bahk J, June KJ, Kim S, Chang WJ: "Working hours and depressive symptomatology among full-time employees: results from the fourth Korean National Health and Nutrition Examination Survey (2007–2009)." *Scand J Work Environ Health* 2013, 39(5):515–520.
20. Korea Labor Institute: *Korean Labor and Income Panel Study 1–11th User's Guide*. Korea Labor Institute, 2013:1–4. Available: http://www.kli.re.kr/klips/ko/datadown/lst.klips0700;jsessionid=AB176B56A72EBFE173E7E657EB366996#none [cited on March 25, 2013]. Korean.
21. Won JW, Kim SK, Lim HJ, Kim HR: "A study on approval criteria of cardiovascular disease from overwork." In *Ministry of Employment and Labor*. Seoul, Korea: Institute for Occupational Health, Yonsei University College of Medicine, 2008:100–101. Korean.

22. Phelan J: "The paradox of the contented female worker: an assessment of alternative explanations." *Soc Psychol Q* 1994, 57(2):95–107.
23. Siegrist J, Rödel A: "Work stress and health risk behavior." *Scand J Work Environ Health* 2006, 32(6):473–481.
24. van der Hulst M: "Long workhours and health." *Scand J Work Environ Health* 2003, 29(3):171–188.
25. Taris TW, Ybema JF, Beckers DG, Verheijden MW, Geurts SA, Kompier MA: "Investigating the associations among overtime work, health behaviors, and health: a longitudinal study among full-time employees." *Int J Behav Med* 2011, 18(4):352–360.
26. Meijman TF, Mulder G: "Psychological aspects of workload." In *Handbook of Work and Organizational Psychology, Volume 2. Work Psychology.* 2nd edition. Edited by Drenth PJD, Thierry H, de Wolff CJ. Hove, United Kingdom: Psychology Press, 1998:5–33.
27. Dahlgren A, Kecklund G, Akerstedt T: "Overtime work and its effects on sleep, sleepiness, cortisol and blood pressure in an experimental field study." *Scand J Work Environ Health* 2006, 32(4):318–327.
28. Nakashima M, Morikawa Y, Sakurai M, Nakamura K, Miura K, Ishizaki M, Kido T, Naruse Y, Suwazono Y, Nakagawa H: "Association between long working hours and sleep problems in white-collar workers." *J Sleep Res* 2011, 20(1 Pt 1):110–116.
29. Totterdell P, Spelten E, Smith L, Baron J, Folkard S: "Recovery from work shifts: how long does it take?" *J Appl Psychol* 1995, 80(1):43–57.
30. Geurts SA, Sonnentag S: "Recovery as an explanatory mechanism in the relation between acute stress reactions and chronic health impairment." *Scand J Work Environ Health* 2006, 32(6):482–492.
31. Härmä M: "Workhours in relation to work stress, recovery and health." *Scand J Work Environ Health* 2006, 32(6):502–514.
32. Hayashi T, Kobayashi Y, Yamaoka K, Yano E: "Effect of overtime work on 24-hour ambulatory blood pressure." *J Occup Environ Med* 1996, 38(10):1007–1011.
33. Virtanen M, Ferrie JE, Singh-Manoux A, Shipley MJ, Vahtera J, Marmot MG, Kivimäki M: "Overtime work and incident coronary heart disease: the Whitehall II prospective cohort study." *Eur Heart J* 2010, 31(14):1737–1744.
34. Steptoe A, Wardle J, Lipsey Z, Mills R, Oliver G, Jarvis M, Kirschbaum C: "A longitudinal study of work load and variations in psychological well-being, cortisol, smoking, and alcohol consumption." *Ann Behav Med* 1998, 20(2):84–91.
35. Mizoue T, Fujino Y, Yamato H, Tokunaga S, Kubo T, Reijula K: "Overtime work, cigarette consumption, and addiction to cigarette among workers subject to mild smoking restrictions." *Ind Health* 2006, 44(2):244–249.
36. Artazcoz L, Cortès I, Escribà-Agüir V, Cascant L, Villegas R: "Understanding the relationship of long working hours with health status and health-related behaviours." *J Epidemiol Commun Health* 2009, 63(7):521–527.
37. Maruyama S, Morimoto K: "Effects of long workhours on life-style, stress and quality of life among intermediate Japanese managers." *Scand J Work Environ Health* 1996, 22(5):353–359.

38. Oliver G, Wardle J, Gibson EL: "Stress and food choice: a laboratory study." *Psychosom Med* 2000, 62(6):853–865.
39. Korean Statistical Information Service: *Social Survey. Health 2012*. Available: http://kosis.kr/common/meta_onedepth.jsp?vwcd=MT_CTITLE&listid=MT_CTITLE_g [cited June 19, 2013]. Korean.
40. Rimm EB, Klatsky A, Grobbee D, Stampfer MJ: "Review of moderate alcohol consumption and reduced risk of coronary heart disease: is the effect due to beer, wine, or spirits." *BMJ* 1996, 312(7033):731–736.
41. Lippi G, Franchini M, Favaloro EJ, Targher G: "Moderate red wine consumption and cardiovascular disease risk: beyond the 'French paradox'." *Semin Thromb Hemost* 2010, 36(1):59–70.
42. Korean Statistical Information Service: *Time Use Survey. Average Time 2009*. Available: http://kosis.kr/common/meta_onedepth.jsp?vwcd=MT_CTITLE&listid=MT_CTITLE_i [cited June 19, 2013]. Korean.
43. Karasek R, Theorell T: *Healthy Work: Stress, Productivity, and the Reconstruction of Working Life*. New York, NY: Basic Books, 1990.
44. Kivimäki M, Nyberg ST, Batty GD, Fransson EI, Heikkilä K, Alfredsson L, Bjorner JB, Borritz M, Burr H, Casini A, Clays E, de Bacquer D, Dragano N, Ferrie JE, Geuskens GA, Goldberg M, Hamer M, Hooftman WE, Houtman IL, Joensuu M, Jokela M, Kittel F, Knutsson A, Koskenvuo M, Koskinen A, Kouvonen A, Kumari M, Madsen IE, Marmot MG, Nielsen ML, Nordin M, Oksanen T, Pentti J, Rugulies R, Salo P, Siegrist J, Singh-Manoux A, Suominen SB, Väänänen A, Vahtera J, Virtanen M, Westerholm PJ, Westerlund H, Zins M, Steptoe A, Theorell T, IPD-Work Consortium: "Job strain as a risk factor for coronary heart disease: a collaborative meta-analysis of individual participant data." *Lancet* 2012, 380(9852):1491–1497.
45. Nyberg ST, Fransson EI, Heikkilä K, Alfredsson L, Casini A, Clays E, de Bacquer D, Dragano N, Erbel R, Ferrie JE, Hamer M, Jöckel KH, Kittel F, Knutsson A, Ladwig KH, Lunau T, Marmot MG, Nordin M, Rugulies R, Siegrist J, Steptoe A, Westerholm PJ, Westerlund H, Theorell T, Brunner EJ, Singh-Manoux A, Batty GD, Kivimäki M, IPD-Work Consortium: "Job strain and cardiovascular disease risk factors: meta-analysis of individual-participant data from 47,000 men and women." *PLoS One* 2013, 8(6):e67323.
46. Yamaoka K, Tango T: Effects of lifestyle modification on metabolic syndrome: a systematic review and meta-analysis. *BMC Med* 2012, 10:138.
47. Nisbeth O, Klausen K, Andersen LB: "Effectiveness of counselling over 1 year on changes in lifestyle and coronary heart disease risk factors." *Patient Educ Couns* 2000, 40(2):121–131.
48. Shah D: "Healthy worker effect phenomenon." *Indian J Occup Environ Med* 2009, 13(2):77–79.

Chapter 6

The Relationship between Night Work and Involuntary Weight Change

Data from the Fifth Korea National Health and Nutrition Examination Survey (KNHANES 2010–2012)

Jongho Kwon, Jung-Woo Park, Jin-Soo Park, Seyoung Kim, Hyunrim Choi, and Sinye Lim

BACKGROUND

It[1] has been proposed that adjustments in working time are necessary with human activity hours expanding to twenty-four hours and the society becoming complex with the development of technology. The form of shift work using time other than normal day work hours based on economic rationality has come to the fore with shift work carried out in many industry fields as a method to improve productivity and to secure business competitiveness [1]. Although a clear definition for shift work has not been defined, all types of work outside the day work hours of 6:00 a.m. to 6:00 p.m. are considered as shift work which in many cases include night work. International Labour Organization (ILO) defines night work as "all work which is performed during a period of not less than seven consecutive hours, including the interval from midnight to 5 a.m." [2].

According to the fifth European Working Conditions Survey (EWCS), 19 percent of workers in twenty-seven countries are engaged in shift work including night work, while in the United States, around 15 percent of full-time workers are engaged in shift work [3, 4]. In South Korea, the survey carried out by the Ministry of Employment and Labor in 2011 showed that 15.2 percent of 3,414 companies with ten or more workers are engaged in shift work. According to the 2010 Korean Working Conditions Survey (KWCS), a high percentage of shift work was found in assembly of machinery and machine operation workers (24.3 percent) and service workers (13.6 percent) [5, 6].

Shift work is known to disturb the normal circadian rhythm causing sleep disorders and sleepiness during everyday life and work [7]. Such sleep disorders and sleepiness lower productivity during work and increase incidence of accidents [8], heighten job stress and depressed mood [9, 10], increase smoking and alcohol consumption, result in lack of exercise, and bring about changes in eating habits [11, 12]. In addition to these, it has been reported that disturbance of autonomic nervous system, inflammatory responses, and lipid and glucose metabolism resulting from shift work increased the incidence of cardiovascular and gastrointestinal diseases [13, 14]. There is also a limited evidence that shift work increased breast cancer incidence rates in female shift workers [15] and it has also been reported that it increases the risks of spontaneous abortion, low birth weight, and preterm birth [16]. Crucially, the effect of shift work is more pronounced in shift work including night work [17].

Modest weight change can be considered as a process of maintaining homeostasis; however, imbalance of weight like continuous weight gain or weight loss can cause obesity or underweight. In addition, weight changes are known to work as an independent factor in increasing the mortality [18, 19]. Weight gain is a risk factor of coronary heart disease, type 2 diabetes, and breast cancer [20–22]. In the case of weight loss, it can lead a decline in load of weight-bearing skeleton and it may cause changes in bone remodeling leading to bone loss. As a result, weight loss is a risk factor of hip fracture. Furthermore, weight loss can be an indicator of malnutrition or poor health state, and it was significantly associated with poor self-reported health [23, 24]. Therefore, the study on weight change associated with occupational factors is being performed in various viewpoints [25, 26].

Previous studies on weight change associated with shift or night work have been mostly performed to examine the risk of weight gain caused by shift or night work. However, such relationship failed to show consistent results due to limitations of cross-sectional study design and insufficient adjusting for confounders [27]. Therefore, the possibility of weight loss from shift or night work has also been raised [28]. To examine the association between shift or night work and weight change accurately, it is needed to evaluate the effect of weight change by dividing into weight gain and weight loss. In addition, to exclude the positive health effect of voluntary weight change, it is necessary to explore only involuntary weight change. And a clear definition for shift work has not been defined, it is necessary to evaluate limited night work group that work a substantial number of hours in night (from midnight to 5:00 a.m). In this study, we aimed to explore the possibility of involuntary weight gain or weight loss associated with night work separately by applying the definition of night work by ILO with using a nationwide representative data.

METHODS

Study Subjects

The KNHANES is a survey used as a basis in calculating the statistical data needed in determining the status of health and nutrition of Koreans nationwide and in health policy establishment and evaluation. This survey was carried out from 1998 and conducted up to the fifth survey (2010–2012) with the sixth survey currently in progress. In the fifth KNHANES (2010–2012), the number of survey participants in each year was 8,958 (participation rate; 81.9 percent), 8,518 (participation rate; 80.4 percent), and 8,058 (participation rate; 80.0 percent), respectively. The fifth KNHANES applied Rolling Sampling Survey method; therefore, the study participants became a probability sample representing Koreans nationwide. Sampling frameworks have been divided into ordinary residential and apartment areas with the residential registration data used for ordinary residential areas and the apartment market price trends used for apartment areas. Accordingly, 576 areas were selected with twenty households chosen per area through table of random numbers, amounting to 11,400 households. Interviews for questionnaire survey, nutritional examinations, and medical examinations were carried out on the 25,534 members of the selected households to produce total of around 600 types of socioeconomic, occupational, nutritional, and health status information.

Among the fifth KNHANES total survey participants of 25,534 people, we restricted the study population of this study to full-time wage workers between the age of twenty and sixty-nine and excluded voluntary weight changers, soldiers, pregnant women, and short-time workers working less than ten hours per week. Finally, 1,605 people were selected as the final analysis group.

General Characteristics

The gender-stratified analysis was performed through classification of male and female. Age was classified into units of ten years between the age of twenty and sixty-nine and the education level classified into less than high school, graduated from high school, and graduation from college or university. The socioeconomic status was classified into four levels by using the obtained data in household income quartiles, while the marital status was classified into single, married, and others (separated, divorced, and widow/widower).

Smoking was classified into current smoker for participants currently smoking and have smoked 100 cigarettes or more in the entire life, while the rest of the participants were classified as none or exsmoker. For the alcohol consumption condition, men drinking seven glasses (five glasses for women) per occasion on average of once or more a week were classified as moderate or heavy alcohol consumption group, while those not applicable were classified as none or social. Exercise status was classified into light, moderate, and vigorous exercise according to the intensity and frequency of exercise. Moderate exercise was defined as five times or more a week and more than thirty minutes of moderate intensity of exercise (e.g., swimming, volleyball). Vigorous exercise was defined as three times or more a week and more than twenty minutes of vigorous intensity of exercise (e.g., soccer, basketball). The other was defined as light exercise.

Occupational Characteristics

The labor status was classified into nonmanual work for government officials, managers, professionals, and office workers, while those working in services, sales and agriculture and fishery industries, and factory workers were classified as manual work. Working more than forty-eight hours per week were defined as long working hours by ILO standard [29], therefore, the work hours per week was classified into forty-eight hours or less group and more than forty-eight hours group.

Night Work

In KNHANES, shift work group was decided by the question, "Do you work mostly during the day time (between 6:00 a.m. and 6:00 p.m.)? Or do you work at a different time period?" Participants who answered "Mostly at day time" were classified as day workers, while the rest of the participants who answered "Evening shift (between 2:00 p.m. and midnight), night shift (between 9:00 p.m. and 8:00 a.m. next day), regular day and night rotating shift, 24-hour rotating shift, split shift (working two shifts in one day), irregular rotating shift, and others" were classified as shift workers. In this study, evening shift group, split shift group, and others which are unlikely to meet the definition of night work have been eliminated from the final analysis to explore the health effects associated with shift work including night work (working over seven consecutive hours including the interval from midnight and 5:00 a.m.) defined by the ILO [2]. In the final analysis, the day-work group was decided as the control group, while participants who answered night shift, regular day and night rotating shift, twenty-four–hour rotating shift, and irregular shift were decided as the night-work group. In the case of irregular shift, there is no more intensive information about irregular shift system in KNHANES. However, most train drivers and controllers with irregular shift systems participating in one study in Finland included night work in their shift schedules, therefore, we included irregular shift in the night work group [30].

Involuntary Weight Change

Weight change is considered clinically significant if there is a loss of over 5 percent of one's weight within six months to a year [31], whereas weight gain of more than two kilograms in a year has been suggested as a significant weight gain, although there is no clinical consensus on weight gain other than Body Mass Index (BMI) standard for obesity [32]. We used two questions in KNHANES to evaluate weight change and voluntariness: "Were there any changes in weight compared to the previous year?" and "Have you ever tried to control weight voluntarily in the previous year?" For the question about weight change, the answer was categorized with "No changes (Weight changes of less than 3 kg)," "Lost weight," and "Gained weight" and for the question about voluntariness, the answer was classified as "Tried to lose weight," "Tried to maintain current weight," "Tried to gain weight," and "Never tried to control weight."

In this study, we excluded the subjects that answered with "Tried to maintain current weight," "Tried to lose weight," and "Tried to gain weight." The reasons are that these subjects voluntarily changed or maintained their weight. As the final analysis subjects, among the subjects that answered "Never tried to control weight," the subjects that answered with "No changes (weight changes of less than 3 kg)" were classified as the no weight change group, while the subjects that answered with "Lost weight" as the weight loss group, and "Gained weight" as the weight gain group.

Statistical Analysis

The fifth KNHANES applied complex sampling design to improve the sample's representativeness and the accuracy of the estimation. To estimate unbiased outcomes in the average, prevalence rate, and risk ratio, stratified variables, cluster variables, and weights should be applied. Weight used in fifth KNHANES has two levels to represent total households and population of South Korea: household weight for household-level analysis and individual weight for individual-level analysis. Final weights were created through several steps, such as calculating the base design weight, adjusting for nonresponse, poststratification adjustment, and extreme value trimming. This study used complex sample module of SPSS. The module was operated to estimate the frequency of a population from the sampling data by using stratified variables, cluster variables, and weights. After applying statistical algorithms in the module, total subjects of this study became 4,077,302.

To figure out the general characteristics of the study participants, the frequency and the configuration fraction of each variable were presented through the stratification of total participants, male, and female. Then chi-square tests were conducted on weight loss and weight gain, respectively, and compared to the no weight change group to analyze the relationship between several relating factors associated with weight loss and weight gain. Odds ratio (OR) was calculated by using logistic regression analysis to determine the association between night work and involuntary weight change. It was constructed into a three-level model, with the first model using unadjusted logistic regression analysis and the second model using multivariate logistic regression analysis with adjusted sociodemographic factors (age, education, household income, and marital status). Sociodemographic factors, health behavior-related factors (smoking, alcohol drinking, and physical activity), and occupational factors (type of job and working hours per week) were all adjusted in the final model. Then, the average working hours per week have been stratified by forty-eight hours or less group and more than forty-eight hours group and logistic regression analysis conducted to explore OR influenced by long working hours. SPSS version 19.0 was used for the statistical analysis and the statistical significance level was set at $p < 0.05$.

Ethics Statement

This study was performed by using the open data of the fifth KNHANES. All study participants of the fifth KNHANES signed a consent form agreeing to the purposes of the survey, and this survey has been approved by the Institutional Review Board (IRB) of the Korea Centers for Disease Control and Prevention (KCDC).

RESULTS

General Characteristics of the Study Participants

Among the total study participants, male participants accounted for 72.6 percent and female 27.4 percent. In terms of occupational characteristics, the percentage of manual work for male was slightly higher than that of female.

Workers who worked more than forty-eight hours per week on average as long working hours accounted for 41.6 percent of the total study participants, and the percentage of long working hours in male was 46.3 percent and significantly higher than that of female (29.1 percent) (table 6.1).

The participants working in night work accounted for 10.6 percent of total study participants with the percentage of night work in male (11.9 percent) higher than female (7.4 percent). The percentage of night work by shift type was 46.5 percent for regular shift work, 21.4 percent for twenty-four–hour shift work, 17.2 percent for night shift work, and 15.0 percent for irregular shift work, in order. In terms of distinguishing differences between male and female participants, female showed a lower percentage in the twenty-four–hour shift work compared to male (male:24.2 percent, female: 9.6 percent) and a higher percentage in night shift work (male: 13.8 percent, female: 31.5 percent) (table 6.1).

The male participants working in night work was significant in the age group of sixties, low level of educational attainment, manual workers, and working more than forty-eight hours a week. The female participants working in night work was significant in moderate or heavy alcohol consumption group (table 6.2).

Involuntary Weight Change and Its Association with Relevant Variables

In regards to involuntary weight change, weight loss in male participants was significant in the age group of twenties and thirties and manual workers. Weight gain in male was significant in the age group of twenties and thirties, high level of educational attainment, single, and moderate or heavy alcohol consumption group (table 6.3).

Weight loss in female was significant in the age group of thirties. Weight gain in female participants was significant in the age group of thirties and forties, low educational attainment, moderate or heavy alcohol consumption group, and current smokers (table 6.4).

The Relationship between Night Work and Involuntary Weight Change

To explore the relationship between weight change and night work, logistic regression analysis in conformity with the three-level model was carried out after stratification by gender. In addition to this, the average working hours per week were stratified by forty-eight hours or less group and more than forty-eight hours group to figure out OR influenced by long working hours and conducted logistic regression analysis (table 6.5).

Table 6.1 General Characteristics of the Study Subjects

	Total		Male		Female	
Variable	n[a]	n[b](%[c])	n[a]	n[b](%[c])	n[a]	n[b](%[c])
Total	1,605	4,077,302(100.0)	1,075	2,960,342(100.0)	530	1,116,959(100.0)
Age(years)						
20–29	216	821,331(20.1)	116	529,449(17.9)	100	291,882(26.1)
30–39	474	1,230,449(30.2)	343	980,278(33.1)	131	250,171(22.4)
40–49	401	1,068,241(26.2)	285	794,654(26.8)	116	273,587(24.5)
50–59	315	654,930(16.1)	205	458,585(15.5)	110	196,345(17.6)
60–69	199	302,351(7.4)	126	197,377(6.7)	73	104,974(9.4)
Education						
≤ Middle school	347	782,262(19.2)	192	493,489(16.7)	155	288,773(25.9)
High school	540	1,500,737(36.8)	366	1,120,342(37.8)	174	380,394(34.1)
≥ University	718	1,794,303(44.0)	517	1,346,511(45.5)	201	447,792(40.1)
Income						
First quartile	137	328,103(8.0)	74	196,406(6.6)	63	131,697(11.8)
Second quartile	443	1,204,464(29.5)	313	927,339(31.3)	130	277,125(24.8)
Third quartile	552	1,445,150(35.4)	371	1,043,236(35.2)	181	401,914(36.0)
Fourth quartile	473	1,099,584(27.0)	317	793,362(26.8)	156	306,223(27.4)
Marital status						
Single	262	934,340(22.9)	154	630,167(21.3)	108	304,173(27.2)
Married	1,252	2,931,100(71.9)	893	2,243,410(75.8)	359	687,690(61.6)
Others	91	211,862(5.2)	28	86,766(2.9)	63	125,096(11.2)
Alcohol drinking						
None or social	1,159	2,837,667(69.6)	674	1,832,693(61.9)	485	1,004,975(90.0)
Moderate or heavy	446	1,239,634(30.4)	401	1,127,650(38.1)	45	111,985(10.0)
Smoking						
None or exsmoker	999	2,322,062(57.0)	503	1,289,687(43.6)	496	1,032,375(92.4)
Current smoker	606	1,755,240(43.0)	572	1,670,656(56.4)	34	84,585(7.6)
Physical activity						
Light	1,383	3,462,054(84.9)	918	2,484,421(83.9)	465	977,633(87.5)
Moderate	91	242,915(6.0)	52	155,782(5.3)	39	87,133(7.8)
Vigorous	131	372,332(9.1)	105	320,139(10.8)	26	52,193(4.7)
Type of job						
Nonmanual	713	1,771,262(43.4)	479	1,257,519(42.5)	234	513,743(46.0)
Manual	892	2,306,040(56.6)	596	1,702,823(57.5)	296	603,217(54.0)
Working hours per week						
≤ 48	957	2,380,084(58.4)	570	1,588,447(53.7)	387	791,637(70.9)
> 48	648	1,697,218(41.6)	505	1,371,896(46.3)	143	325,322(29.1)
Work schedule						
Day work	1,418	3,643,616(89.4)	923	2,609,320(88.1)	495	1,034,295(92.6)
Night work	187	433,686(10.6)	152	351,022(11.9)	35	82,664(7.4)
Night shift	28	74,393(17.2)	18	48,319(13.8)	10	26,074(31.5)
Regular shift	78	201,489(46.5)	62	164,707(46.9)	16	36,781(44.5)
Twenty-four hour shift	51	92,821(21.4)	46	84,865(24.2)	5	7,956(9.6)
Irregular shift	30	64,983(15.0)	26	53,130(15.1)	4	11,853(14.3)

(Continued)

Table 6.1 General Characteristics of the Study Subjects *(Continued)*

	Total		Male		Female	
Variable	n[a]	n[b](%[c])	n[a]	n[b](%[c])	n[a]	n[b](%[c])
Weight change						
No weight change	1,248	3,042,783(74.6)	847	2,219,990(75.0)	401	822,794(73.7)
Weight loss	142	381,040(9.3)	92	278,769(9.4)	50	102,270(9.2)
Weight gain	215	653,478(16.0)	136	461,583(15.6)	79	191,895(17.2)

a Unweighted count
b Estimated population size
c Column and estimated percentage

Weight loss in male workers associated with night work showed that the risk was significantly low in night work group (OR 0.34, 95 % CI 0.16–0.76) after controlling for several related factors. However, OR for weight gain associated with night work was not significant in male workers. In the case of female workers, ORs for weight loss and weight gain associated with night work were not significant. However, the results after stratifying by average weekly working hours revealed that ORs were higher than 1.0 in more than forty-eight hours working group with 1.95 (95 percent CI 0.47–80.86) in weight loss group and 2.83 (95 percent CI 0.12–69.83) in weight gain group.

DISCUSSION

This study evaluated the risk of involuntary weight change associated with night work in Korean full-time wage workers from the nationwide representative data and revealed that night work may lower the risk of weight loss in male workers and induce weight change (loss or gain) in female workers with long working hours.

Most previous studies stated that there was a high risk of weight gain or obesity development resulting from shift or night work. Antunes [33] reviewed numerous articles related to metabolic syndrome, dyslipidemia, unhealthy eating habits, and increase in BMI and waist-hip ratio (WHR) associated with shift work and argued the risk of weight gain related with shift work [33]. Also, Drongelen [34] suggested a relationship between shift work and weight gain which was consistent to the statement presented earlier by Antunes [33] in a review article restricting with longitudinal studies on shift work exposed to night work between midnight and 6:00 a.m. [34]. Weight gain associated with shift work can be explained through the complex mechanisms brought on by the disturbance of circadian rhythm. First of all, changes in night and day patterns associated with shift work will reduce the production of the appetite-suppressing hormone, leptin, which is produced

Table 6.2 General Characteristics of Male and Female by Work Schedule

	Male		*Female*	
Variable	*Day Work* n[a](*%*[b])	*Night Work* n[a](*%*[b])	*Day Work* n[a](*%*[b])	*Night Work* n[a](*%*[b])
Total	2,609,320(100.0)	351,022(100.0)	1,034,295(100.0)	82,664(100.0)
Age(years)[c]				
20–29	468,087(17.9)	61,363(17.5)	261,607(25.3)	30,275(36.6)
30–39	875,124(33.5)	105,154(30.0)	232,659(22.5)	17,512(21.2)
40–49	738,135(28.3)	56,519(16.1)	253,412(24.5)	20,175(24.4)
50–59	404,736(15.5)	53,848(15.3)	185,802(18.0)	10,543(12.8)
60–69	123,239(4.7)	74,138(21.1)	100,814(9.7)	4,160(5.0)
Education[c]				
≤ Middle school	422,070(16.2)	71,419(20.3)	277,763(26.9)	11,010(13.3)
High school	945,666(36.2)	174,676(49.8)	342,680(33.1)	37,714(45.6)
≥ University	1,241,584(47.6)	104,927(29.9)	413,852(40.0)	33,940(41.1)
Income				
First quartile	178,888(6.9)	17,518(5.0)	128,559(12.4)	3,138(3.8)
Second quartile	835,447(32.0)	91,892(26.2)	253,419(24.5)	23,706(28.7)
Third quartile	902,113(34.6)	141,123(40.2)	370,488(35.8)	31,426(38.0)
Fourth quartile	692,873(26.6)	100,489(28.6)	281,829(27.2)	24,394(29.5)
Marital status				
Single	538,421(20.6)	91,746(26.1)	274,416(26.5)	29,757(36.0)
Married	1,988,519(76.2)	254,890(72.6)	645,458(62.4)	42,232(51.1)
Others	82,380(3.2)	4,386(1.2)	114,422(11.1)	10,674(12.9)
Alcohol drinking[d]				
None or social	1,592,309(61.0)	240,384(68.5)	944,300(91.3)	60,675(73.4)
Moderate or heavy	1,017,012(39.0)	110,638(31.5)	89,995(8.7)	21,989(26.6)
Smoking				
None or exsmoker	1,111,880(42.6)	177,806(50.7)	964,964(93.3)	67,411(81.5)
Current smoker	1,497,440(57.4)	173,216(49.3)	69,331(6.7)	15,253(18.5)
Physical activity				
Light	2,174,814(83.3)	309,607(88.2)	910,681(88.0)	66,952(81.0)
Moderate	147,376(5.6)	8,406(2.4)	82,729(8.0)	4,405(5.3)
Vigorous	287,130(11.0)	33,010(9.4)	40,886(4.0)	11,307(13.7)
Type of job[c]				
Nonmanual	1,212,165(46.5)	45,354(12.9)	487,665(47.1)	26,078(31.5)
Manual	1,397,155(53.5)	305,668(87.1)	546,630(52.9)	56,586(68.5)

(Continued)

Table 6.2 General Characteristics of Male and Female by Work Schedule (*Continued*)

	Male		*Female*	
Variable	*Day Work* n[a](%[b])	*Night Work* n[a](%[b])	*Day Work* n[a](%[b])	*Night Work* n[a](%[b])
Working hours per week[c]				
≤ 48	1,471,445(56.4)	117,002(33.3)	734,250(71.0)	57,386(69.4)
> 48	1,137,876(43.6)	234,020(66.7)	300,045(29.0)	25,278(30.6)
Weight change				
No weight change	1,938,500(74.3)	281,489(80.2)	764,035(73.9)	58,759(71.1)
Weight loss	259,215(9.9)	19,554(5.6)	96,299(9.3)	5,971(7.2)
Weight gain	411,605(15.8)	49,978(14.2)	173,961(16.8)	17,934(21.7)

[a] Estimated population size.
[b] Column and estimated percentage.
[c] Significantly different between day work and night work in male subjects ($p < 0.05$).
[d] Significantly different between day work and night work in female subjects ($p < 0.05$).

normally during the night while sleeping, and instead increase the production of the appetite enhancing hormone, ghrelin, resulting in stimulation of the appetite. As a result of this, the weight increases due to increased high calorie diet and late-night meals. Also, the disturbance of circadian rhythm leads to weight gain by increasing insulin resistance and bringing changes in the glucose and lipid homeostasis. In addition to this, the effects of reduction in physical activity during spare time, reduced social and family relationship, and job stress accelerate weight gain [33, 34].

Despite various evidences on weight gain associated with shift work suggested in the previous studies, weight loss associated with shift work has been reported in a one-year follow-up cohort study observing 377 new workers in the Netherlands [28]. In this Dutch study, Amelsvoort [28] assumed that the growth in smoking rate, the change in the neuroendocrine secretion of hormones due to sleep problems, and the disturbance of the metabolic system increased the risk of weight loss. In addition to these interpretations, Amelsvoort [28] pointed out that the growth in smoking rate was not sufficient to explain the total effect, the disturbance of the metabolic system could induce weight loss only in short term, and BMI could increase after several years of shift work with increasing energy intake. Furthermore, Amelsvoort [28] assumed that the result was influenced by a behavioral change of the participants caused by the realization of the study itself.

On the contrary, some studies evaluated weight change with using the average value of BMI or by conducting long-term follow-up observations

Table 6.3 Involuntary Weight Change According to Characteristics in Male Subjects

Variable	*No Weight Change* n[a](%[b])	*Weight Loss* n[a](%[b])	*Weight Gain* n[a](%[b])
Total	2,219,990(100.0)	278,769(100.0)	461,583(100.0)
Age(years)[c,d]			
20–29	309,365(13.9)	61,956(22.2)	158,128(34.3)
30–39	638,936(28.8)	129,157(46.3)	212,184(46.0)
40–49	687,560(31.0)	48,748(17.5)	58,346(12.6)
50–59	416,913(18.8)	15,891(5.7)	25,780(5.6)
60–69	167,216(7.5)	23,016(8.3)	7,145(1.5)
Education[d]			
≤ Middle school	415,384(18.7)	41,724(15.0)	36,381(7.9)
High school	809,988(36.5)	121,416(43.6)	188,938(40.9)
≥ University	994,617(44.8)	115,629(41.5)	236,265(51.2)
Income			
First quartile	128,890(5.8)	37,409(13.4)	30,107(6.5)
Second quartile	690,811(31.1)	81,863(29.4)	154,665(33.5)
Third quartile	784,316(35.3)	109,728(39.4)	149,192(32.3)
Fourth quartile	615,973(27.7)	49,770(17.9)	127,619(27.6)
Marital status [d]			
Single	406,539(18.3)	80,784(29.0)	142,844(30.9)
Married	1,749,396(78.8)	188,786(67.7)	305,228(66.1)
Others	64,055(2.9)	9,199(3.3)	13,512(2.9)
Alcohol drinking[d]			
None or social	1,410,436(63.5)	177,538(63.7)	244,719(53.0)
Moderate or heavy	809,553(36.5)	101,232(36.3)	216,864(47.0)
Smoking			
None or exsmoker	1,022,453(46.1)	96,115(34.5)	171,118(37.1)
Current smoker	1,197,536(53.9)	182,654(65.5)	290,465(62.9)
Physical activity			
Light	1,848,629(83.3)	219,257(78.7)	416,536(90.2)
Moderate	123,131(5.5)	21,311(7.6)	11,341(2.5)
Vigorous	248,230(11.2)	38,202(13.7)	33,707(7.3)
Type of job[c]			
Nonmanual	965,184(43.5)	74,162(26.6)	218,173(47.3)
Manual	1,254,805(56.5)	204,607(73.4)	243,411(52.7)
Working hours per week			
≤ 48	1,183,501(53.3)	119,901(43.0)	285,045(61.8)
> 48	1,036,489(46.7)	158,868(57.0)	176,538(38.2)
Work schedule			
Day work	1,938,500(87.3)	259,215(93.0)	411,605(89.2)
Night work	281,489(12.7)	19,554(7.0)	49,978(10.8)

[a] Estimated population size.
[b] Column and estimated percentage.
[c] Significantly different between no weight change and weight loss subjects ($p < 0.05$).
[d] Significantly different between no weight change and weight gain subjects ($p < 0.05$).

Table 6.4 Involuntary Weight Change According to Characteristics in Female Subjects

Variable	*No Weight Change* n[a](%[b])	*Weight Loss* n[a](%[b])	*Weight Gain* n[a](%[b])
Total	822,794(100.0)	102,270(100.0)	191,895(100.0)
Age(years)[c,d]			
20–29	216,836(26.4)	25,752(25.2)	49,294(25.7)
30–39	148,273(18.0)	39,560(38.7)	62,338(32.5)
40–49	191,374(23.3)	18,203(17.8)	64,009(33.4)
50–59	174,512(21.2)	10,948(10.7)	10,886(5.7)
60–69	91,799(11.2)	7,807(7.6)	5,368(2.8)
Education[d]			
≤ Middle school	245,145(29.8)	23,029(22.5)	20,599(10.7)
High school	241,590(29.4)	31,565(30.9)	107,239(55.9)
≥ University	336,059(40.8)	47,676(46.6)	64,057(33.4)
Income			
First quartile	96,039(11.7)	13,273(13.0)	22,386(11.7)
Second quartile	202,988(24.7)	30,086(29.4)	44,051(23.0)
Third quartile	299,364(36.4)	32,570(31.8)	69,980(36.5)
Fourth quartile	224,403(27.3)	26,341(25.8)	55,478(28.9)
Marital status			
Single	235,649(28.6)	19,664(19.2)	48,860(25.5)
Married	489,691(59.5)	69,149(67.6)	128,851(67.1)
Others	97,454(11.8)	13,458(13.2)	14,184(7.4)
Alcohol drinking[d]			
None or social	766,987(93.2)	93,006(90.9)	144,982(75.6)
Moderate or heavy	55,807(6.8)	9,264(9.1)	46,913(24.4)
Smoking[d]			
None or exsmoker	775,650(94.3)	94,836(92.7)	161,889(84.4)
Current smoker	47,144(5.7)	7,435(7.3)	30,006(15.6)
Physical activity			
Light	714,667(86.9)	81,249(79.4)	181,717(94.7)
Moderate	65,375(7.9)	16,373(16.0)	5,385(2.8)
Vigorous	42,752(5.2)	4,649(4.5)	4,793(2.5)
Type of job			
Nonmanual	384,975(46.8)	44,607(43.6)	84,161(43.9)
Manual	437,819(53.2)	57,663(56.4)	107,734(56.1)
Working hours per week			
≤ 48	588,048(71.5)	68,562(67.0)	135,026(70.4)
> 48	234,745(28.5)	33,708(33.0)	56,869(29.6)
Work schedule			
Day work	764,035(92.9)	96,299(94.2)	173,961(90.7)
Night work	58,759(7.1)	5,971(5.8)	17,934(9.3)

[a] Estimated population size
[b] Column and estimated percentage
[c] Significantly different between no weight change and weight loss subjects ($p < 0.05$)
[d] Significantly different between no weight change and weight gain subjects ($p < 0.05$)

Table 6.5 OR and 95 % Confidence Intervals (CI) for Involuntary Weight Change

		Male			Female		
		Model 1[a]	*Model 2*[b]	*Model 3*[c]	*Model 1*[a]	*Model 2*[b]	*Model 3*[c]
Weight loss							
	Day work	1.00	1.00	1.00	1.00	1.00	1.00
	Night work	0.52(0.24–1.11)	0.44(0.20–0.95)	0.34(0.16–0.76)	0.81(0.22–2.93)	0.66(0.15–2.84)	0.58(0.14–2.40)
Stratification by working hours per week							
≤48	Day work	1.00	1.00	1.00	1.00	1.00	1.00
	Night work	0.25(0.42–1.45)	0.23(0.36–1.50)	0.22(0.03–1.50)	0.60(0.12–3.05)	0.57(0.10–3.16)	0.47(0.08–2.93)
>48	Day work	1.00	1.00	1.00	1.00	1.00	1.00
	Night work	0.56(0.24–1.34)	0.44(0.16–1.20)	0.35(0.12–1.00)	1.64(0.17–16.07)	1.43(0.08–27.08)	1.95(0.47–80.86)
Weight gain							
	Day work	1.00	1.00	1.00	1.00	1.00	1.00
	Night work	0.84(0.44–1.59)	0.92(0.46–1.84)	0.98(0.48–2.02)	1.34(0.40–4.54)	1.19(0.33–4.30)	0.80(0.22–2.85)
Stratification by working hours per week							
≤48	Day work	1.00	1.00	1.00	1.00	1.00	1.00
	Night work	0.57(0.17–1.90)	0.53(0.15–1.93)	0.49(0.13–1.92)	0.57(0.12–2.76)	0.53(0.10–2.67)	0.34(0.40–2.87)
>48	Day work	1.00	1.00	1.00	1.00	1.00	1.00
	Night work	1.19(0.55–2.61)	1.75(0.70–4.28)	1.55(0.57–4.18)	5.04(0.77–32.89)	9.58(0.83–110.20)	2.83(0.12–69.83)

[a] Model 1: crude model.
[b] Model 2: adjusted with sociodemographic factors (age, education, household income, and marital status).
[c] Model 3: adjusted with sociodemographic factors (age, education, household income, and marital status), health behavior-related factors (smoking, alcohol drinking, and physical activity), and occupational factors (type of job and working hours per week).

[35, 36]. However, such studies had the problem of not being able to determine the risk of weight gain and weight loss separately in shift workers, because the average value of BMI or the amount of weight change was used. For example, participants showing weight gain accounted for 42.9 percent in the fourteen-year follow-up study of Suwazono [35] observing the changes in weight. This finding explained the reason why the impact of weight gain may be relatively significant when examining the risk of weight change with applying the average value of weight change. However, in the study of Kivimäki [25] for the association between job stress and weight change, the risk of weight gain and weight loss was separately evaluated. For five to eight years of follow-up, 29.2 percent of male participants were weight loss and 70.7 percent of them were weight gain. Among male participants, lower control group was significantly high risk in weight loss with bottom quintile in baseline BMI and higher strain group was significantly high risk in weight gain with top quintile in baseline BMI [25].

This cross-sectional study showed that night work may effect differently by gender on body weight. According to this study for male workers, night work may decrease the risk of weight loss with statistical significance compared with day work and increase the risk of weight gain with long working hours without statistical significance. In a previous study, Roos [37] reported that the risk of weight gain associated with shift work including night shift was elevated (OR 1.25, 95 percent CI 0.81–1.82) in male workers and OR of weight gain associated with shift work with no night shift was similar. However, long working hours (>50 hours) may lower the risk of weight gain (OR 0.87, 95 percent CI 0.41–1.83) without statistical significance in Finnish male workers. The results of Roos's study were different from this study because some difference between Roos's study and this study. The study design of Roos's study was a prospective cohort study with a questionnaire survey, and this study is a cross-sectional survey. Furthermore, industrial history of the country as well as working hours is quite different between Finland and Korea. Because of this different nature of the societies, the results might not be the same direction. Besides, the combined effect of both shift work and long working hours was not evaluated in Roos's study, but this study. Long working hours as well as shift work is an established risk factor of workers' health. Shift work with long working hours may more aggravate workers' health compared with day workers without overtime work. In most previous studies, both factors were analyzed separately. As shown in Liu's study (2002), the proportion of shift workers was highest in the long working hour group (more than sixty hours per week) in Japan [38]. However, the combined health effects of both long working hours and shift work were not assessed in this study, even though the short sleeping time was included as a proxy of shift work. Korea is one of the longest working countries in OECD countries. Therefore, future studies are needed to elucidate the combined aggravating health effects of both long working and shift work in Korea.

On the contrary, in the case of female workers, night work may induce weight change (weight loss or weight gain) with long working hours, even though the results were not statistically significant. In the aspect of weight gain, we suggest the possibility of weight gain caused by job stress as a medium. Kivimäki [25] already argued this by using the Whitehall II study, and there can be bidirectional results for weight gain and weight loss associated with job stress [25]. In female participants, the higher follow-up BMI was slightly associated with higher job demand after adjusting with age, grade, and baseline BMI. Previous studies revealed that such job stress was more significant in shift work group than day work group, especially in a low level of job control [39, 40]. Therefore, there is a possibility of weight gain resulting from shift work in association with low job control. In Roos's study (2013), the authors reported that the risk of weight gain associated with shift work including night shift was higher than that of male workers and showed a statistical significance. OR of weight gain associated with shift work with night shift was 1.37 (95 percent CI 1.08–1.74) and the risk of weight gain associated with shift work with no night shift was decreased in female workers [37]. In addition, the risk of weight gain was slightly increased (OR 1.03, 95 percent CI 0.64–1.65) in female workers with long working hours (>fifty hours), even though the risk was statistically insignificant. Furthermore, female shift workers with long working hours have no time to rest, exercise, and have social relationships with their friends and families.

For explaining the possibility of the weight loss with night work, we suggest several hypotheses related to weight loss associated with night work in female workers with long working hours. First explanation is the possibility of weight loss caused by depressive symptoms and gastrointestinal disorders known to occur highly in shift workers. Driesen [9] reported that OR for depressive symptoms in shift workers was 2.05 in male (95 % CI 1.52–2.77) and 5.96 in female (95 % CI 2.83–12.56), compared to day workers. According to studies with Korean workers, Kim [41] reported a higher prevalence of irritable bowel syndrome and functional dyspepsia in female shift workers and Cho [42] reported depressive symptoms related with job stress and sleep quality in female workers. Knutsson [14] announced that shift workers showed increased incidence for gastrointestinal symptoms and peptic ulcer through the review about shift work and gastrointestinal disorders. Such a series of health effects related to shift work has been reported as a common cause of weight loss [31]. Therefore, depressive symptoms and gastrointestinal disorders caused by shift work may contribute to weight loss in shift workers. Second explanation is the suggestion in Kivimäki's study

(2006) for explaining the significant higher risk of weight loss in the low control group in bottom quintile in baseline BMI, even though the results were from male participants [25]. Kivimäki explained that it was influenced by the loss of appetite due to stress and suppression of upper gastrointestinal motility caused by activation of the sympathetic nervous system. In spite of these possibilities, the increased risk of weight loss related to night work was limited to long working female workers in our study without statistical significance. Furthermore, the risk of weight loss associated with night work was significantly low in male workers. Therefore, further studies are needed to explain these findings in this country.

We suggest several hypotheses to explain gender difference in the effect on weight associated with night work with long working hours. We present two factors related with the characteristics of Korean society. First factor is that women have experienced higher domestic labor burden than men. According to Korea's Time Use Survey conducted in 2009, among double-income households, women used 185 minutes for housework, while men used twenty-seven minutes. Therefore, Korean women disproportionately lack in time for sleep and recovery from work compared to Korean men [43], showing increased vulnerability to stress caused by long working hours. Second factor is that women are subject to discrimination in terms of promotion and wage and the risk of depressive symptoms related to organization injustice is higher for female than male [44]. According to previous studies, disturbances of circadian rhythm and sleep associated with shift work could cause weight gain. However, gender difference in weight gain associated with sleep disturbance was unclear [45]. In Korean society that have forced high domestic labor burden on women, sleep disturbance is more likely to occur in female workers with night work with long working hours and the effects have been reflected in our results.

This study has several limitations. First, this study used data of the fifth KNHANES with a cross-sectional design to explore the current status of the population. Therefore, the participant's weight change during the previous year was assessed instead of following of body weight of participants. Second, the participant's period of time engaged in night work was not considered. In KNHANES, the only information available for shift work is the work schedule and work type, and there is no data on duration of shift work. In the study of Amelsvoort [28], although weight loss was shown for one-year follow-up after starting shift work, there is also the possibility of weight gain after many years of shift work [28]. So the risk of weight change in night workers shown in this study may be a short-term effect like in the study of Amelsvoort [28], especially about the risk of weight loss. Therefore, the risk of weight gain and weight loss should be figured out by considering the period engaged in night work in follow-up studies in the future. Third, there is the possibility of information bias resulting from the use of participant's self-report survey data on weight change during the previous year. However, we excluded participants with intentional weight change (loss or gain or maintenance) to overcome the limitation of a cross-sectional study design. In spite of these limitations, this study has secured the representativeness and credibility by using the KNHANES which determines the status of health and nutrition of Koreans nationwide. In addition, this study evaluated the risk of involuntary weight change associated with night work in Korean full-time wage workers, considering several related factors with weight, sociodemographic variables, health behavior-related variables, and occupational variables. Besides, we examined the risk of weight change caused by night work by dividing into weight loss and weight gain group and further analysis after stratification by working hours in male and female workers.

CONCLUSIONS

In this cross-sectional study with national representative sample, night work may lower the risk of weight loss in male workers and induce weight change (weight loss or weight gain) in female workers with long working hours. Therefore, future studies with cohort study design for night workers are needed to reveal the mechanisms and health effects of weight change associated with night work through monitoring health risk behaviors including smoking, drinking, nutrition intake, physical activities, and consideration of other related occupational factors and establish proper management solutions with health and labor policies for Korean night workers.

NOTE

1. This chapter was previously published as Kwon, Jongho, Jung-Woo Park, Jin-Soo Park, Seyoung Kim, Hyunrim Choi, and Sinye Lim. "The relationship between night work and involuntary weight change: data from the fifth Korea National Health and Nutrition Examination Survey (KNHANES 2010–2012)." *Annals of Occupational and Environmental Medicine* 28, no. 1 (2016): 4.

REFERENCES

1. Costa G. "Shift work and occupational medicine: an overview." *Occup Med (Lond)*. 2003;53:83–8.
2. Kogi K, Thurman JE. "Trends in approaches to night and shiftwork and new international standards." *Ergonomics*. 1993;36:3–13.

3. Parent-Thirion A, Vermeylen G, Van Houten G, Lyly-Yrjänäinen M, Biletta I, Cabrita J, et al. *Fifth European Working Conditions Survey*. Luxembourg: Eurofound, Publications Office of the European Union, 2012. http://www.eurofound.europa.eu/sites/default/files/ef_files/pubdocs/2011/82/en/1/EF1182EN.pdf. Accessed 21 February 2015.
4. Caruso C, Rosa RR. "Shift work and long work hours." In: *Environmental and Occupational Medicine*, Rom WN, editor. 4th ed. Philadelphia, PA: Lippincott Williams & Wilkins, 2007. p. 1359–72.
5. Park TJ, Pack DM, Joh KO, Park JS, Cho SI. "The relationship between shift work and work-related injuries among Korean workers." *Korean J Occup Environ Med.* 2012;24:52–60.
6. Wang JH, Lee G, Song JT, Kwon J, Choi H, Lim S, et al. "The association between shift work and bone mineral density : analysis of 2008–2009 Korean National Health and Nutrition Examination Survey." *Korean J Occup Environ Med.* 2012;24:274–86.
7. Sallinen M, Kecklund G. "Shift work, sleep, and sleepiness-differences between shift schedules and systems." *Scand J Work Environ Health.* 2010;36:121–33.
8. Wagstaff AS, Sigstad Lie JA. "Shift and night work and long working hours—a systematic review of safety implications." *Scand J Work Environ Health.* 2011;37:173–85.
9. Driesen K, Jansen NW, Kant I, Mohren DC, van Amelsvoort LG. "Depressed mood in the working population: associations with work schedules and working hours." *Chronobiol Int.* 2010;27:1062–79.
10. Härmä M. "Workhours in relation to work stress, recovery and health." *Scand J Work Environ Health.* 2006;32:502–14.
11. Lowden A, Moreno C, Holmbäck U, Lennernäs M, Tucker P. "Eating and shift work-effects on habits, metabolism, and performance." *Scand J Work Environ Health.* 2010;36:150–62.
12. Tenkanen L, Sjöblom T, Härmä M. "Joint effect of shift work and adverse life-style factors on the risk of coronary heart disease." *Scand J Work Environ Health.* 1998;24:351–7.
13. Frost P, Kolstad HA, Bonde JP. "Shift work and the risk of ischemic heart disease—a systematic review of the epidemiologic evidence." *Scand J Work Environ Health.* 2009;35:163–79.
14. Knutsson A, Bøggild H. "Gastrointestinal disorders among shift workers." *Scand J Work Environ Health.* 2010;36:85–95.
15. Kolstad HA. "Nightshift work and risk of breast cancer and other cancers—a critical review of the epidemiological evidence." *Scand J Work Environ Health.* 2008;34:5–22.
16. Knutsson A. "Health disorders of shift workers." *Occup Med (Lond).* 2003;53:103–8.
17. Costa G. "The impact of shift and night work on health." *Appl Ergon.* 1996;27:9–16.
18. Wannamethee SG, Shaper AG, Walker M. "Weight change, weight fluctuation, and mortality." *Arch Intern Med.* 2002;162:2575–80.

19. Mikkelsen KL, Heimann BL, Keiding N, Sorensen TI. "Independent effects of stable and changing body weight on total mortality." *Epidemiology*. 1999;10:671–8.
20. Willett WC, Manson JE, Stampfer MJ, Colditz GA, Rosner B, Speizer FE, et al. "Weight, weight change, and coronary heart disease in women: risk within the 'normal' weight range." *JAMA*. 1995;273:461–5.
21. Ford ES, Williamson DF, Liu S. "Weight change and diabetes incidence: findings from a national cohort of US adults." *Am J Epidemiol*. 1997;146:214–22.
22. Huang Z, Hankinson SE, Colditz GA, Stampfer MJ, Hunter DJ, Manson JE, et al. "Dual effects of weight and weight gain on breast cancer risk." JAMA. 1997;278:1407–11.
23. Ensrud KE, Ewing SK, Stone KL, Cauley JA, Bowman PJ, Cummings SR. "Intentional and unintentional weight loss increase bone loss and hip fracture risk in older women." *J Am Geriatr Soc*. 2003;51:1740–7.
24. Sahyoun N, Serdula M, Galuska D, Zhang X, Pamuk E. "The epidemiology of recent involuntary weight loss in the United States population." *J Nutr Health Aging*. 2003;8:510–7.
25. Kivimäki M, Head J, Ferrie J, Shipley M, Brunner E, Vahtera J, et al. "Work stress, weight gain and weight loss: evidence for bidirectional effects of job strain on body mass index in the Whitehall II study." *Int J Obes (Lond)*. 2006;30:982–7.
26. Quist HG, Christensen U, Christensen KB, Aust B, Borg V, Bjorner JB. "Psychosocial work environment factors and weight change: a prospective study among Danish health care workers." *BMC Public Health*. 2013;13:43.
27. Esquirol Y, Perret B, Ruidavets JB, Marquie JC, Dienne E, Niezborala M, et al. "Shift work and cardiovascular risk factors: new knowledge from the past decade." *Arch Cardiovasc Dis*. 2011;104:636–68.
28. van Amelsvoort LG, Schouten EG, Kok FJ. "Impact of one year of shift work on cardiovascular disease risk factors." *J Occup Environ Med*. 2004;46:699–706.
29. Lee S, McCann D, Messenger JC. *Working Time around the World*. Geneva: ILO, 2007.
30. Sallinen M, Härmä M, Mutanen P, Ranta R, Virkkala J, Müller K. "Sleep–wake rhythm in an irregular shift system." *J Sleep Res*. 2003;12:103–12.
31. Wong CJ. "Involuntary weight loss." *Med Clin North Am*. 2014;98:625–43.
32. Kroke A, Liese AD, Schulz M, Bergmann MM, Klipstein-Grobusch K, Hoffmann K, et al. "Recent weight changes and weight cycling as predictors of subsequent two year weight change in a middle-aged cohort." *Int J Obes Relat Metab Disord*. 2002;26:403–9.
33. Antunes L, Levandovski R, Dantas G, Caumo W, Hidalgo M. "Obesity and shift work: chronobiological aspects." *Nutr Res Rev*. 2010;23:155–68.
34. van Drongelen A, Boot CR, Merkus SL, Smid T, van der Beek AJ. "The effects of shift work on body weight change-a systematic review of longitudinal studies." *Scand J Work Environ Health*. 2011;37:263–75.
35. Suwazono Y, Dochi M, Sakata K, Okubo Y, Oishi M, Tanaka K, et al. "A longitudinal study on the effect of shift work on weight gain in male Japanese workers." *Obesity (Silver Spring)*. 2008;16:1887–93.

36. Hannerz H, Albertsen K, Nielsen ML, Tüchsen F, Burr H. "Occupational factors and 5-year weight change among men in a Danish national cohort." *Health Psychol.* 2004;23:283–8.
37. Roos E, Lallukka T, Rahkonen O, Lahelma E, Laaksonen M. "Working conditions and major weight gain—a prospective cohort study." *Arch Environ Occup Health.* 2013;68:166–72.
38. Liu Y, Tanaka H, Fukuoka Heart Study Group. "Overtime work, insufficient sleep, and risk of non-fatal acute myocardial infarction in Japanese men." *Occup Environ Med.* 2002;59:447–51.
39. Bøggild H, Burr H, Tüchsen F, Jeppesen HJ. "Work environment of Danish shift and day workers." *Scand J Work Environ Health.* 2001;27:97–105.
40. Tenkanen L, Sjöblom T, Kalimo R, Alikoski T, Härmä M. "Shift work, occupation and coronary heart disease over 6 years of follow-up in the Helsinki Heart Study." *Scand J Work Environ Health.* 1997;23:257–65.
41. Kim HI, Jung S, Choi JY, Kim S-E, Jung H-K, Shim K-N, et al. "Impact of shiftwork on irritable bowel syndrome and functional dyspepsia." *J Korean Med Sci.* 2013;28:431–7.
42. Cho HS, Kim YW, Park HW, Lee KH, Jeong BG, Kang YS, et al. "The relationship between depressive symptoms among female workers and job stress and sleep quality." *Ann Occup Environ Med.* 2013;25:12.
43. Song JT, Lee G, Kwon J, Park JW, Choi H, Lim S. "The association between long working hours and self-rated health." *Ann Occup Environ Med.* 2014;26:2.
44. Park SG, Min KB, Chang SJ, Kim HC, Min JY. "Job stress and depressive symptoms among Korean employees: the effects of culture on work." *Int Arch Occup Environ Health.* 2009;82:397–405.
45. Bayon V, Leger D, Gomez-Merino D, Vecchierini M-F, Chennaoui M. "Sleep debt and obesity." *Ann Med.* 2014;46:264–72.

Chapter 7

The Association between Korean Employed Workers' On-Call Work and Health Problems and Injuries

Chulin Baek, Jae Bum Park, Kyungjong Lee, and Jaehyuk Jung

BACKGROUND

On-call[1] work, by definition, is a form of work that requires the person to work at any time during the on-call period. Therefore, a person often has to work during both daytime and nighttime hours, leading to stressful situations for the worker [1]. Thus, on-call work is often regarded as one of the most severe stress factors [2–4]. This was reflected in a European Working Conditions Survey (EWCS) performed to establish the foundation for creating a healthy work environment; on-call work assessment was first introduced in the fifth European EWCS performed in 2010. Similarly, in Korea, assessment of on-call work was first included the second Korean Working Conditions Survey in 2010, which defined on-call work as "immediately providing work or service if contacted or called." The present study also used this definition.

Previous studies have reported the various effects of on-call work on workers. The health-related effects of on-call work include stress-related symptoms such as exhaustion, irritation, sleep disorders, memory disorders, and headache [4]. A previous study on nurses reported that on-call work was associated with musculoskeletal symptoms including pain in back and muscles of the upper limbs [5]. The neuropsychological effects of on-call work include depressed mood [6], sleep deprivation and insomnia [7], sleepiness during the daytime [7, 8], reduced cognitive function [9, 10], and difficulty in concentrating [10]. Furthermore, a study on residents showed that long on-call work periods were associated with occupational injuries and malpractice [11].

On-call work may also affect sociopsychological stress. A previous study of Korean physicians showed an association between the frequency of on-call duty during the week and work-related stress [12]. Another study showed the relationship between on-call work and job dissatisfaction [2, 13] and also between on-call work and turnover intention [14], suggesting that job dissatisfaction from on-call work can affect turnover intention. In the United States, the annual loss of operating budget due to job change is an estimated 5 percent [15]. Therefore, increased turnover of employees from on-call work may also become a social cost problem. Moreover, irregular working hours due to on-call work is associated with work-life imbalance [16], and a study of on-call workers and their spouses demonstrated the negative effects of on-call work on family life including constraints in their lives, forced sacrifice by spouses, and communication issues among family members [17]. These results clearly showed that on-call work affects not only work life but also life outside of work. In addition, the negative effects of on-call work on other family members were clearly demonstrated. Thus, on-call work not only has negative effects both physically and psychologically but may also result in sociopsychological stress, eventually affecting the quality of life of workers and their family members in addition to the social costs.

However, there are very few studies about on-call work in Korea. Moreover, previous studies generally focused on specific occupations (i.e., nurses and physicians), and no previous study on the effect of on-call work on health and other aspects has included a broad range of the job spectrum. This study aimed to investigate the possible associations between on-call work and its possible negative effects on health and other injuries by utilizing data from the third Korean Working Conditions Survey performed in 2011 regarding on-call work-related personal and occupational characteristics and work environment in a large sample of workers representative of Korean workers nationwide.

METHODS

Study Population

This study was based on the third Korean Working Conditions Survey performed by Korean Occupational Safety and Health Research Institute in 2011. The survey was conducted on a representative sample of workers (≥15 years). A worker was defined as "a person who during the reference week did any work for pay or profit." A total of 50,032 subjects were included in the study, and in-person interviews were performed by professional interviewers from professional survey services after obtaining informed consent. This study focused on employed workers from the entire of 50,032 subjects.

An employed worker was defined as "a person who signed either expressed or implied employment contract with individual, family, or business and is receiving salary or daily wage or spot goods in return for their labor." Furthermore, since we aimed to investigate the effect of on-call work on the workers, only the employed workers who had been working for at least one year were included. Eventually, a total of 29,246 subjects were included in this study. Although the age limit for the Working Conditions Survey was fifteen years, since the subjects included in this study had been working for at least one year, the subjects in this study were at least sixteen years of age.

On-Call Work

The subject was defined as working on-call if they responded "Yes" to the question "Do you work on-call (immediately providing work or service if contacted or called)?"

Health Problems and Injuries

For health problems and injuries, the subject was defined as having health problems and injuries if they answered "Yes" to the question "Over the last 12 months, did you suffer from any of the following health problems?" The questionnaire contained subcategories for questions regarding health problems and injuries including hearing problems, skin problems, back pain, muscular pains in upper limbs, muscular pains in lower limbs, headaches or eyestrain, abdominal pain, respiratory difficulties, cardiovascular diseases, injuries, depression or anxiety, fatigue, insomnia, and general sleep difficulties. Any report of hearing problems, skin problems, backache, muscular pains in upper limbs, muscular pains in lower limbs, headaches or eyestrain, abdominal pain, respiratory difficulties, cardiovascular diseases, and fatigue was defined as a physical health problem. Similarly, if the subject had depression or anxiety, insomnia, and general sleep difficulties, the subject was defined as having a psychological health problem.

General and Occupational Characteristics

The general characteristics of the subjects investigated in this study included gender, age, education level, income level, alcohol consumption, smoking, obesity, and hypertension. For obesity and hypertension, the subject was defined as having a chronic condition if they answered "Yes" to the question "Were you ever diagnosed with chronic obesity or hypertension by your physician?" However, for obesity, if the subject answered "Not obese" to the additional question "What is your current status in terms of obesity?" the subject was not considered obese.

The occupational characteristics included job type, employment type, working hours, and shift work. Two methods were used to categorize the job types. First, the subjects were asked, "What is the job type that best describes your current occupation?" Based on their responses, professional workers and senior managers were defined as "Professional," general office workers as "Office," sales workers and service providers as "Service," and skilled/ semi-skilled/unskilled occupations and agricultural/ forestry/fishery workers as "Physical." Second, based on the middle categorization of the Korean Employment Classification of Occupation (KECO), the subjects' occupations were categorized into twenty-four job groups. Employment type was defined as regular or temporary, and working hours were categorized as $\leq$ 40 h, 41 – 60 h, or > 60 h per week.

Work Environment and Work-Related Stress

Work environment was assessed in terms of exposures to physical, chemical, and ergonomic factors. If the subject answered "All of the time," "Almost all of the time," "Around 3/4 of the time," "Around half of the time" or "Around 1/4 of the time" to the question "Are you exposed at work to . . . ?" the subject was considered to be exposed to the factor. However, if the subject answered "Almost never" or "Never" to the same question, the subject was not considered to be exposed to the factor. The physical factors included the vibrations, noise, high temperatures, and low temperatures. The chemical factors included breathing in smoke, fumes, powder or dust, vapors such as solvents and thinners, handling or being in skin contact with chemical products or substances, and tobacco smoke from other people. Lastly, the ergonomic factors included tiring or painful positions, lifting or moving people, carrying or moving heavy loads, standing, and repetitive hand or arm movements.

For work-related stress, if the subject answered "Always," "Most of the time," or "Sometimes" to the question "For each of the following statements, please select the response which best describes your work situation—You experience stress in your work," the subject was defined as having work-related stress. If the answer was "Rarely" or "Never," the subject was defined as being free of work-related stress.

Data Analysis

This study utilized IBM SPSS Statistics for Windows version 19.0 (IBM Corp: Armonk, NY, USA) for analysis of the data after applying weighting adjustments. Personal and occupational characteristics, work environment, and work-related stress were analyzed using frequency analysis. Chi-square analysis was used to determine the associations between on-call work and characteristics of the subject and on-call work and health problems and injuries. In order to determine the risk of health problems and injuries due to on-call work, bivariate logistic regression analysis was performed to calculate the odds ratios. Model I was the analysis after adjusting for personal characteristics, while Model II was additionally adjusted for occupational characteristics including job type, employment type, working hours, and shift work. Model III further adjusted for physical, chemical, and ergonomic factors of the work environment, while Model IV had additional adjustment for work-related stress in addition to all controls from Model III.

RESULTS

General and Occupational Characteristics of the Study Participants

A total of 29,246 subjects were included in this study. Frequency analysis and descriptive statistics were used to analyze the personal and occupational characteristics, work environment, and work-related stress. The personal characteristics of the subjects included the following: 60.9 percent of the subjects were male; 59.1 percent were between thirty and forty-nine years of age; 55.7 percent had education levels higher than college graduation; 53.5 percent were nonsmokers; 51.5 percent drank alcohol once a week or less; 98.2 percent were not obese; and 95.3 percent were not diagnosed with hypertension. A majority of the subjects were "physical" workers (33.6 percent), and only 8.7 percent were "professional" workers. Moreover, a majority of the subjects were regular employees, and 51.5 percent worked between forty-one and sixty hours per week, while 39.6 percent worked forty hours or less per week. Most of the subjects were not working on a rotating basis (i.e., no shift work). More than half of the subjects responded that they did not have exposure to physical, chemical, or ergonomic factors in their work environment, but 72.1 percent reported that they suffered from work-related stress.

Difference of General Occupational Characteristics According to On-Call Work

A total of 2,722 subjects (9.3 percent) were on-call workers; the remaining 26,524 (90.7 percent) were not on-call workers. Chi-square analysis was used to analyze the differences in each factor according to the on-call work status. The results revealed significant differences between on-call workers and non- on-call workers in all factors except for hypertension and working hours. Assessment of the general characteristics revealed a higher rate of on-call workers in the following groups: male, ≥50 years, high school graduates, monthly income ≥2 million won, smokers, and obese subjects. Among job types, there were more on-call workers in the "physical" group, while the "professional" group had fewer on-call workers. The rate of on-call workers was also higher for temporary and shift workers. Assessment of work environment revealed a higher rate of on-call workers exposed to physical, chemical, or ergonomic factors, as well as work-related stress (table 7.1).

The subjects were divided into twenty-four job classifications based on KECO categorizations and were analyzed for on-call work. The highest rate of on-call workers (31.7 percent) were those in the law, police, firefighting, and prison-related job group. The job classifications that had higher rates of on-call workers than health care and medical-related jobs (12.8 percent) include soldiers (30.2 percent), driver and transportation-related jobs (14.6 percent), information and communications-related jobs (13.4 percent), and construction-related jobs (12.9 percent). Moreover, although the proportions of on-call workers were low for management, accounting, and office-related (8.7 percent) and sales (8.1 percent) jobs, the absolute number of on-call workers in these job classifications were quite high, at 21.2 percent (578 subjects) and 7.8 percent (214 subjects) of the entire on-call workers, respectively (table 7.2).

On-call Work and Its Association with Health Problems and Injuries

Chi-square analysis was performed to determine the relationship between on-call work and health problems and injuries. The results indicated that all health problems except for cardiovascular disease had statistically significant higher prevalence among on-call workers (table 7.3).

Bivariate logistic regression analysis was performed to determine the effect of on-call work on the risk of health problems and injuries. The risks were higher for on-call workers than those for non-on-call workers for the majority of health problems and injuries. This outcome did not change even after adjusting for personal and occupational characteristics, work environment, and work-related stress. The odds ratios for on-call workers in terms of physical health problems, psychological health problems, and injuries were 1.33 (95% confidence interval [CI] 1.22–1.44), 1.31 (95% CI 1.08–1.60), and 2.76 (95% CI 2.26–3.37), respectively. Analysis of the detailed symptoms revealed odds ratios in on-call workers of 2.06 for hearing problems (95% CI 1.63–2.62); 1.71 for skin problems (95% CI 1.38–2.12); 1.22 for back pain (95% CI 1.08–1.38); 1.23 for muscular pains in upper limbs (95% CI 1.12–1.34); 1.27 for muscular pains in lower limbs (95% CI 1.15–1.40); 1.46 for headache, eye fatigue (95% CI 1.32–1.60); 1.37 for abdominal pain (95% CI 1.02–1.85); 1.43 for depression or anxiety disorders (95% CI 1.07–1.93);

Table 7.1 Comparisons of the Characteristics of the Study Subjects According to the On-call Work

		On-call Work n(%)		
		Yes	*No*	
Characteristics		*2,722(9.3)*	*26,524(90.7)*	P-*value*
Sex	Male	1,813(10.2)	15,999(89.8)	< 0.001
	Female	909(7.9)	10,525(92.1)	
Age(years)	15–29	417(8.2)	4,684(91.8)	0.004
	30–49	1,621(9.4)	15,651(90.6)	
	≥ 50	684(10.0)	6,189(90.0)	
Education	Below middle school	261(9.5)	2,489(90.5)	0.008
	High school	1,018(10.0)	9,174(90.0)	
	College and beyond	1,443(8.9)	14,861(91.1)	
Income (10,000won/month)	< 100	156(6.7)	2,183(93.3)	< 0.001
	100–199	948(8.7)	9,962(91.3)	
	200–299	945(10.4)	8,161(89.6)	
	≥ 300	673(9.8)	6,208(90.2)	
Smoking	Never	1,376(8.8)	14,263(91.2)	< 0.001
	Quit	273(8.5)	2,957(91.5)	
	Current	1,073(10.3)	9,304(89.7)	
Drinking	No	608(9.8)	5,576(90.2)	0.004
	≤ 1/week	1,318(8.8)	13,732(91.2)	
	≥ 2/week	796(9.9)	7,216(90.1)	
Obesity	No	2,658(9.3)	26,063(90.7)	0.022
	Yes	64(12.2)	461(87.8)	
Hypertension	No	2,597(9.3)	25,278(90.7)	0.794
	Yes	125(9.1)	1,246(90.9)	
Employment type	Regular	2,266(9.1)	22,651(90.9)	0.003
	Temporary	456(10.5)	3,873(89.5)	
Working time (Hours/week)	≤ 40	1,034(8.9)	10,553(91.1)	0.159
	41–60	1,432(9.5)	13,631(90.5)	
	> 60	256(9.9)	2,340(90.1)	
Job type	Professional	185(7.3)	2,356(92.7)	< 0.001
	Office	860(9.1)	8,607(90.9)	
	Service	677(9.1)	6,749(90.9)	
	Physical	1,000(10.2)	8,812(89.8)	
Shift work	No	2,200(8.3)	24,247(91.7)	< 0.001
	Yes	522(18.6)	2,277(81.4)	
Physical exposure	No	1,580(8.5)	16,953(91.5)	< 0.001
	Yes	1,142(10.7)	9,571(89.3)	
Chemical exposure	No	1,719(8.1)	19,563(91.9)	< 0.001
	Yes	1,003(12.6)	6,961(87.4)	
Ergonomic exposure	No	2,199(9.0)	22,285(91.0)	< 0.001
	Yes	523(11.0)	4,239(89.0)	
Work-related stress	No	673(8.3)	7,481(91.7)	< 0.001
	Yes	2,049(9.7)	19,043(90.3)	

Table 7.2 Comparisons of the On-call Work of the Study Subjects According to the Job Classification

	On-call Work n (%)	
Job Classification (KECO[a])	*Yes 2,722(9.3)*	*No 26,524(90.7)*
Law, police, firefighting, prison	117(31.7)	252(68.3)
soldier	26(30.2)	60(69.8)
Drivers and transportation	243(14.6)	1,412(85.4)
Information and communications	74(13.4)	478(86.6)
Construction	241(12.9)	1,625(87.1)
Public healthcare, medical	206(12.8)	1,406(87.2)
Management	68(11.2)	538(88.8)
Agriculture, forestry, and fishing	17(10.5)	145(89.5)
Security and janitorial staff and cleaning	166(9.6)	1,563(90.4)
Electricity and electronics	96(9.4)	927(90.6)
Culture, art, design, broadcasting	53(9.3)	517(90.7)
Management, accounting, office job	579(8.6)	6,181(91.4)
Machine	129(8.4)	1,404(91.6)
Sales	214(8.1)	2,444(91.9)
Finance and insurance	80(7.6)	967(92.4)
Environment, printing, woodworking, Furniture, crafts, simple manufacturing	79(7.6)	959(92.4)
Food processing	15(7.1)	197(92.9)
Social welfare and religion	41(6.8)	562(93.2)
Food service	90(6.6)	1,265(93.4)
Chemistry	16(6.6)	228(93.4)
Beauty, accommodations, tourism, entertainment, and sports	50(6.3)	741(93.7)
Fabrics and clothing	23(5.6)	390(94.4)
Materials (metal, glass, clay, cement)	26(5.4)	455(94.6)
Research (Education, natural/social sciences)	73(3.9)	1,808(96.1)

[a] *KECO* Korean Employment Classification of Occupation.

1.36 for fatigue (95% CI 1.24–1.49); and1.41 for insomnia and general sleep difficulties (95% CI 1.13–1.76). However, there were no statistically significant differences between groups for the risks of respiratory difficulties or cardiovascular diseases (table 7.4).

DISCUSSION

This study utilized data from the third Korean Working Conditions Survey on employed workers and analyzed the relationships between their characteristics and health problems and injuries as well as the impact of on-call work on health problems and injuries.

Table 7.3 Comparisons of the Health Problems and Injuries of the Study Subjects According to the On-call Work

Health problems and injuries		*On-call Work n (%)* Yes 2,722(9.3)	*On-call Work n (%)* No 26,524(90.7)	P-value
Physical health problems	Yes	1,540(10.6)	13,051(89.4)	< 0.001
	No	1,182(8.1)	13,473(91.9)	
Hearing problems	Yes	92(18.8)	397(81.2)	< 0.001
	No	2,630(9.1)	26,127(90.9)	
Skin problems	Yes	108(15.3)	598(84.7)	< 0.001
	No	2,614(9.2)	25,926(90.8)	
Back pain	Yes	368(11.9)	2,723(88.1)	< 0.001
	No	2,354(9.0)	23,801(91.0)	
Muscular pains in upper limbs	Yes	927(10.5)	7,905(89.5)	< 0.001
	No	1,795(8.8)	18,619(91.2)	
Muscular pains in lower limbs	Yes	609(10.8)	5,008(89.2)	< 0.001
	No	2,113(8.9)	21,516(91.1)	
Headache, eyestrain	Yes	661(12.4)	4,672(87.6)	< 0.001
	No	2,061(8.6)	21,852(91.4)	
Abdominal pain	Yes	53(12.8)	361(87.2)	0.014
	No	2,669(9.3)	26,163(90.7)	
Respiratory difficulties	Yes	27(14.1)	164(85.9)	0.021
	No	2,695(9.3)	26,360(90.7)	
Cardiovascular diseases	Yes	28(8.5)	300(91.5)	0.629
	No	2,694(9.3)	26,224(90.7)	
Fatigue	Yes	765(11.9)	5,680(88.1)	< 0.001
	No	1,957(8.6)	20,844(91.4)	
Psychological health problems	Yes	128(13.1)	847(86.9)	< 0.001
	No	2,594(9.2)	25,677(90.8)	
Depression or anxiety	Yes	54(13.0)	360(87.0)	0.008
	No	2,668(9.3)	26,164(90.7)	
Insomnia and sleep difficulties	Yes	102(14.4)	608(85.6)	< 0.001
	No	2,620(9.2)	25,916(90.8)	
Injuries	Yes	144(24.2)	457(75.8)	< 0.001
	No	2,578(9.0)	26,067(91.0)	

Analysis of the subjects' characteristics according to the on-call work showed differences in both personal characteristics—gender, age, education, income, smoking, alcohol consumption, and obesity—and occupational characteristics—job type, employment type, and shift work. Especially for the employment type, temporary workers were more often on-call workers. Unstable employment status in these temporary workers likely forces them to cope with stressful work environments. Moreover, previous studies reported that on-call workers have extended working hours (both daytime and nighttime) [1] and are exposed to both shift and nighttime work [14], which may explain why on-call workers feel more fatigued in general. In fact, the analysis findings of the current study revealed a higher rate of on-call workers for shift work. However, there was no statistically significant difference in the rate of on-call workers based on working hours. On-call workers had increased exposure to all analyzed physical, chemical, and ergonomic factors, suggesting that these workers tend to work in worse work environments. The rate of on-call workers was also higher in the group that experienced work-related stress, further supporting the previous finding that on-call work is a key factor of work-related stress [2–4]. The rates of on-call workers were higher in law, police, firefighting, and prison-related jobs; soldiers; driving and transportation-related jobs; information and communications-related jobs; and construction-related jobs, compared to the rate in health care and medical-related jobs, which was traditionally thought as a job category with a high rate of on-call workers. This result indicates that in addition to traditional studies of on-call workers that focus on health care and medical-related jobs, additional studies are necessary in order to analyze other job groups.

Analysis of the effects of on-call work on health problems and injuries showed higher odds ratios for the majority of health-related issues and injuries in on-call workers compared to those of non-on-call workers, with exceptions of respiratory difficulties, cardiovascular diseases. These results did not change even after adjusting for personal and occupational characteristics, work environment, and work-related stress.

To our knowledge, no previous study has investigated the relationship between on-call work and hearing problems, skin problems, or abdominal pain. A potential explanation that could explain the relevance of on-call work with these problems is circadian disruption. In a study on sudden sensorineural hearing loss patients, 61.8 percent of the subjects reported insomnia before suffering from hearing loss, and the circadian clock gene was reduced compared to the control group [18]. It is thought that circadian disruption can be caused by irregular sleeping patterns that may occur during on-call work, which may cause hearing problems. Previous study has shown that exposure to light at night causes circadian disruption and decreased melatonin synthesis [19]. Melatonin may protect against psoriasis because it regulates the inflammatory response and antioxidant activity [20]. Previous study on shift workers has also shown that circadian disruption and decreased melatonin are associated with psoriasis [21]. In addition, in a mouse-based experiment, it was possible to regulate the circadian clock to control psoriasis-like skin inflammation by controlling the IL-23 expression in T cells [22], suggesting that circadian disruption may be related to inflammatory skin problems. Our

Table 7.4 Odds Ratios of Health Problems and Injuries on On-call Work from Logistic Regression Models

	Model I *OR[a] (95%CI[b])*	*Model II* *OR(95%CI)*	*Model III* *OR(95%CI)*	*Model IV* *OR(95%CI)*
Physical health problems	1.35(1.25–1.47)	1.35(1.25–1.47)	1.34(1.23–1.45)	1.33(1.22–1.44)
Hearing problems	2.18(1.73–2.75)	2.20(1.74–2.78)	2.07(1.63–2.63)	2.06(1.63–2.62)
Skin problems	1.80(1.46–2.23)	1.83(1.48–2.26)	1.72(1.39–2.13)	1.71(1.38–2.12)
Back pain	1.25(1.11–1.41)	1.22(1.09–1.38)	1.22(1.08–1.38)	1.22(1.08–1.38)
Muscular pains in upper limbs	1.22(1.12–1.33)	1.23(1.13–1.34)	1.23(1.13–1.34)	1.23(1.12–1.34)
Muscular pains in lower limbs	1.26(1.14–1.39)	1.27(1.15–1.40)	1.27(1.15–1.41)	1.27(1.15–1.40)
Headache, eyestrain	1.50(1.36–1.64)	1.50(1.36–1.65)	1.47(1.33–1.61)	1.46(1.32–1.31)
Abdominal pain	1.44(1.07–1.93)	1.47(1.09–1.98)	1.37(1.02–1.85)	1.37(1.02–1.85)
Respiratory difficulties	1.59(1.05–2.39)	1.51(1.00–2.29)	1.38(0.91–2.10)	1.39(0.91–2.11)
Cardiovascular diseases	0.93(0.63–1.39)	0.91(0.61–1.36)	0.89(0.60–1.34)	0.90(0.60–1.34)
Fatigue	1.42(1.30–1.55)	1.39(1.27–1.52)	1.37(1.25–1.50)	1.36(1.24–1.49)
Psychological health problems	1.52(1.26–1.85)	1.38(1.13–1.67)	1.32(1.08–1.61)	1.31(1.08–1.60)
Depression or anxiety	1.50(1.12–2.00)	1.49(1.11–2.00)	1.44(1.07–1.93)	1.43(1.07–1.93)
Insomnia and sleep difficulties	1.68(1.35–2.08)	1.46(1.17–1.82)	1.41(1.13–1.77)	1.41(1.13–1.76)
Injuries	3.00(2.47–3.65)	3.07(2.52–3.74)	2.76(2.26–3.37)	2.76(2.26–3.37)

Model I: Adjusted for personal characteristics (gender, age group, education, income, smoking, drinking, obesity, hypertension) Model II: Model I + Adjusted for occupational characteristics (job type, employment type, working hours, shift work).
Model III: Model II + Adjusted for working environment (physical, chemical, ergonomic exposure).
Model IV: Model III + Adjusted for work-related stress.
[a]OR Odds ratio
[b]CI Confidence interval

study shows that the risk of skin problems is higher for on-call workers even after adjusting for the shift work. This may be due to on-call workers also having disrupted circadian rhythm, which may be caused by their irregular working hours, and light exposure at night. Previous studies have demonstrated the relationship between on-call work and indigestion [4] and possible induction of gastrointestinal tract diseases due to an imbalanced lifestyle from irregular eating habits and lack of sleep [23]. Thus, on-call workers who have irregular eating habits—since they are expected to work when needed—were expected to have various gastrointestinal tract-related issues and diseases. However, similar to hearing problems, additional studies are necessary in order to identify the potential mediating factors of skin problems and abdominal pain. However, this is only one potential explanation that could explain the relevance of on-call work with hearing problems, skin problems, and abdominal pain, so further studies are required.

A previous study reported that on-call work is associated with musculoskeletal pain (i.e., back and shoulder pain) [5], a result in agreement with our findings that on-call work is associated with back and upper/lower limb muscle pain. Furthermore, one possible explanation for these musculoskeletal symptoms was a lack of a rest and recovery period [24]. On-call workers have a shorter time for rest and recovery due to irregular working hours, which could lead to musculoskeletal symptoms in these workers.

A previous study of Finnish anesthesiologists reported that on-call work is associated with exhaustion, frustration, sleep disorders, memory disorders, and headache. Greater work-related burdens from on-call work resulted in an increased severity of these symptoms, and these symptoms disappeared during vacation [4]. These results indicate a strong relationship between on-call work and symptoms such as headache or fatigue. From our study of Korean workers, on-call work was associated with headache, eye fatigue, and general fatigue.

A previous study discussed depressed mood in on-call workers [6], and another suggested the possible relationship between on-call work and negative emotions [25]. Furthermore, on-call work was associated with daytime sleepiness, insomnia, and sleep deprivation [7, 8], and possibly dysthymic disorder from continued sleep deprivation [26]. These results suggest that on-call work may be a cause of sleep deprivation and sleep disorders as well as for negative emotions in on-call workers who are constantly sleep-deprived due to the nature of their work. Moreover, previous studies showed the association between on-call work and work dissatisfaction [2, 13] and the result of a study on the relationship between work dissatisfaction and general mental health (i.e., depression and anxiety) [27] indicated that work dissatisfaction from on-call work might cause depression or anxiety. These results were further supported by the findings of this study showing that on-call work increases the risks of depression or anxiety disorder, insomnia, or sleep disorders.

A previous study suggested the association between on-call work and work-related injuries [11]; the present study also found this association in Korean workers. On-call work is associated with reduced cognitive function and concentration [9, 10], and studies have shown that sleep deprivation can cause reduced cognitive function [28, 29]. Therefore, reduced cognitive function and concentration from on-call work can increase the risk of injuries.

This study has many strengths. To our knowledge, it is the first Korean study to determine the association between on-call work and health problems and injuries. Furthermore, unlike traditional studies that focused on a specific job group, this study included a wide range of job groups in order to investigate the relationship between on-call work and health problems, injuries. In the present study, higher rates of on-call workers were found in other job groups compared to that of the healthcare-related job group, which was the target job group in previous studies. This finding suggests the need for future studies focusing on other job groups. Second, this study utilized data from the Korean Working Conditions Survey, and the 29,246 subjects included in this study were representative of Korean employed workers nationwide. In addition, the utilization of trained investigators to perform the survey minimized arbitrary interpretation of the survey responses.

This study had several limitations. First, the cross-sectional study design based on data from the Korean Working Conditions Survey made it difficult to identify the clear causal relationship between on-call work and health problems and injuries. Future studies are needed to identify the clear causal relationships. Second, the only measurement tools for variables were the responses to the Korean Working Conditions Survey. More specifically, for the work environment, exposures were determined by dichotomous measures of the survey responses rather than actual assessments of work the environments. Furthermore, instead of objective measurements such as physician interviews, blood test, or medical imaging, self-reporting was used to assess health problems. And there may be a misclassification of the job types because there were only four job types, so jobs of different character may belong to same category. Lastly, the assessed medical history of the subjects included only the presence of obesity and hypertension.

CONCLUSION

This is one of the first studies identified a significant relationship between on-call work in Korean workers and health problems and injuries. Moreover, this study included a wide range of job groups in order to investigate the relationship between on-call work and health problems, injuries. Future studies are required to identify clear causal relationships; similarly, additional discussions are needed in order to reduce the adverse effects of on-call work.

NOTE

1. This chapter was previously published as Baek, Chulin, Jae Bum Park, Kyungjong Lee, and Jaehyuk Jung. "The association between Korean employed workers' on-call work and health problems, injuries." *Annals of Occupational and Environmental Medicine* 30, no. 1 (2018): 19.

REFERENCES

1. Akerstedt T. "Altered sleep/wake patterns and mental performance." *Physiol Behav*. 2008;90:209–18.
2. Dowell A, Hamilton S. "Job satisfaction, psychological morbidity, and job stress among New Zealand general practitioners." *N Z Med J*. 2000;113:269–72.
3. Chong A, Killeen O, Clarke T. "Work-related stress among paediatric non-consultant hospital doctors." *Ir Med J*. 2004;97:203–5.
4. Lindfors PM, Nurmi KE, Meretoja OA, et al. "On call stress among Finnish anaesthetists." *Anaesthesia*. 2006;61:856–66.
5. Alison MT, Rong L, Jeanne GB, Jane L, Gary L. "Longitudinal relationship of work hours, mandatory overtime, and on-call to musculoskeletal problems in nurses." *Am J Ind Med*. 2006;49:964–71.
6. Rankin HJ, Serieys NM, Elliott-Binns CP. "Determinants of mood in general practitioners." *Br Med J (Clin Res Ed)*. 1987;294:618–20.
7. Kaneita Y, Ohida T. "Association of current work and sleep situations with excessive daytime sleepiness and medical incidents among Japanese physicians." *J Clin Sleep Med*. 2011;7(5):512–22.
8. Wali SO, Qutah K, Abushanab L, Basamh R, Abushanab J, Krayem A. "Effect of on-call-related sleep deprivation on physicians' mood and alertness." *Ann Thorac Med*. 2013;8:22–7.
9. Rubin R, Orris P, Lau SL, Hryhorczuk DO, Furner S, Letz R. "Neurobehavioral effects of the on-call experience in housestaff physicians." *J Occup Med*. 1991;33:13–8.
10. Florian E, Markus R, Heinz Z, et al. "Effects of 24h working on-call on psychoneuroendocrine and oculomotor function: a randomized cross-over trial." *Psychoneuroendocrinology*. 2014;47:221–31.
11. Lockley SW, Barger LK, Ayas NT, et al. "Effects of health care provider work hours and sleep deprivation on safety and performance." *Jt Comm J Qual Patient Saf*. 2007;33:7–18.
12. Kang YS, Kam S, Lee SW, Chun BY, Yeh MH. "Job stress and its related factors in south Korean doctors." *J Prev Med Public Health*. 2001;34(2):141–8.

13. Van HI, Verhoeven AA, Groenier KH, Groothoff JW, De HJ. "Job satisfaction among general practitioners: a systematic literature review." *Eur J Gen Pract.* 2006;12:174–80.
14. Heponiemi T, Kouvonen A, Vanska J, et al. "Effects of active on-call hours on physicians' turnover intentions and well-being." *Scand J Work Environ Health.* 2008;34:356–63.
15. Waldman JD, Kelly F, Aurora S, Smith HL. "The shocking cost of turnover in health care." *Health Care Manag Rev.* 2004;29:2–7.
16. Yildirim D, Aycan Z. "Nurses' work demands and work-family conflict: a questionnaire survey." *Int J Nurs Stud.* 2008;45:1366–78.
17. Emmett BM, Dovey SM, Wheeler BJ. "After-hours on-call: the effect on paediatricians' spouses and families." *J Paediatr Child Health.* 2013;49:246–50.
18. Yang CH, Hwang CF, Lin PM, Chuang JH, Hsu CM, Lin SF, Yang MY. "Sleep disturbance and altered expression of circadian clock genes in patients with sudden sensorineural hearing loss." *Medicine.* 2015;94(26):e978.
19. Scheer FA, Hilton MF, Mantzoros CS, Shea SA. "Adverse metabolic and cardiovascular consequences of circadian misalignment." *Proc Natl Acad Sci U S A.* 2009;106(11):4453–8.
20. Bonnefont-Rousselot D, Collin F. "Melatonin: action as antioxidant and potential applications in human disease and aging." *Toxicology.* 2010;278(1):55–67.
21. Li WQ, Qureshi AA, Schernhammer ES, Han J. "Rotating night-shift work and risk of psoriasis in US women." *J Invest Dermatol.* 2013;133(2):565–7.
22. Ando N, Nakamura Y, Aoki R, Ishimaru K, Ogawa H, Okumura K, Shibata S, Shimada S, Nakao A. "Circadian gene clock regulates psoriasis-like skin inflammation in mice." *J Invest Dermatol.* 2015;135:3001–8.
23. Konturek PC, Brzozowski T, Konturek SJ. "Gut clock: implication of circadian rhythms in the gastointestinal tract." *J Physiol Pharmacol.* 2011;62(2):139–50.
24. Nicole J, IJmert K, Ludovic VA, Frans N, Piet VDB. "Need for recovery from work: evaluating short-term effects of working." *Ergonomics.* 2003;46(7):664–80.
25. Rose M, Manser T, Ware JC. "Effects of call on sleep and mood in internal medicine residents." *Behav Sleep Med.* 2008;6:75–88.
26. Birchler-Pedross A, Schroder CM, Munch M, et al. "Subjective well-being is modulated by circadian phase, sleep pressure, age, and gender." *J Biol Rhythm.* 2009;24:232–42.
27. Faragher EB, Cass M, Cooper CL. "The relationship between job satisfaction and health: a meta-analysis." *Occup Environ Med.* 2005;62:105–12.
28. Wertz AT, Ronda JM, Czeisler CA, WrightJr KP. "Effects of sleep inertia on cognition." *J Am Med Assoc.* 2006;295:163–4.
29. Goel N, Rao H, Durmer JS, Dinges DF. "Neurocognitive consequences of sleep deprivation." *Semin Neurol.* 2009;29:320–39.

Chapter 8

Factors Associated with Health-Related Quality of Life in Korean Older Workers

Sujin Hong, Harin Jeong, Yunjeong Heo, Hosun Chun, Jongtae Park, and Daeseong Kim

BACKGROUND

An[1] aging society is defined as a prevalence of >7 percent of those ≥65 years of age [1]. The prevalence of this age group in an aged society and super-aged society is >14 and >20 percent, respectively [1]. By these definitions, Korea is an aging society, with 7.25 percent of the total population ≥65 years of age in 2000 [2]. By 2017–2018, Korea will become a postaged society, with the prevalence of aged Koreans rising to 14 percent (Statistics Korea, 2011 [3]).

Of note, the economically active segment of Korean society <65 years of age is shrinking. As Korean society continues to disproportionately age, workers in the thirties who represent the most economically active segment of society will further diminish. By 2025, the most economically active segment of Korean society will be those fifty to sixty years of age [3].

The overall decrease in manpower and the decline in productivity due to societal aging portend serious social problems in Korea that include elderly poverty, which can diminish welfare and quality of life of the elderly. To prevent a rapid decrease in the workforce, countermeasures to raise the rate of participation in overall economic activities and rate of employment should be formulated. As well, measures need to be taken to maintain an elderly workforce and to vitalize employment.

Studies of older workers have focused mainly on industrial accidents and injuries [4–7]. But the prevalence of chronic diseases also increases, which is another factor in the exit from the workforce. To maintain the working ability of workers, their health should be managed. To achieve this, older workers' health status first needs to be determined.

Also, as the period of old age grows longer, the quality of life of the aged must be enhanced beyond the simple goal of survival. In particular, the health-related quality of life (HRQL) of the aged must be improved.

Measuring the HRQL of a population group is important because such data can be used as evidence in making decisions on health and medical treatment policies and can be indicators of the outcomes of related projects. Many studies have been conducted in the past ten years in Korea on the relationships between HRQL and a number of factors including disease [8–12], sex [13], age [11, 13–16], income bracket [16, 17], daily life skills [15], subjective health awareness, and health behavior [18]. However, few studies have involved older workers from the viewpoint of occupation.

Using the fifth (2010–2012) Korea National Health and Nutrition Examination Survey (KNHANES), we report the current health status and working conditions of older workers of Korea and confirm the effects of the aforementioned factors on the HRQL of older workers.

MATERIALS AND METHODS

Subjects

Of the 25,534 participants, 6,383 wage workers were selected. From these wage workers, older workers ≥55 years of age (n = 1,413) were selected based on the criterion presented in the Employment Promotion for the Aged Act and the Employment Protection Act. Forty-five individuals were excluded for missing sociodemographic factor values (n = 15), missing health-related factors (n = 14), missing working condition-related values (n = 12), and missing health status and HRQL values (n = 4). The remaining 1,368 persons were analyzed.

Methods

General Characteristics

Sociodemographic factors included sex, age, education, household income, and marital status (having a spouse). Age groups were divided into 55–64 years, 65–74 years, and ≥75 years. Level of education was classified into elementary school graduate and below, middle school graduate, high school graduate, and college graduate and above. Income level according to household income quartile was classified into low, below middle, above middle, and high. Drinking (none, 1–4 times a month, >2 times a week), smoking (current smoker, ex-smoker, nonsmoker), and obesity (body mass index 18.5, 18.5–22.9, 23.0–24.9, 25.0–29.9, ≥30.0 kg/m2) were classified, respectively.

Health Status

Chronic diseases were examined because of their appreciable effects on older workers' health status. Questions concerned cardiovascular diseases, musculoskeletal diseases, and mental health. Cardiovascular diseases included the presence of hypertension, hyperlipidemia, stroke, myocardial infarction, angina, and diabetes. The prevalence of diseases like diabetes was determined based on the reported diagnosis. Musculoskeletal diseases or symptoms included the presence of osteoarthritis and knee, hip and back pain, with subjects queried whether they had experienced knee, hip and back pain for thirty days or more in the prior three months. Assessment of mental health status included the presence of depression and stress recognition rate. The stress recognition rate was classified based on responses to the occurrence of daily stress (high = very much or much, low = little or rarely).

Working Conditions

Types of occupation, types of employment by employment status and working time, weekly average working hours, and shift work were examined. The types of occupation were classified into office work (administrators, specialists and related workers, and office workers), service work (service and sales employees), manufacturing work (skilled agriculture workers, forestry and fishery workers, functional employees and related functional employees, and equipment, machine operation, and assembly workers), and elementary occupations. The subjects were classified according to their employment status into regular employees, temporary employees, and daily employees, and whether they worked part-time or full-time. The weekly average working hours was classified as <40, 40–52, 52–60, and <60. Shift work, except for day duty workers, comprised all workers who worked in the afternoon (2:00 p.m. to midnight), at night (9:00 p.m. to 8:00 a.m.), in regular rotation of shifts between the day and the nightshifts, in twenty-four-hour shifts, in segmented shifts (working more than two shifts a day), and in irregular shifts.

Health-Related Quality of Life (HRQL)

The World Health Organization (WHO) defines quality of life as the degree of realization of a person's interests, expectations, ideals, and hopes according to his or her current value and cultural system, in his or her life [19, 20]. Quality of life is so comprehensive and extensive that it is sometimes classified into nonhealth-related quality of life (NHRQL) and HRQL. HRQL represents general well-being as well as elements that have direct effects on the individual's physical, psychological, and mental health [21]. There are many instruments for evaluating HRQL. They include the Quality of Well-Being (QWB) scale [22], HUI-II [23] and -III [24], EQ-5D [25], and SF-6D [26]. EQ-5D, developed by the EuroQoL Group to measure general health status, has advantages that include simple questions, applicability to diverse clinical situations, and easy and quick preparation [25]. The fifth KNHANES also used EQ-5D to measure HRQL. The analysis in this study was conducted based on the results of the survey. In the survey, the subjects were asked to choose one of the following three responses, for each of the five given dimensions, that best explained their current health status: "1 = no problem," "2 = some problems," and "3 = severe problems." The five questions concerning health status expressed health status between 1, which represents perfect health status, and −1, which represents a health status that is no better than death. In this research, the EQ-5D index, which Nam et al. calculated using their estimated weighted quality value for Koreans [27], was used. The formula for the EQ-5D index is

$$\begin{aligned}\text{EQ-5D index} = 1 - (&0.05 + 0.096 \times \text{M2} + 0.418 \times \text{M3} + 0.046 \times \text{SC2} \\ &+ 0.136 \times \text{SC3} + 0.051 \times \text{UA2} + 0.208 \times \text{UA3} \\ &+ 0.037 \times \text{PD2} \mp 0.151 \times \text{PD3} \\ &+ 0.043 \times \text{AD2} + 0.158 \times \text{AD3} + 0.05 \times \text{N3}).\end{aligned}$$

where M2 – Mobility "level 2" = 1; otherwise, 0; M3 – Mobility "level 3" = 1; otherwise, 0; SC2 – Self-care "level 2" = 1; otherwise, 0; SC3 – Self-care "level 3" = 1; otherwise, 0; UA2 – Usual activities "level 2" = 1; otherwise, 0 ; UA3 – Usual activities "level 3" = 1; otherwise, 0; PD2 – Pain/discomfort "level 2" = 1; otherwise, 0; PD3 – Pain/discomfort "level 3" = 1; otherwise, 0; AD2 – Anxiety/ depression "level 2" = 1; otherwise, 0; AD3 – Anxiety/ depression "level 3" = 1; otherwise, 0; N3 – Only one "level 3" = 1, and the rest = 0.

Data Analysis

The subjects' characteristics were presented using their frequency and percentage. To compare the HRQL values according to the subjects' sociodemographic characteristics, working conditions, and health status, *t*-test and ANOVA were used with a statistical significance level of $\alpha = 0.05$. To adjust for the effect of confounders and to understand reciprocal action, logistic regressions were conducted. Because there is no standard point that can be used as a standard dichotomy in EQ-5D index, and EQ-5D index score is calculated by using their estimated weighted quality value of response to each of the five dimensions, and the weighted quality values are different for each country, we concluded that it is a more fundamental and concrete method to see response to each dimension rather than EQ-5D index score in logistic regression analysis. We used the response of EQ-5D dimensions as dependent variable. For all five dimensions levels 2 and 3 on the EQ-5D dimensions were merged and thus dichotomized to "no problem" (0: level 1) or "some or extreme problem" (1: level 2 and 3). All analyses were performed in SPSS version 18.0 (SPSS, Chicago, IL, USA).

RESULTS

General Characteristics, Health Status, and Working Conditions Distribution

Of the 1,368 older wage workers, 712 (52 percent) were male and 656 (48 percent) were female. Workers fifty to sixty-four years of age comprised the majority of older age workers (64.7 percent males, 60.4 percent female). The percentages decreased with increasing age, with the respective percentage of males and females being 30.9 and 32.2 percent in the sixty-five to seventy-four age group, and 4.4 and 7.5 percent in the ≥74-year-old group. Of all male and female older wage workers, the highest percentage groups in education level were high school graduates (32.4 percent) and elementary school graduates (63.7 percent), respectively. Concerning household income quartile, of the male and female older workers, the highest percentage was in the second quartile (32.3 percent) and first quartile (36.3 percent), respectively (table 8.1).

Concerning smoking behavior, the percentage of ex-smokers among the male older workers was the highest (53.1 percent). Among females, the percentage of nonsmokers was the highest (94.7 percent). The most frequent health problem of male older workers was hypertension (37.4 percent), followed by musculoskeletal pain (19.2 percent), stress (16.2 percent), diabetes (15.2 percent), and hyperlipidemia (14.7 percent). The most frequent health problem of female older workers was musculoskeletal pain (45.3 percent), followed by hypertension (39.7 percent), osteoarthritis (29.0 percent), stress (22.7 percent), and hyperlipidemia (18.8 percent) (table 8.1).

Regarding the distribution of occupations, among the male older workers, the percentage of elementary occupations was the highest at 42.0 percent, followed by office work (28.7 percent), manufacturing work (26.0 percent), and service work (6.4 percent). Among female older workers, the percentage

Table 8.1 General Characteristics and Health Status of Older Wage Workers According to Sex

	Total (%)	*M (%)*	*F (%)*
	1,368 (100.0)	712 (52.0)	656 (48.0)
Age			
55–64	857 (62.6)	461 (64.7)	396 (60.4)
65–74	431 (31.5)	220 (30.9)	211 (32.2)
75–	80 (5.8)	31 (4.4)	49 (7.5)
Education			
<elementary school	609 (44.5)	191 (26.8)	418 (63.7)
Middle school	263 (19.2)	139 (19.5)	124 (18.9)
High school	316 (23.1)	231 (32.4)	85 (13.0)
>College	180 (13.2)	151 (21.2)	29 (4.4)
Household Income (quartile)			
First (lowest)	344 (25.1)	106 (14.9)	238 (36.3)
Second	424 (31.0)	230 (32.3)	194 (29.6)
Third	309 (22.6)	186 (26.1)	123 (18.8)
Fourth (highest)	291 (21.3)	190 (26.7)	101 (15.4)
Existence of spouse			
Yes	1,123 (82.1)	676 (94.9)	447 (68.1)
No	245 (17.9)	36 (5.1)	209 (31.9)
Drinking	448 (32.7)	137 (19.2)	311 (47.4)
None			
1–4/month	599 (43.8)	295 (41.4)	304 (46.3)
2–/week	321 (23.5)	280 (39.3)	41 (6.3)
Smoking			
nonsmoker	749 (54.8)	128 (18.0)	621 (94.7)
ex-smoker	395 (28.9)	378 (53.1)	17 (2.6)
current smoker	224 (16.4)	206 (28.9)	18 (2.7)
BMI			
< 18.5	35 (2.6)	22 (3.1)	13 (2.0)
18.5–22.9	493 (36.0)	269 (37.8)	224 (34.1)
23.0–24.9	391 (28.6)	197 (27.7)	194 (29.6)
25.0–29.9	413 (30.2)	213 (29.9)	200 (30.5)
30.0–	36 (2.6)	11 (1.5)	25 (3.8)
Hypertension			
Yes	523 (38.2)	266 (37.4)	257 (39.2)
No	845 (61.8)	446 (62.6)	399 (60.8)
Hyperlipidemia			
Yes	228 (16.7)	105 (14.7)	123 (18.8)
No	1,140 (83.3)	607 (85.3)	533 (81.3)
Cerebrocardiovascular event (stroke, myocardial infarction, angina)			
Yes	90 (6.6)	49 (6.9)	41 (6.3)
No	1,278 (93.4)	663 (93.1)	615 (93.8)
Diabetes			
Yes	170 (12.4)	108 (15.2)	62 (9.5)
No	1,198 (87.6)	604 (84.8)	594 (90.5)
Osteoarthritis			
Yes	249 (18.2)	59 (8.3)	190 (29.0)
No	1,119 (81.8)	653 (91.7)	466 (71.0)

(Continued)

Table 8.1 General Characteristics and Health Status of Older Wage Workers According to Sex *(Continued)*

	Total (%)	M (%)	F (%)
Musculoskeletal pain (knee, hip, back)			
Yes	434 (31.7)	137 (19.2)	297 (45.3)
No	934 (68.3)	575 (80.8)	359 (54.7)
Depression			
Yes	54 (3.9)	13 (1.8)	41 (6.3)
No	1,314 (96.1)	699 (98.2)	615 (93.8)
Stress			
High	264 (19.3)	115 (16.2)	149 (22.7)
Low	1,104 (80.7)	597 (83.8)	507 (77.3)

of elementary occupations was also the highest at 66.0 percent, followed by service work (20.4 percent), office work (9.5 percent), and manufacturing work (4.1 percent). Concerning the employment status, over half of the male older workers were regular employees, with more females having temporary and daily employment than regular employment. The percentage of part-time workers was higher (36.4 percent) among the female older workers than males (11.9 percent). The average number of weekly working hours of male and female older workers was 45.00 ± 21.18 and 31.63 ± 19.37, respectively. The percentage of male older workers with forty to fifty-two weekly working hours was the highest at 36.2 percent, and the percentage of female older workers with less than forty weekly working hours was the highest at 60.4 percent. The percentage of shiftwork was higher among the male older workers (29.5 percent) than among female older workers (13.1 percent) (table 8.2).

Health-Related Quality of Life (HRQL)

EQ-5D index scores for male and female older workers were 0.956 ± 0.087 and 0.917 ± 0.124, respectively; the difference was significant ($p < 0.001$). As age increased for both genders, the EQ-5D index significantly decreased ($p < 0.001$). There were significant differences in the EQ-5D index according to the level of education. Among the male older workers, increasing level of education was associated with increased EQ-5D index ($p < 0.001$). Among the female older workers, the scores of elementary school graduates were the lowest; scores did not tend to increase according to the education level. For both genders, the EQ-5D index tended to significantly increase according to the income level ($p < 0.001$). Smoking behavior showed statistically significant differences in the EQ-5D index of the male older workers; EQ-5D index of the smokers was significantly lower than that of the nonsmokers and

Table 8.2 Working Conditions of Older Wage Workers According to Sex

	Total (%)	*M (%)*	*F (%)*
Occupation			
Office work	266 (19.4)	204 (28.7)	62 (9.5)
Service work	158 (11.5)	24 (3.4)	134 (20.4)
Manufacturing work	212 (15.5)	185 (26.0)	27 (4.1)
Elementary occupations	732 (53.5)	299 (42.0)	433 (66.0)
Employment status			
Regular employees	756 (55.3)	478 (67.1)	278 (42.4)
Temporary employees	305 (22.3)	121 (17.0)	184 (28.0)
Daily employees	307 (22.4)	113 (15.9)	194 (29.6)
Full-/Part-time			
Full-time worker	1044 (76.3)	627 (88.1)	417 (63.6)
Part-time worker	324 (23.7)	85 (11.9)	239 (36.4)
Working hour/week			
Mean ± S.D	38.60 ± 21.40	45.00 ± 21.18	31.63 ± 19.37
<40	623 (45.5)	227 (31.9)	396 (60.4)
40–52	426 (31.1)	258 (36.2)	168 (25.6)
52–60	87 (6.4)	54 (7.6)	33 (5.0)
≥60	232 (17.0)	173 (24.3)	59 (9.0)
Shift work			
Yes	1072 (78.4)	210 (29.5)	86 (13.1)
No	296 (21.6)	502 (70.5)	570 (86.9)
Total	1368 (100.0)	712 (100.0)	656 (100.0)

SD standard deviation

ex-smokers ($p < 0.001$). The health status items associated with statistically significant differences in the EQ-5D index of both the male and the female older workers were cerebrocardiovascular events, osteoarthritis, musculoskeletal pain, and stress (table 8.3).

The EQ-5D index according to the occupation was highest in the service work (0.984 ± 0.038) among the male older workers and in the office work (0.984 ± 0.038) among the female older workers. Elementary occupations among both the male and female older workers had the lowest scores, which significantly differed from the highest scores. For the employment status, the EQ-5D index was significantly high among both the male and the female regular employees ($p < 0.001$). For the working hours, the EQ-5D index was lowest in the group of males and females who worked for less than forty hours weekly (table 8.4).

The percentage of male older workers who reported problems related to "mobility," "self-care," "usual activities," "pain/discomfort, and "anxiety/depression" was 13.4, 3.5, 4.6, 17.3, and 7.7 percent, respectively. The respective percentages for female older workers were 27.1, 4.4, 11.9, 30.5, and 15.4 percent (table 8.5).

Table 8.3 General Characteristics, Health Status, and Health-Related Quality of Life Instruments (EQ-5D index) of Older Wage Workers According to Sex

	M			F		
	N	Mean ± S.D	P-value	N	Mean ± S.D	P-value
	712	0.956 ± 0.087		656	0.917 ± 0.124	0.000
Age						
55–64	461	0.966 ± 0.082	0.000	396	0.936 ± 0.106	0.000
65–74	220	0.940 ± 0.091		211	0.893 ± 0.139	
75–	31	0.925 ± 0.094		49	0.863 ± 0.152	
Education						
<Elementary school	191	0.939 ± 0.093	0.000	418	0.899 ± 0.137	0.000
Middle school	139	0.944 ± 0.119		124	0.953 ± 0.081	
High school	231	0.963 ± 0.069		85	0.937 ± 0.098	
> College	151	0.978 ± 0.055		29	0.958 ± 0.070	
Household Income (quartile)						
First (lowest)	106	0.919 ± 0.138	0.000	238	0.882 ± 0.147	0.000
Second	230	0.950 ± 0.083		194	0.928 ± 0.109	
Third	186	0.968 ± 0.062		123	0.944 ± 0.101	
Fourth (highest)	190	0.972 ± 0.065		101	0.944 ± 0.095	
Existence of spouse						
Yes	676	0.956 ± 0.087	0.753	447	0.929 ± 0.112	0.001
No	36	0.952 ± 0.084		209	0.890 ± 0.142	
Drinking						
None	137	0.957 ± 0.088	0.866	311	0.906 ± 0.132	0.082
1–4/month	295	0.958 ± 0.093		304	0.928 ± 0.112	
2–/week	280	0.954 ± 0.079		41	0.924 ± 0.134	
Smoking						
Nonsmoker	128	0.969 ± 0.066	0.001	621	0.915 ± 0.125	0.416
Ex-smoker	378	0.961 ± 0.073		17	0.953 ± 0.065	
Current smoker	206	0.938 ± 0.114		18	0.932 ± 0.127	
BMI						
< 18.5	22	0.968 ± 0.072	0.701	13	0.912 ± 0.114	0.612
18.5–22.9	269	0.952 ± 0.084		224	0.922 ± 0.112	
23.0–24.9	197	0.958 ± 0.079		194	0.922 ± 0.129	
25.0–29.9	213	0.960 ± 0.097		200	0.905 ± 0.133	
30.0–	11	0.934 ± 0.107		25	0.924 ± 0.104	
Hypertension						
Yes	266	0.954 ± 0.079	0.684	257	0.903 ± 0.127	0.027
No	446	0.957 ± 0.091		399	0.926 ± 0.120	
Hyperlipidemia						
Yes	105	0.954 ± 0.073	0.819	123	0.901 ± 0.151	0.179
No	607	0.956 ± 0.089		533	0.921 ± 0.116	
Cerebrocardiovascular event (Stroke, Myocardial infarction, Angina)						
Yes	49	0.915 ± 0.110	0.008	41	0.848 ± 0.186	0.017
No	663	0.959 ± 0.084		615	0.921 ± 0.117	

(Continued)

Table 8.3 General Characteristics, Health Status, and Health-Related Quality of Life Instruments (EQ-5D index) of Older Wage Workers According to Sex *(Continued)*

	M			*F*		
	N	*Mean ± S.D*	P-*value*	*N*	*Mean ± S.D*	P-*value*
Diabetes						
Yes	108	0.940 ± 0.089	0.040	62	0.887 ± 0.161	0.122
No	604	0.959 ± 0.086		594	0.920 ± 0.119	
Osteoarthritis						
Yes	59	0.920 ± 0.092	0.001	190	0.860 ± 0.160	0.000
No	653	0.959 ± 0.085		466	0.940 ± 0.096	
Musculoskeletal pain (knee, hip, back)						
Yes	137	0.892 ± 0.132	0.000	297	0.858 ± 0.149	0.000
No	575	0.971 ± 0.063		359	0.966 ± 0.065	
Depression						
Yes	13	0.941 ± 0.099	0.534	41	0.865 ± 0.145	0.005
No	699	0.956 ± 0.086		615	0.920 ± 0.121	
Stress						
High	115	0.942 ± 0.080	0.049	149	0.878 ± 0.153	0.000
Low	597	0.959 ± 0.088		507	0.928 ± 0.111	

SD standard deviation

Regression Analyses

Logistic regression analysis was done on chosen variables (age, education, household income, smoking, hypertension, diabetes, musculoskeletal pain, stress, occupation, working hours, and employment status) which showed meaningful difference by EQ-5D index score. In the case of the male older workers (table 8.6), age-associated problems in all the dimensions (OR 1.03–1.07) and musculoskeletal pain had effects in all the dimensions except in the "anxiety/depression" dimensions (OR 3.45–7.01). And education (OR 0.55, 95 % CI 0.33–0.93), smoking (OR 2.36, 95 % CI 1.45–3.85), diabetes (OR 1.94, 95 % CI 1.05–3.85), and occupation had statistically significant effects in the "mobility" dimension (OR 0.38, 95 % CI 0.22–0.64). The employment status had effects in the "usual activities" dimension (OR 2.78, 95 % CI 1.11–6.96); the type of occupation, in the "pain/discomfort" dimension (OR 0.60, 95 % CI 0.38–0.95); and education and stress, in the "anxiety/depression" dimension. In the case of the female older workers (table 8.7), age and musculoskeletal pain had statistically significant effects in all dimensions (OR 1.02–1.07 and OR 2.62–12.43, respectively). The working hours had statistically significant effects in all dimensions except in the "anxiety/

Table 8.4 Working Conditions and HRQL Instruments (EQ-5D index) of Older Wage Workers

	M			*F*		
	N	*Mean ± S.D°*	P-*value*	*N*	*Mean ± S.D°*	P-*value*
Occupation						
Office work	204	0.975 ± 0.058	0.000	62	0.961 ± 0.065	0.008
Service work	24	0.984 ± 0.038		134	0.927 ± 0.133	
Manufacturing work	185	0.962 ± 0.078		27	0.928 ± 0.096	
Elementary occupations	299	0.938 ± 0.105		433	0.907 ± 0.127	
Employment status						
Regular employee	478	0.966 ± 0.067	0.000	278	0.941 ± 0.088	0.000
Temporary employee	121	0.942 ± 0.097		184	0.900 ± 0.153	
Daily employee	113	0.928 ± 0.131		194	0.898 ± 0.130	
Full-/Part-Time						
Full-time worker	627	0.957 ± 0.079	0.481	417	0.920 ± 0.119	0.009
Part-time worker	85	0.950 ± 0.129		239	0.911 ± 0.131	
Working hour/week						
< 40	227	0.946 ± 0.106	0.043	396	0.905 ± 0.133	0.024
40–52	258	0.967 ± 0.069		168	0.930 ± 0.112	
52–60	54	0.965 ± 0.085		33	0.940 ± 0.090	
≥ 60	173	0.952 ± 0.081		59	0.945 ± 0.095	
Shift work						
Yes	210	0.957 ± 0.080	0.788	86	0.932 ± 0.096	0.217
No	502	0.956 ± 0.089		570	0.915 ± 0.127	

SD standard deviation

Table 8.5 Distribution of Levels of Perceived Problem in Each of the Dimensions of the EQ-5D Descriptive System, According to Sex in Older Wage Workers

	M (n = 712)			*F (n = 656)*		
	Level of perceived problem (%)					
Dimension	1[a]	2[a]	3[a]	1[a]	2[a]	3[a]
Mobility	616 (86.5)	95 (13.3)	1 (0.1)	478 (72.9)	176 (268)	2 (0.3)
Self-care	694 (97.5)	15 (2.1)	3 (0.4)	627 (95.6)	27 (4.1)	2 (0.3)
Usual activities	679 (95.4)	32 (4.5)	1 (0.1)	578 (88.1)	74 (11.3)	4 (0.6)
Pain/discomfort	589 (82.7)	113 (15.9)	10 (1.4)	456 (69.5)	178 (27.1)	22 (3.4)
Anxiety/ depression	657 (92.3)	54 (7.6)	1 (0.1)	555 (84.6)	93 (14.2)	8 (1.2)

[a]Level 1 implies no problem, 2 moderate problem, 3 severe problem.

depression" dimensions (OR 0.98–0.98). Stress had significant effects in the "self-care," "usual activities" and "anxiety/depression" dimensions (OR 2.31, 2.34 and 4.09, respectively).

Table 8.6 Logistic Regression Analyses of the Responses to the EQ-5D Items by the Male Older Workers

	Mobility OR (95% CI)	*Self-Care OR (95% CI)*	*Usual Activities OR (95% CI)*	*Pain/ Discomfort OR (95% CI)*	*Anxiety/ Depression OR (95% CI)*
Age	1.03 (1.04 – 1.01)***	1.06 (1.1 – 1.03)***	1.07 (1.1 – 1.04)***	1.03 (1.05– 1.02)***	1.05 (1.07– 1.03)***
Education (/<Elementary school)	0.55 (0.33– 0.93)*	0.57 (0.21– 1.57)	0.66 (0.31– 1.44)	0.80 (0.50– 1.27)	0.52 (0.28– 0.98)*
Household Income (quartile) (/4th(highest))					
1st (lowest)	0.96 (0.41– 2.26)	1.97 (0.39– 10.08)	2.21 (0.54– 9.02)	1.84 (0.85– 4.01)	2.02 (0.64– 6.33)
2nd	0.78 (0.38– 1.60)	0.86 (0.19– 3.92)	1.96 (0.56– 6.91)	1.62 (0.86– 3.05)	2.42 (0.95– 6.20)
3rd	0.71 (0.34– 1.51)	0.19 (0.02– 1.96)	0.87 (0.2– 3.78)	1.17 (0.61– 2.23)	1.56 (0.61– 3.98)
Smoking (current/ non & ex-smoker)	2.36 (1.45– 3.85)***	1.11 (0.40– 3.07)	1.96 (0.92– 4.17)	1.14 (0.73– 1.79)	0.79 (0.41– 1.50)
Hypertension (/no)	1.13 (0.68– 1.88)	0.74 (0.24– 2.24)	1.28 (0.57– 2.87)	1.30 (0.84– 2.01)	1.26 (0.68– 2.33)
Diabetes (/no)	1.94 (1.05– 3.58)*	0.19 (0.02– 1.56)	1.41 (0.53– 3.76)	1.30 (0.74– 2.27)	1.62 (0.78– 3.36)
Musculoskeletal pain (/no)	7.01 (4.26– 11.56)***	3.45 (1.28– 9.34)*	5.82 (2.74– 12.36)***	5.26 (3.38– 8.17)***	1.62 (0.84– 3.12)
Stress (/low)	0.79 (0.40– 1.56)	2.12 (0.69– 6.54)	0.32 (0.09– 1.20)	1.18 (0.68– 2.05)	4.95 (2.71– 9.03)***
Occupation (/Elementary occupations)	0.38 (0.22– 0.64)***	0.35 (0.11– 1.13)	0.49 (0.22– 1.10)	0.60 (0.38– 0.95)*	0.73 (0.39– 1.38)
Working hour/week	1.00 (0.98– 1.01)	1.01 (0.99– 1.04)	1.00 (0.98– 1.02)	1.00 (0.99– 1.01)	1.00 (0.98– 1.01)
Employment status (/Regular employee)	1.20 (0.67– 2.17)	1.97 (0.59– 6.57)	2.78 (1.11– 6.96)*	1.03 (0.62– 1.73)	1.25 (0.62– 2.52)
R^2_N	0.702	0.927	0.882	0.579	0.789

Some variables were reclassified because of small group size. Education (0: elementary school, 1: middle and high school, and collage); occupation (0: elementary occupations, 1: office, service and manufacturing work)

OR odds ratio, *CI* confidence intervals

*$p < 0.05$, ***$p < 0.001$

Table 8.7 Logistic Regression Analyses of the Responses to the EQ-5D Items by the Female Older Workers

	Mobility OR (95 % CI)	*Self-Care OR (95 % CI)*	*Usual Activities OR (95 % CI)*	*Pain/ Discomfort OR (95 % CI)*	*Anxiety/ Depression OR (95 % CI)*
Age	1.02 (1.04–1.01)***	1.07 (1.1–1.04)***	1.06 (1.08–1.04)***	1.02 (1.03–1.01)***	1.04 (1.05–1.02)***
Education (/<Elementary school)	0.64 (0.40–1.02)	0.37 (0.12–1.15)	0.61 (0.31–1.21)	0.9 (0.59–1.40)	0.92 (0.54–1.58)
Household Income (quartile) (/4th(highest))					
1st (lowest)	1.43 (0.71–2.87)	1.42 (0.32–6.32)	2.05 (0.70–6.02)	1.06 (0.55–2.03)	0.92 (0.41–2.02)
2nd	1.03 (0.53–2.00)	0.91 (0.20–4.06)	1.85 (0.64–5.37	0.87 (0.48–1.59)	0.78 (0.37–1.64)
3rd	0.65 (0.31–1.37)	0.8 (0.14–4.50)	1.06 (0.31–3.61)	0.62 (0.32–1.21)	0.65 (0.29–1.48)
Smoking (current/ non and ex-smoker)	0.52 (0.13–2.10)	2.44 (0.44–13.63)	0.99 (0.18–5.49)	0.45 (0.12–1.71)	1.57 (0.45–5.41)
Hypertension (/ no)	1.26 (0.84–1.90)	0.69 (0.30–1.59)	1.17 (0.68–2.03)	0.86 (0.58–1.27)	1.02 (0.63–1.65)
Diabetes (/no)	0.99 (0.51–1.92)	3.64 (1.36–9.70)**	1.64 (0.74–3.63)	0.96 (0.51–1.81)	1.13 (0.53–2.41)
Musculoskeletal pain (/no)	7.18 (4.68–11.02)***	6.13 (2.17–17.33)***	12.43 (5.79–26.7)***	6.01 (4.04–8.93)***	2.62 (1.61–4.27)***
Stress (/low)	1.53 (0.98–2.41)	2.31 (1.02–5.24)*	2.34 (1.31–4.17)**	1.29 (0.84–1.99)	4.09 (2.55–6.56)***
Occupation (/ Elementary occupations)	0.65 (0.41–1.04)	0.78 (0.30–2.04)	0.46 (0.23–0.91)*	1.09 (0.71–1.68)	0.85 (0.50–1.45)
Working hour/ week	0.98 (0.97–0.99)**	0.98 (0.96–0.99)*	0.97 (0.96–0.99)***	0.98 (0.98–0.99)**	0.99 (0.98–1.00)
Employment status (/Regular employee)	0.76 (0.48–1.20)	1.87 (0.66–5.27)	1.37 (0.71–2.65)	1.28 (0.83–1.95)	1.23 (0.72–2.10)
R^2_N	0.473	0.879	0.748	0.382	0.618

Some variables were reclassified because of small group size. Education (0: elementary school, 1: middle and high school, and collage); occupation (0: elementary occupations, 1: office, service and manufacturing work).

OR odds ratio, CI confidence intervals.

$^{*}p < 0.05$, $^{**}p < 0.01$, $^{***}p < 0.001$.

DISCUSSION

Korea is aging much more rapidly than other countries. The aging includes those in the productive work force. In Korea, the percentage of older workers ≥50 years of age has increased from 22.6 percent of all employed persons in 2000 to 27.7 percent in 2013. Approximately 77 percent of wage-earning wage workers from 2009 to 2013 was ≥50 years of age [28].

Aging has significant effects on production [29, 30]. The aging of current employees is decreasing their productivity due to the decrease in their physical abilities. Enterprises are trying to restructure to reduce their wage burden on account of the aged, and the vicious cycle of productivity deterioration is likely to continue. Also, with the increase in senile disorders, its cost burden on Korean society is increasing. Regional population is experiencing discrimination due to age, so central and local governments need to formulate policies supporting the welfare of the aged. To achieve this, the health status of current older workers must be determined. Based on this, national government must formulate plans to maintain and extend the working abilities of older workers.

It is important to measure the HRQL of older workers. This information can be used in decisions concerning older worker-related health and medical policies and can be indicators of the outcomes of related projects. The factors that produced significant differences in the older workers" EQ-5D index were age, education, household income, cerebrocardiovascular event, and presence of osteoarthritis, musculoskeletal pain, and stress (table 8.3). Past studies of HRQL have identified age, education, income, stress, and number of chronic diseases as factors affecting the EQ-5D index [8–12]. This was confirmed presently, and the associated occupational factors were occupation type, employment status, and working hours (table 8.4). In prior studies that analyzed workers" employment status and HRQL [31], the tendency for the average EQ-5D index to be lower among temporary and daily employees than among regular employees was reported. This was also evident in the present study.

And as seen in table 8.2, differences were evident according to gender in the distributions of the occupations and the employment status. More female older workers were engaged in elementary occupations than male older workers, and most of the female older workers were temporary or daily employees rather than regular employees. The data indicate a more unstable working environment for female older workers.

The response frequency at level 1 at each area of EQ-5D was minimum 69.5 percent (pain/discomfort with older female workers) and maximum 69.5 percent (pain/discomfort with older female workers). Because EQ-5D questionnaire divides the perceived problem levels into three levels at each item, slight problems cannot be reported; this is called as ceiling effect. This has been pointed out as an inherent problem of EQ-5D because the purpose of developing EQ-5D was to measure HRQL easily [32]. Compared with the studies from other countries, it was turned out that 59.2 percent (pain/discomfort) at minimum and 95.9 percent (self-care) at maximum in America [33] and 78.0 percent (pain/discomfort) at minimum and 96.7 percent (self-care) at maximum in China [34]. Ceiling effect was seen in this research as well, but it seems to be lower than in that of general population. Ceiling effect of EQ-5D is often pointed out as a flaw of the tool. However, EQ-5D normally shows a high response rate because it is easy to use [34], and ceiling effect tends to decrease in elder population than in general population. With this regard, we believe that it is an appropriate tool to use for a research toward massive group.

The OR of problems with each of the EQ-5D items was determined with binary logistic regression (tables 8.6 and 8.7). The variables which remained meaningful in both male and female were age and musculoskeletal pain. Age related in all dimensions both male and female, with ORs exceeding 1. It is well known that the probability of problem in EQ-5D increases as the age increases. However, it turned out not to affect as much as expected as ORs were nearly 1.

Musculoskeletal pain showed the highest OR compared with the other factors. Musculoskeletal pain seldom has fatal results, so little attention is paid to early symptoms. However, among the dimensions of EQ-5D, problems were most frequently appealed to "'pain/discomfort" dimension (table 8.5), and it was indicated that the more older workers feel this kind of pain, the more they appeal their problems in the other EQ-5D dimensions (tables 8.6 and 8.7). Repeated mitigation of the symptoms and consequent muscle deterioration become more deleterious with increasing age. The symptoms can become chronic. This greatly affects productivity due to short-term cessation, absence from work, and significant lessening of the quality of life. Musculoskeletal pain must be continuously managed, especially in older workers.

Presently, stress was closely associated with the "anxiety/depression" dimension between both the male and the female older workers. In related prior studies [13], stress has been documented to have more significant effects on HRQL of the female elderly than male elderly. Management of mental health including stress is nonetheless important for older workers.

Smoking among male older workers caused problems in the dimension of "mobility" (table 8.6). The average EQ-5D index was lowest among the current smokers, followed by ex-smokers and nonsmokers (table 8.3). It appears that older workers must be educated on the benefits of not smoking and their smoking habit must be managed.

Compared with the other factors, hypertension did not produce statistically significant changes in its OR, but the OR of diabetes significantly rose in the "mobility" dimension of male older workers (OR 1.94; 95 % CI, 1.05–3.85) and in the "self-care" dimension of female older workers (OR 3.64; 95 % CI 1.36–9.70). Hypertension itself is asymptomatic and blood pressure regulation is relatively easy with medication. However, diabetes should be treated with medication and strict dietary control, and complications can occur easily, so it can be more problematic than hypertension.

Factors closely related to the working conditions included the type of occupations and employment status in male older workers and the type of occupations and the working hours in female older workers. Occupation type related in "mobility" (OR 0.38; 95 % CI 0.22–0.64) and "pain/discomfort" dimension (OR 0.60; 95 % CI 0.38–0.95) of male and in "usual activities" dimension of female (OR 0.46; 95 % CI 0.23–0.91), with ORs < 1. In other dimensions, the average ORs were <1, too; nevertheless, those were included 1 in confidence interval. This shows that people who fall into the categories of elementary occupations are more vulnerable to their health-related issues. And the ratio of elementary occupations took up the largest part of older workers (table 8.2). We will have to come up with countermeasures and methods of care for those vulnerable occupations.

The employment status displayed increased OR in the "usual activities" dimension of the male older workers (OR 2.78; 95% CI 1.11–6.96). In other dimensions, the average ORs were exceeding 1, yet those were included 1 in confidence interval. Generally, the working conditions of the nonregular workers is less stable than that of the regular workers, and nonregular (temporary and daily) workers are more liable to be assigned dangerous tasks. This may make nonregular workers injured, and it may have made their usual activities bad. Presently, thirty-three male older workers (4.6 percent) responded that they had problems with their "usual activities" dimension. As the sample size was small, the small difference may have been manifest as significant problems. Further study is needed to exclude the selection bias that by chance many of the subjects who had problems with their usual activities were in nonregular employees.

The working hours made the OR < 1 in all dimensions except "anxiety/depression" dimension of female older workers. More studies have been addressing the effects of long working hours on health. Long working hours can raise the occurrence of work-related injuries [35] and affect cardiac disease [36–38], sleep disturbance [39], and mental health [40]. In this study, however, unlike prior studies, the longer the working hours were, the lower was the probability of occurrence of problems with these dimensions. Those who have problems with these dimensions may have chosen jobs with short working hours because they have realized that long working hours aggravate their symptoms or problems. Or it could be because those who have these types of problems might be not hired in long-time labor market because they were not preferred by the employers. Since the OR is close to 1, it can show an insignificant difference. But the appropriate number of hours of work can be a means of raising the quality of life of older workers, so it is necessary to examine the effects of the working hours on older workers and to confirm the appropriate working hours.

To sum up the results of this study, to eventually raise the quality of life of older workers through health maintenance and management, it is necessary to manage musculoskeletal diseases including musculoskeletal pain, mental health factors like stress, difficult chronic diseases including diabetes, and living habits like smoking, as well as paying attention to relatively vulnerable workers, such as nonregular employees and female workers.

The present study determined the health status of older workers, established HRQL and associated factors, examined the relationships between the factors known to have effects on HRQL, and determined the extent of the effects. This research is significant because it clarifies HRQL and presents basic data needed to establish related policies.

There are limitations. First, a cross-sectional research method was used. Thus, correlations between variables do not always show causal relationships. Second, the KNHANES results could have been affected by the differences in the subject selection method, questionnaire survey method, and survey period. The EQ-5D survey results could have been affected by the differences in the health levels and the cultural differences in the attitude toward and awareness of health. By supplementing these factors, more in-depth studies are needed concerning diverse and comprehensive disease structures and subjective health status.

CONCLUSIONS

Using the data from the fifth KNHANES, health status, working conditions, and HRQL of Korean older workers were examined. Factors that influenced the EQ-5D dimensions of older workers were age, musculoskeletal pain, stress, diabetes, smoking, occupation type, employment status, and working hours.

In this aging era, health management of older workers is absolutely necessary. For efficient health management for older workers, their health must be continuously managed through the development of diverse policies and health promotion programs that reflect sociodemographic characteristics, health-related characteristics, and work-related factors. Studies geared toward increasing the quality of life of older workers should be conducted.

NOTE

1. This chapter was previously published as Hong, Sujin, Harin Jeong, Yunjeong Heo, Hosun Chun, Jongtae Park, and Daeseong Kim. "Factors associated with health-related quality of life in Korean older workers." *Annals of Occupational and Environmental Medicine* 27, no. 1 (2015): 25.

REFERENCES

1. The Korean Society for Preventive Medicine. *Preventive Medicine and Public Health.* 2/e ed. Korea: Gyechuk, 2013.
2. *Korean Statistical Information Service: 2000 Census*, 2000. http://kosis.kr. Accessed: 20 January 2015.
3. Statistics Korea. *Population Projections for Korea: 2010–2060 (Based on the 2010 Census).* Daejeon: Statistics Korea, 2011.
4. Choi DW. *Accident Characteristics and Safety Measures for Aging Workers in Korea* [Master's Thesis]. Seoul: Seoul National University of Science and Technology, 2013. p. 106.
5. Kim YS, Kim BH, Kim HM. "A study on occupational accident of older workers and vulnerable working condition." *Health Soc Sci.* 2014;35:309–29.
6. Lee JC, Shin SW, Lee CS. "Accident analysis of middle-aged & advanced-aged construction workers." *J Archit Inst Korea.* 2007;27(1):797–800.
7. Park SY. *Risk Factors for Occupational Injuries: A Comparison of Older and Younger Workers in Korea* [Master's Thesis]. Seoul: Catholic university of Korea, 2009. p. 31.
8. Lee JJ, Lee HJ, Park EJ. "Effect of staged education program for hypertension, diabetes patients in a community (assessment of quality of life using EQ-5D)." *J Agric Med Commun Health.* 2014;39(1):37–45.
9. Jo MW, Kim SK, Lee JY, Lee KS. "Estimating quality adjusted life year loss of persons disabled by stroke using EQ-5D in Korea." *J Agric Med Commun Health.* 2011;36(2):120–9.
10. Shin S. "A study on health related quality of life in people living with HIV/AIDS in Korea." *Health Welf Rev.* 2011;31(4):424–53.
11. Oh KA, Park J, Jeon DJ, Han MA, Choi SW. "Relationship between low back pain and health-related quality of life among some elderly." *J Agric Med Commun Health.* 2012;37(3):156–66.
12. Kim JG, Kwon LS. "Measurement of quality of life related to health by demographic characteristics of adult patients with cancer using EQ-5D index-focused on the Korea health & nutrition examination survey." *J Digit Convergence.* 2013;11(8):281–91.
13. Lee SH. "Gender difference in influencing factors on health related quality of life among the elderly in community." *J Digit Convergence.* 2013;11(12):523–35.
14. Kim JY. *Factors Affecting Health Related Quality of Life among Aged* [Master's Thesis]. Kimhae: Inje University, 2014. p. 54.

15. Shin KR, Byeon YS, Kang Y, Oak J. "A study on physical symptom, activity of daily living, and health-related quality of life (HRQoL) in the community-dwelling older adults." *Taehan Kanho Hakhoe Chi*. 2008;38(3):437–44.
16. Kim Y. "Factors influencing the health-related quality of life by age among vulnerable elderly women." *J Korea Acad-Ind Soc*. 2013;14(3):1342–9.
17. Lee JH, Yoon BJ, Jeong H-S. "Decomposition of the health concentration index by health dimensions applied on EQ-5D." *Health Soc Sci*. 2009;26:67–87.
18. Choi H, Lee E-O, Kim B-W, Kim I-J. "Stage of change for exercise and health-related quality of life in Korean adults." *Korean J Adult Nurs*. 2004;16(2):191–201.
19. Taylor WJ, Myers J, Simpson RT, McPherson KM, Weatherall M. "Quality of life of people with rheumatoid arthritis as measured by the World Health Organization Quality of Life Instrument, short form (WHOQOL-BREF): score distributions and psychometric properties." *Arthritis Rheum*. 2004;51(3):350–7. doi:10.1002/art.20398.
20. The WHOQOL Group. "The World Health Organization Quality of Life assessment (WHOQOL): position paper from the World Health Organization." *Soc Sci Med*. 1995;41(10):1403–9.
21. Spiker B, Revicki DA. "Quality of life and pharmacoeconomics in clinical trials." In: *Taxonomy of Quality of Life*, Spiker B, editor. 2nd ed. Philadelphia, PA: Lippincott-Raven Publishers, 1996. p. 25–31.
22. Kaplan RM, Ganiats TG, Sieber WJ. *The Quality of Well-Being Scale – Self Administered (QWB-SA)*, 1996. https://hoap.ucsd.edu/qwb-info. Accessed: 3 January 2015.
23. Torrance GW, Feeny DH, Furlong WJ, Barr RD, Zhang Y, Wang Q. "Multiattribute utility function for a comprehensive health status classification system. Health utilities index mark 2." *Med Care*. 1996;34(7):702–22.
24. Feeny D, Furlong W, Torrance GW, Goldsmith CH, Zhu Z, DePauw S, et al. "Multiattribute and single-attribute utility functions for the health utilities index mark 3 system." *Med Care*. 2002;40(2):113–28.
25. Group EQ. "EuroQol – a new facility for the measurement of health-related quality of life." *Health Policy*. 1990;16(3):199–208.
26. Brazier JE, Fukuhara S, Roberts J, Kharroubi S, Yamamoto Y, Ikeda S, et al. "Estimating a preference-based index from the Japanese SF-36." *J Clin Epidemiol*. 2009;62(12):1323–31. doi:10.1016/j.jclinepi.2009.01.022.
27. Nam HS, Kim KY, Kwon SS, Koh KW, Kind P. *EQ-5D Korean Valuation Study Using Time Trade Off Method*. Seoul: Korea Centers for Disease Control and Prevention, 2007.
28. *Economically Active Population Survey*. Statistics Korea, 2013. http://kosis.kr. Accessed: 3 January 2015.
29. Ryu JY. *A Study on the Ways of Activating Elderly Labor Forces in the Aging Society* [Master's Thesis]. Seongnam: Kyoungwon University, 2005. p. 135.
30. Lee S-L. "Labor force shortage projection and policy implications: impact of demographic transition in Korea." *Korea J Popul*. 2012;35(2):1–28.
31. Kim KH. *Comparison of Health-Related Quality of Life by Occupational Status using EQ-5D Index* [Master's Thesis]. Seoul: Catholic University of Korea, 2010. p. 34.

32. Coons SJ, Rao S, Keininger DL, Hays RD. "A comparative review of generic quality-of-life instruments." *Pharmacoeconomics*. 2000;17(1):13–35.
33. Luo N, Johnson JA, Shaw JW, Feeny D, Coons SJ. "Self-reported health status of the general adult U.S. Population as assessed by the EQ-5D and health utilities index." *Med Care*. 2005;43(11):1078–86.
34. Wang HM, Patrick DL, Edwards TC, Skalicky AM, Zeng HY, Gu WW. "Validation of the EQ-5D in a general population sample in urban China." *Qual Life Res*. 2012;21(1):155–60. doi:10.1007/s11136-011-9915-6.
35. Dembe AE, Erickson JB, Delbos RG, Banks SM. "The impact of overtime and long work hours on occupational injuries and illnesses: new evidence from the United States." *Occup Environ Med*. 2005;62(9):588–97. doi:10.1136/oem.2004.016667.
36. Iwasaki K, Sasaki T, Oka T, Hisanaga N. "Effect of working hours on biological functions related to cardiovascular system among salesmen in a machinery manufacturing company." *Ind Health*. 1998;36(4):361–7.
37. Jeong I, Rhie J, Kim I, Ryu I, Jung PK, Park YS, et al. "Working hours and cardiovascular disease in Korean workers: a case–control study." *J Occup Health*. 2014;55(5):385–91.
38. Choi B, Schnall PL, Dobson M, Garcia-Rivas J, Kim H, Zaldivar F, et al. "Very long (>48 hours) shifts and cardiovascular strain in firefighters: a theoretical framework." *Ann Occup Environ Med*. 2014;26(1):5. doi:10.1186/2052-4374-26-5.
39. Virtanen M, Ferrie JE, Gimeno D, Vahtera J, Elovainio M, Singh-Manoux A, et al. "Long working hours and sleep disturbances: the Whitehall II prospective cohort study." *Sleep*. 2009;32(6):737–45.
40. Kleppa E, Sanne B, Tell GS. "Working overtime is associated with anxiety and depression: the hordaland health study." *J Occup Environ Med*. 2008;50(6):658–66. doi:10.1097/JOM.0b013e3181734330.

Chapter 9

Hazards and Health Problems in Occupations Dominated by Aged Workers in South Korea

Jungsun Park, Soo Geun Kim, Jong-shik Park, Boyoung Han, Kab Bae Kim, and Yangho Kim

BACKGROUND

South[1] Korea's population is aging more rapidly than any other country [1, 2]. It became an aging society in 2000, will be an aged society by 2018, and a super-aged society by 2026 [1]. Labor shortages and a lack of skilled workers are expected due to reductions in the size of the productive population (fifteen to sixty-four years old) in 2017 and the mass retirement of "baby boomers," who were born after the Korean War. Further, the most economically active age group (thirty to forty-nine years old) will decline continuously, from 49 percent in 2005, to 42 percent in 2020, and to 37 percent in 2050. Thus, aging of the productive population will reach the point when most current baby boomers have left the labor market, probably by 2030 [1]. Similarly, the percentage of elderly people (at least fifty years old) was 25 percent in 2010, and is expected to exceed 33 percent in 2020 [1, 3]. The aging of the workforce will likely increase the rate of workplace accidents because more elderly workers than young workers have degradations of physiological functions, such as sensory systems, sense of equilibrium, and motor control [4, 5]. The increased prevalence of chronic and degenerative diseases due to aging will also lead to a decreased quality of the labor force [6]. Health-care strategies that seek to maintain and promote the work ability of elderly employees are needed to meet the impending shortage of labor and the decreasing quality of the labor force in South Korea.

Thus, South Korea needs long-term and short-term strategies that maintain and promote the work ability of aged individuals. One long-term strategy is to prevent noncommunicable diseases (NCDs) through workplace health promotion activities, while workers are still actively employed. These activities require the collaboration of governmental agencies at the central and local levels. First, the common goal of central governmental agencies should be reinforcement of follow-up measures in general medical examinations and promotion of healthy lifestyles for workers. Second, collaboration at the local level should be performed at the Worker's Health Center, the Health Promotion Center, and community health centers [7]. One short-term strategy is to support the establishment of work environments that are appropriate for elderly workers who have reduced physical capacity. Long- and short-term strategies should focus on workplaces that are dominated by aged workers, rather than the entire population of aged workers, because the work ability of aged workers can be efficiently and effectively maintained and promoted when employers take the responsibility to lead such activities, and workers will then be more likely to participate. Thus, we must first identify the occupations that employ the most aged workers and the prevalence of different occupational hazards at these workplaces. Second, we must improve the health and safety of the elderly workers in their workplaces by developing and disseminating age-friendly occupational health and safety guidelines, based on job-specific information.

As a short-term strategy, the present study aims to identify occupations that are dominated by aged workers and assess the exposure to hazards and work-related health problems of aged workers in these occupations.

METHODS

Materials and Subjects

We defined aged workers as those who were at least fifty-five years old, according to Enforcement Decree of the Act on Prohibition of Age Discrimination in Employment and Aged Employment Promotion in Korea.

Selection of Occupations

Study subjects were aged workers and young workers in occupations that were dominated by aged workers, based on raw data of the 2014 Employment Survey by Area (A type) [8]. We initially identified 20 of 149 occupations, in descending order of the number of aged workers. These are minor categories (identified by three digits), as defined by the Korean Standard Classification of Occupations (KSCO) [9].

Source of Data on Hazards and Health Problems

We analyzed the results of the fourth Working Conditions Survey of 2014 by the Korea Occupational Safety and Health Agency to evaluate the characteristics of working conditions, exposure to hazards, and work-related health problems in these twenty occupations. The survey population was a representative sample of those who were aged fifteen years or older. Individuals who were retired, unemployed, housewives, or students were excluded. The basic design was a multistage random sampling of the enumeration districts used for the 2010 population and housing census. A total of 50,007 interviews were conducted, but we only included the responses of 30,751 employees who had worked in their current workplaces for more than one year prior to the survey. Among the 6,502 aged workers (fifty-five or older), there were 3,482 males (53.6 percent) and 3,020 females (46.4 percent) (total 6,502 workers). Among the 24,249 workers younger than fifty-five, there were 12,260 males (50.6 percent) and 11,989 females (49.4 percent).

Survey data were weighted with reference to the economically active population. The questionnaire assessed exposure to physical and chemical agents, including vibration, noise, high and low temperatures, fumes and dust, solvents, skin contact with chemicals, and passive smoking. The methodology and questionnaire were almost identical to those of the European Working Conditions Survey [10]. We defined exposure as "exposure to hazards during at least a half of the work time" and a work-related health problem as any of thirteen conditions, including hearing loss, skin problems, muscle pain, depression, sleeping disturbance, and others, that may be work-related. After explanation of the survey, all participants provided written informed consent.

Statistical Analysis

Differences between aged workers (total) and those younger than fifty-five (total) in working conditions, exposure to hazards, and work-related health problems were analyzed using a chi-squared test. STATA (ver. 12) was used for all statistical analyses, and a p-value below 0.05 was considered significant.

RESULTS

General Characteristics of Study Subjects

Aged workers, defined as those older than fifty-five, worked at places with fewer employees, accounted for a smaller proportion of regular workers, received lower salaries, and accounted for a higher percentage of those employed in

Elementary Occupations, relative to workers younger than fifty-five (table 9.1). This tendency was particularly strong in workers older than sixty-five.

Occupations Dominated by Aged Workers

Table 9.2 shows twenty occupations, in descending order of the total number of aged workers, among the 149 occupations defined as minor categories (identified by three digits) by the KSCO. In 2014, there were 3,428,823 aged workers, and this accounted for 18.1 percent of the 18,945,403 workers in South Korea. A total of 2,439,330 of these aged workers (71.1 percent) were employed in the twenty listed occupations. "Elementary Occupations," which the KSCO classifies as a major category (nine), accounted for the largest proportion of aged workers among the twenty occupations (45 percent), and workers employed in the nine "Elementary Occupations" accounted for 42.3 percent of all 3,428,823 aged workers. These "Elementary Occupations" were "Cleaner and Sanitation Workers" (941), "Guards and Ticket Examiners" (942), "Elementary Occupations Related to Food" (952), "Elementary Occupations Related to Construction and Mining" (910), "Domestic Chores and Infant Rearing Helpers" (951), "Elementary Occupations related to Agriculture and Fishery" (991), "Elementary Occupations Related to Production" (930), "Elementary Occupations Related to Other Services" (999), and "Deliverers" (922). There were five occupations of skilled manual workers that accounted for 17.4 percent of the total aged workers: "Automobile Drivers" (873), "Service Workers Related to Medical and Welfare" (421), "Chefs and Cooks" (441), "Technical Worker Related to Construction" (772), and "Technical Workers Related to Construction Finishing" (773). There were also workers in six skilled non-manual occupations that accounted for 11.4 percent of the total aged workers: "Clerks Related to Administration" (312), "Store Sales Workers" (521), "Sales Workers" (510), "Administration Clerks" (311), "Religious Professionals and Associate Professionals" (248), and "Teachers" (252).

Occupations in which aged workers accounted for more than 50 percent of the total workers were "Cleaner and Sanitation Workers" (941), "Guards and Ticket Examiners" (942), "Service Workers Related to Medical and Welfare" (421), "Domestic Chores and Infant Rearing Helpers" (951), "Elementary Occupations Related to Agriculture and Fishery" (991), and "Elementary Occupations Related to Other Services" (999).

Exposure of Aged Workers to Hazards in Different Occupations

Aged workers classified as "Technical Workers Related to Construction" (772) reported the greatest exposure to vibration (61.3 percent), followed by

Table 9.1 General Characteristics of Study Subjects

		Age < 55 Frequency (%)	*≥55 Age < 65 Frequency (%)*	*Age ≥ 65 Frequency (%)*	p-*value*
Workplace size	<5 workers	5,097(21.5)	1,052(25.4)	647(31.2)	*P* < 0.001
	5–<30 workers	9,158(38.5)	1,761(42.6)	1,051(50.7)	
	30–<50 workers	2,774(11.7)	412(10.0)	165(8.0)	
	50–<300 workers	4,583(19.3)	660(16.0)	187(9.0)	
	≥300 workers	2,149(9.0)	254(6.1)	24(1.2)	
	Total	23,761(100.0)	4,139(100.0)	2,074(100.0)	
Type of employment	Regular	19,041(79.0)	2,528(59.2)	602(27.5)	*P* < 0.001
	Temporary	3,782(15.7)	1,052(24.6)	1,037(47.3)	
	Daily	1,280(5.3)	689(16.1)	552(25.2)	
	Total	24,103(100.0)	4,269(100.0)	2,191(100.0)	
Monthly salary (Korean won)	<1,000,000	1,622(9.4)	544(18.2)	1,040(62.0)	*P* < 0.001
	1,000,000–<2,000,000	6,007(35.0)	1,326(44.4)	528(31.5)	
	2,000,000–<3,000,000	5,226(30.4)	549(18.4)	75(4.5)	
	3,000,000–<4,000,000	2,750(16.0)	318(10.6)	22(1.3)	
	≥4,000,000	1,575(9.2)	251(8.4)	12(0.7)	
	Total	17,180(100.0)	2,988(100.0)	1,677(100.0)	
Major categories of occupation (KSCO)	Managers	466(1.9)	120(2.8)	14(0.6)	*P* < 0.001
	Professionals and related workers	3,753(15.5)	268(6.3)	41(1.9)	
	Clerks	7,321(30.3)	420(9.8)	43(2)	
	Service workers	3,353(13.9)	710(16.5)	207(9.4)	
	Sales workers	3,550(14.7)	331(7.7)	43(2)	
	Skilled workers related to agriculture, forestry, and fishery	44(0.2)	37(0.9)	51(2.3)	
	Craft and related trades workers	2,357(9.8)	483(11.3)	92(4.2)	
	Workers related to equipment, machine operating and assembling	1,479(6.1)	366(8.5)	57(2.6)	
	Elementary occupations	1,835(7.6)	1,559(36.3)	1,658(75.2)	
	Total	24,158(100.0)	4,294(100.0)	2,206(100.0)	

Total numbers are not identical due to nonresponse.

Table 9.2 Occupations That Are Dominated by Aged Workers (Unit; Number)

Occupation, Korean Standard Classification of Occupations (No. of minor category)	*Workers Younger than 55*	*Workers Aged 55 or Older*	*Total Workers*	*Proportion of Aged Workers (%)*
Total	15,516,580	3,428,823	18,945,403	18.1
Cleaner and sanitation workers (941)	154,789	514,734	669,523	76.9
Guards and ticket examiners (942)	34,376	206,817	241,193	85.7
Automobile drivers (873)	354,404	174,921	529,325	33.0
Elementary occupations related to food(952)	213,327	154,840	368,167	42.1
Clerks related to administration (312)	1,845,084	149,151	1,994,235	7.5
Service workers related to medical and welfare (421)	142,735	148,189	290,924	50.9
Elementary occupations related to construction and mining (910)	252,974	145,535	398,509	36.5
Domestic chores and infant rearing helpers (951)	65,415	127,163	192,578	66.0
Chefs and cooks (441)	347,880	115,729	463,609	25.0
Elementary occupations related to agriculture and fishery (991)	38,169	102,634	140,803	72.9
Elementary occupations related to production (930)	299,138	93,173	392,311	23.7
Technical worker related to construction (772)	152,831	91,909	244,740	37.6
Elementary occupations related to other services (999)	56,680	72,691	129,371	56.2
Store sales workers (521)	841,347	66,002	907,349	7.3
Technical workers related to construction finishing (773)	151,042	65,353	216,395	30.2
Sales workers (510)	471,593	62,289	533,882	11.7
Administration clerks (311)	362,739	41,447	404,186	10.3
Religious professionals and associate Professionals (248)	88,487	38,701	127,188	30.4
Deliverers (922)	173,066	34,361	207,427	16.6
Teachers (252)	356,014	33,691	389,705	8.6

"Elementary Occupations Related to Construction and Mining" (910) (47.8 percent) (table 9.3). Exposure to noise was also greatest for aged workers classified as "Technical Workers Related to Construction" (772) reported the greatest exposure to vibration (45.1 percent), followed by "Elementary Occupations Related to Construction and Mining" (910) (40.2 percent).

Table 9.3 Proportion of Aged Workers Exposed to Hazards in Different Occupations (%)

Occupation, Korean Standard Classification of Occupations (No. of minor category)	*Vibration*	*Noise*	*High Temperature*	*Low Temperature*	*Fumes and Dust*	*Solvents*	*Skin Contact with Chemicals*	*Passive Smoking*	*Tiring or Painful Positions*	*Lifting or Moving People*	*Carrying or Moving Heavy Loads*	*Standing long*	*Repetitive Movements*
Cleaner and sanitation workers (941)	6.1	4.4	28.3	15.0	17.9	2.1	4.0	3.9	43.9	3.4	20.8	66.1	68.1
Guards and ticket examiners (942)	1.8	2.5	13.9	8.7	4.8	1.0	1.3	3.0	18.3	4.4	12.2	28.1	19.9
Automobile drivers (873)	32.0	11.5	12.7	8.2	22.6	3.0	1.9	5.9	53.7	7.8	14.5	13.5	70.6
Elementary occupations related to food(952)	6.1	7.9	21.2	7.3	3.7	1.2	2.4	2.4	46.7	5.5	23.6	72.4	67.9
Clerks related to administration (312)	10.5	6.1	6.1	3.4	4.4	1.7	1.4	1.0	13.6	4.4	7.8	15.0	30.4
Service workers related to medical and welfare (421)	4.0	1.8	7.1	4.9	2.2	0.5	0.9	0.9	30.9	42.0	15.6	30.8	40.5
Elementary occupations related to construction and mining (910)	47.8	40.2	53.7	25.5	50.2	8.5	6.4	18.3	67.9	8.5	72.2	83.8	69.8

(Continued)

Table 9.3 Proportion of Aged Workers Exposed to Hazards in Different Occupations (%) *(Continued)*

Occupation, Korean Standard Classification of Occupations (No. of minor category)	*Vibration*	*Noise*	*High Temperature*	*Low Temperature*	*Fumes and Dust*	*Solvents*	*Skin Contact with Chemicals*	*Passive Smoking*	*Tiring or Painful Positions*	*Lifting or Moving People*	*Carrying or Moving Heavy Loads*	*Standing long*	*Repetitive Movements*
Domestic chores and infant rearing helpers (951)	1.7	2.2	5.6	5.0	1.1	1.7	1.7	1.1	34.8	32.6	8.4	21.7	35.6
Chefs and cooks (441)	8.3	9.2	30.7	8.9	7.6	1.0	1.6	1.6	47.5	7.0	24.1	84.2	71.2
Elementary occupations related to agriculture and fishery (991)	6.9	4.6	40.0	13.1	14.6	1.5	2.3	0.8	66.4	3.8	29.0	41.9	78.5
Elementary occupations related to production (930)	36.4	25.6	25.6	10.1	21.7	7.8	7.0	3.1	56.6	6.3	32.0	50.4	85.2
Technical worker related to construction (772)	61.3	45.1	48.6	23.2	51.4	10.6	5.7	24.1	65.3	6.3	58.2	88.0	83.8
Elementary occupations related to other services (999)	7.9	7.9	11.1	7.9	12.7	0.0	0.0	6.4	30.7	1.6	7.9	65.1	49.2

Store sales workers (521)	3.8	6.9	8.8	9.3	5.6	1.3	0.6	1.9	42.6	7.5	24.2	71.6	55.9
Technical workers related to construction finishing (773)	42.0	36.0	46.0	22.0	50.0	31.0	28.3	27.0	61.0	14.0	52.0	70.0	76.0
Sales workers (510)	2.1	2.0	4.8	3.4	0.7	0.7	0.0	2.0	9.6	0.0	4.1	21.2	21.9
Administration clerks (311)	4.0	4.0	9.1	2.6	2.6	0.0	0.0	0.0	15.8	2.6	6.6	13.2	38.2
Religious professionals and associate professionals (248)	0.0	0.0	0.0	0.0	0.0	0.0	0.0	0.0	9.1	0.0	4.6	36.4	27.3
Deliverers (922)	12.3	7.0	26.3	10.5	7.0	0.0	0.0	3.5	38.6	0.0	63.2	56.1	52.6
Teachers (252)	8.2	8.2	9.8	4.9	9.8	0.0	1.6	1.6	19.7	5.0	3.3	88.5	57.4
Workers 55 or older (total)	17.3	13.0	22.9	11.6	16.0	3.6	3.8	5.0	38.4	7.4	23.4	50.7	55.9
Workers younger than 55 (total)	14.6	11.0	11.5	6.9	8.8	2.7	2.9	3.3	27.9	5.1	15.7	41.9	49.9
P-value#	< 0.001	< 0.001	< 0.001	< 0.001	< 0.001	< 0.001	< 0.001	< 0.001	< 0.001	< 0.001	< 0.001	< 0.001	< 0.001

#Differences between aged workers (total) and those younger than fifty-five (total) using a chi-squared test.

Table 9.4 Proportion of Aged Workers Having Work-related Health Problems in Different Occupations (%)

Occupation, the Korean Standard Classification of Occupations (No. of minor category)	*Hearing Loss*	*Skin Problems*	*Back pain*	*Upper Extremity Pain*	*Lower Extremity Pain*	*Headache and Eye Fatigue*	*Abdominal Pain*	*Breathing Difficulty*	*Cardiovascular Disease*	*Injury Due to Accident*	*Depression and Anxiety Disorder*	*General Fatigue*	*Sleep Disturbance*
Cleaner and sanitation workers (941)	0.9	1.1	21.2	38.6	33.3	7.9	0.6	0.2	0.7	0.3	0.4	20.7	0.6
Guards and ticket examiners (942)	0.5	0.5	7.6	20.4	16.5	9.9	0.5	0.2	0.5	0.5	0.5	20.2	4.0
Automobile drivers (873)	1.5	1.8	17.7	44.1	32.7	24.6	0.7	0.7	0.0	0.4	0.7	22.8	1.8
Elementary occupations related to food (952)	0.0	0.6	17.6	47.3	42.4	6.7	0.0	0.6	1.2	2.4	0.0	27.3	0.0
Clerks related to administration (312)	0.0	0.0	3.0	13.1	5.4	15.2	0.0	0.0	0.3	0.0	0.0	32.7	1.7
Service workers related to medical and welfare (421)	0.4	0.8	21.7	41.5	28.5	7.9	0.0	0.0	0.4	1.6	1.2	29.6	2.4
Elementary occupations related to construction and mining (910)	1.7	1.0	22.9	58.9	49.2	9.1	0.7	0.7	0.3	4.0	1.0	31.7	0.7
Domestic chores and infant rearing helpers (951)	0.6	0.6	27.5	41.8	27.5	6.0	1.1	0.0	0.0	0.6	1.7	26.9	2.2
Chefs and cooks (441)	0.3	0.6	23.7	51.3	40.5	10.4	0.3	0.0	1.3	2.2	0.3	29.8	2.2

Elementary occupations related to agriculture and fishery (991)	1.5	2.3	37.9	53.0	46.2	14.4	2.3	3.0	0.8	3.0	0.0	28.8	4.5
Elementary occupations related to production (930)	1.6	3.1	25.6	51.9	38.8	22.5	0.0	0.8	2.3	4.7	0.0	27.9	0.8
Technical worker related to construction (772)	2.8	2.8	26.1	61.3	44.4	12.7	0.0	0.0	0.0	3.5	0.7	32.4	0.0
Elementary occupations related to other services (999)	0.0	0.0	7.9	19.0	14.3	12.7	0.0	0.0	0.0	0.0	0.0	17.5	0.0
Store sales workers (521)	0.0	0.6	17.9	28.4	32.7	13.0	0.0	0.0	0.0	0.6	0.0	25.9	0.6
Technical workers related to construction finishing (773)	1.0	2.0	30.7	54.5	42.6	7.9	0.0	2.0	0.0	5.9	0.0	35.6	3.0
Sales workers (510)	0.0	0.0	2.0	15.6	8.8	18.4	1.4	0.0	0.0	4.1	1.4	21.1	3.4
Administration clerks (311)	0.0	1.3	7.8	11.7	9.1	16.9	1.3	0.0	0.0	0.0	1.3	10.4	1.3
Religious professionals and associate professionals (248)	0.0	0.0	9.1	9.1	9.1	18.2	0.0	0.0	4.5	4.5	0.0	4.5	4.5
Deliverers (922)	0.0	0.0	14.0	49.1	36.8	14.0	0.0	0.0	1.8	0.0	0.0	38.6	0.0
Teachers (252)	0.0	0.0	11.5	19.7	16.4	11.5	1.6	1.6	0.0	0.0	0.0	14.8	0.0
Workers 55 or older (total)	1.2	1.0	16.7	36.2	28.2	11.6	0.5	0.4	0.6	1.4	0.6	22.7	1.6
Workers younger than 55 (total)	1.1	1.2	10.3	25.6	16.1	15.8	0.6	0.3	0.2	1.1	0.7	18.7	1.7
p-value#	0.615	0.110	< 0.001	< 0.001	< 0.001	< 0.001	0.206	0.667	< 0.001	0.041	0.178	< 0.001	0.809

#Differences between aged workers (total) and those younger than fifty-five (total) using a chi-squared test.

Exposure to high temperatures was reported by aged workers who had outdoor jobs, such as "Elementary Occupations Related to Construction and Mining" (910) (53.7 percent), "Technical Workers Related to Construction" (772) (48.6 percent), "Technical Workers Related to Construction Finishing" (773) (46.0 percent), and "Elementary Occupations related to Agriculture and Fishery" (991) (40 percent); exposure to low temperatures was most common in the same occupations. Exposure to fumes and dust was most common in "Technical Workers Related to Construction" (51.4 percent), followed by "Elementary Occupations Related to Construction and Mining" and "Technical Workers Related to Construction Finishing." Exposure to solvents was most common in "Technical Workers Related to Construction Finishing" (31.0 percent), followed by "Technical Workers Related to Construction." Skin contact with chemicals was most common in "Technical Workers Related to Construction Finishing," and then "Elementary Occupations Related to Production." Exposure to passive tobacco smoke was most common in "Technical Workers Related to Construction Finishing," and then "Technical Workers Related to Construction."

Exposure to tiring or painful positions was most common in "Elementary Occupations Related to Construction and Mining" (67.9 percent), followed by "Elementary Occupations related to Agriculture and Fishery" (991) (66.4 percent), "Technical Workers Related to Construction" (65.3 percent), and "Technical Workers Related to Construction Finishing." Exposure to lifting or moving people was most common in "Service Workers Related to Medical and Welfare" (42 percent), and "Domestic Chores and Infant Rearing Helpers" (32.6 percent). Carrying or moving heavy loads was most common in "Elementary Occupations Related to Construction and Mining" (72.2 percent), and then "Deliverers" (63.2 percent), "Technical Workers Related to Construction" (58.2 percent), and "Technical Workers Related to Construction Finishing" (52.0 percent). Exposure to prolonged standing was most common in "Teachers," "Technical Workers Related to Construction," "Chefs and Cooks," and "Elementary Occupations Related to Construction and Mining." Exposure to repetitive movements was most common in "Elementary Occupations Related to Production" (85.2 percent), "Technical Workers Related to Construction" (83.8 percent), and "Elementary Occupations related to Agriculture and Fishery" (78.5 percent). Furthermore, aged workers (total) were more likely to report all of these hazards than young workers (total).

These results showed that aged workers in many occupations reported frequent exposure to ergonomic hazards such as tiring or painful positions, carrying or moving heavy loads, and repetitive movements. These aged workers also reported frequent exposure to physical factors such as noise, vibration, high and low temperatures, and chemical factors, such as solvents and other chemicals, in different specific occupations.

Work-Related Health Problems of Aged Workers in Different Occupations

Hearing loss and skin problems were most common in "Technical Workers Related to Construction" and "Elementary Occupations Related to Production" (2.8 and 3.1 percent, respectively) (table 9.4). Back pain was most common in "Elementary Occupations related to Agriculture and Fishery" (37.9 percent), and was reported about 20 percent, in most occupations. Upper extremity pain and lower extremity pain were reported in most occupations, and the frequencies were about 40 to 50 percent and 30 to 40 percent, respectively. Furthermore, aged workers (total) were more likely to report musculoskeletal symptoms than young workers (total). Headache and eye fatigue were most common in "Automobile Drivers" and "Elementary Occupations Related to Production," each with a frequency of about 20 percent. Aged workers (total) were less likely to report headache and eye fatigue than young workers (total). Abdominal pain and breathing difficulty were most common in "Elementary Occupations related to Agriculture and Fishery." Cardiovascular disease was the most common disease among "Religious Professionals and Associate Professionals." Injury due to accidents was most common in machinery-handling occupations, including "Technical Workers Related to Construction," "Technical Workers Related to Construction Finishing," "Elementary Occupations Related to Construction and Mining," and "Elementary Occupations Related to Production." Injury due to accidents was also common in "Sales Workers" and "Religious Professionals and Associate Professionals." Furthermore, aged workers (total) were more likely to report occupational injuries than young workers (total). Depression and anxiety disorder was most common among "Domestic Chores and Infant Rearing Helpers" (1.7 percent), followed by other occupations that are dominated by women. General fatigue was present in about 20 to 30 percent of aged workers in most occupations, and aged workers (total) were more likely to report this symptom than young workers (total). Sleep disturbance was most common in "Elementary Occupations related to Agriculture and Fishery" (4.5 percent), and "Religious Professionals and Associate Professionals" (248) (4.5 percent) followed by "Guards and Ticket Examiners" (4.0 percent), "Sales Workers," "Technical Workers Related to Construction Finishing," "Service Workers Related to Medical and Welfare," "Domestic Chores and Infant Rearing Helpers," and "Chefs and Cooks," each with a frequency of 2 to 3 percent.

DISCUSSION

The KSCO categorizes occupations based on the skills required to carry out the necessary tasks and duties. Skill has two dimensions: skill level and skill specialization. Skill level is a function of the complexity and range of tasks and duties to be performed. According to the International Standard Classification of Occupations (ISCO), an individual obtains a skill level by formal education, and informally by on-the-job training and from previous experience in a related occupation [11]. Thus, the concept of skill level, applied to the classification of occupations, places more emphasis on the ability to perform a job than the requirement for a formal education. Bearing in mind the international character of the classification, there are four skill levels. Occupations at Skill Level 1 typically require the performance of simple and routine physical or manual tasks and may require physical strength and/or endurance (e.g., the nine Elementary Occupations). Occupations at Skill Level 2 typically require the performance of tasks such as operating machinery and electronic equipment; driving vehicles; maintenance and repair of electrical and mechanical equipment; and manipulation, ordering, and storage of information. Almost all occupations at Skill Level 2 require the ability to read information, make written records of work completed, and accurately perform simple arithmetical calculations. Many occupations at this skill level require a high level of manual dexterity (e.g., the minor categories of 311, 312, 510, 521, 421, 441, 772, 773, and 873). Occupations at Skill Level 3 typically require the performance of complex technical and practical tasks that rely upon an extensive body of factual, technical, and procedural knowledge in a specialized field (e.g., the minor categories of 248 and 252). Occupations at Skill Level 4 typically require the performance of tasks that rely upon complex problem-solving, decision-making, and creativity, and are based on an extensive body of theoretical and factual knowledge in a specialized field (e.g., the minor categories of 248 and 252).

The twenty occupations dominated by aged workers can be classified as: (a) "Elementary Occupations," in which aged workers can perform simple manual tasks without specific training, and (b) Skill Level 2 occupations, in which aged workers can continue to work due to the skills they acquired during their long time of employment. Very few aged workers were in occupations at Skill Levels 3 and 4.

Workers in the nine "Elementary Occupations" accounted for 42.3 percent of all aged workers, and 59.5 percent of aged workers were employed in the twenty occupations analyzed here. In Korea, the average retirement age from primary jobs is about fifty, after which most retirees get a series of second jobs, mostly low-quality "Elementary Occupations" [3]. They also tend to work at places with fewer employees, account for a smaller proportion of regular workers, and receive lower salaries than workers younger than fifty-five (table 9.1). Aged workers employed in Elementary Occupations often perform simple but physically demanding jobs in new environments and thus have increased risk of occupational injury. In addition, age-related musculoskeletal deterioration may increase the risk of occupational injuries in aged workers [12, 13]. Thus, aged workers are most susceptible to injury when employed in "Elementary Occupations."

In occupations at Skill Level 2, the skill and experience that aged workers have acquired over time may offset their decreased performance due to aging. However, aged manual workers in occupations at Skill Level 2 were exposed to job-specific hazards. According to the present study, "Automobile Drivers" are exposed to whole body vibration, compatible with previous studies [14–16], and "Service Workers Related to Medical and Welfare" are exposed to lifting or moving people, in agreement with previous study [17]. The present study also showed that "Chefs and Cooks" were exposed to high temperatures and long standing, compatible with previous studies [18, 19]. "Technical Workers Related to Construction" were exposed to vibrations, noises, awkward postures, carrying heavy loads, and long standing, as reported in a previous study [20]. "Technical Workers Related to Construction Finishing" were exposed to solvents.

However, workers in skilled nonmanual occupations were less likely to report most occupational hazards and work-related health problems. These low-risk occupations were "Clerks Related to Administration" (312), "Administration Clerks" (311), "Store Sales Workers" (521), "Sales Workers" (510), "Religious Professionals and Associate Professionals" (248), and "Teachers" (252).

Taken together, these results indicate we should focus on "Elementary Occupations," and then skilled manual occupations (e.g., "Automobile Drivers," "Service Workers Related to Medical and Welfare," "Chefs and Cooks," "Technical Worker Related to Construction," and "Construction Finishing") to improve the health and safety of aged workers. These target occupations employ about 60 percent of all aged workers, have greater proportions of aged workers, and have more occupational hazards.

The present study indicated that aged workers in the target occupations had more frequent exposure to ergonomic hazards, such as tiring or painful positions, carrying or moving heavy loads, and repetitive movements, and also had more work-related musculoskeletal disorders and general fatigue than the average for all aged workers.

Injury due to accident was frequently reported in machinery-handling occupations, such as "Technical Workers Related to Construction Finishing" and "Elementary Occupations Related to Production." In particular, the frequency of injury due to accident in aged workers who were "Technical Workers Related to Construction Finishing" and "Elementary Occupations Related to Production" were 5.9 and 4.7 percent, respectively, more than three times the average of all aged workers (1.4 percent). The present findings are compatible with those of previous papers [5, 20, 21]. In particular, aged workers who have poor muscle strength and elasticity and limited range of motion in joints, are more likely to complain of musculoskeletal symptoms and suffer from work-related injuries than young workers [4, 22]. The higher frequency of injury due to accident in aged workers who were in "Sales Workers" and "Religious Professionals and Associate Professionals" may be related to traffic accidents.

The present study has several strengths. We focused on high-risk workplaces that are dominated by aged workers, rather than on the entire population of aged workers. The work ability of aged workers can be efficiently and effectively maintained and promoted only when employers take a leadership role in activities that promote their work ability, and when the aged workers themselves actively participate in these activities in high-risk workplaces. In addition, job-specific risks for aged workers can be assessed in these workplaces, and this can provide better management of job-specific occupational hazards and establishment of age-friendly workplaces.

The present study also had several limitations. First, we used self-reported data, instead of objective findings. Second, we did a cross-sectional study. Therefore, we cannot infer causality.

The present study has several practical implications. First, we identified occupations that were dominated by aged workers. These occupations, "Elementary Occupations" in particular, should be the target of interventions that aim to improve the occupational safety and health of aged workers. Second, we assessed job-specific hazards and health problems in the different occupations that employ the most aged workers. This assessment provides a basis on which age-friendly occupational health and safety guidelines can be developed to improve the health and safety of aged workers.

CONCLUSIONS

Employers should try to reduce job-specific hazards to which aged workers are exposed to prevent work-related disorders in occupations dominated by aged workers. In addition, better prevention of ergonomic risk factors and preventive measures, such as a muscle strengthening and stretching program, may help to prevent work-related musculoskeletal disorders.

NOTE

1. This chapter was previously published as Park, Jungsun, Soo Geun Kim, Jong-shik Park, Boyoung Han, Kab Bae Kim, and Yangho Kim. "Hazards and health problems in occupations dominated by aged workers in South Korea." *Annals of Occupational and Environmental Medicine*, 29, no. 1 (2017): 27.

REFERENCES

1. Statistics Korea. *Population Projections*, 2010. Available at: http://kostat.go.kr/portal/korea/kor_nw/2/1/index.board?bmode=read&aSeq=252623. Accessed 29 December 2016.
2. United Nations. *World Population Prospects the 2008 Revision*, 2009. Available at: http://www.un.org/esa/population/publications/wpp2008/wpp2008_highlights.pdf. Accessed 29 December 2016.
3. Statistics Korea. *Economically Active Population Survey*, 2016. Available at: http://www.kostat.go.kr/portal/korea/kor_nw/2/3/2/index.board?bmode=read&aSeq=355178&pageNo=1&rowNum=10&amSeq=&sTarget=&sTxt=. Accessed 29 March 2017.
4. Lockhart TE, Smith JL, Woldstad JC. "Effects of aging on the biomechanics of slips and falls hum factors." *Hum Factors*. 2005;47:708–29.
5. Rhee KY, Seo DU. "Gender-specific incidence rate of industrial accidents and type of accident." *OSH Issue Rep*. 2014;8:2–29.
6. Korean Ministry of Employment and Labor. *Occupational Safety and Health Act*, 2015. Available at: http://www.law.go.kr/eng/engLsSc.do?menuId=&query=Occupational+safety+and+health+act.&x=0&y=0#liBgcolor20. Accessed 29 December 2016.
7. Park J, Park JT, Kim SG, Yoo CI, Son J, Yim J, et al. "Health care strategy for ensuring work ability in an aging Korea." *Ann Occup Environ Med.* 2016;28:42.
8. Statistics Korea. "Employment survey by area." *KOSIS*, 2014. Available at: http://kosis.kr/statisticsList/statisticsList_01List.jsp?vwcd=MT_ZTITLE&parentId=B#SubCont. Accessed 29 December 2016.
9. Statistics Korea. *Korean Standard Classification of Occupations*, 2016. Available at: http://kssc.kostat.go.kr/. Accessed 29 March 2017.
10. Park JS, Lee N. "First Korean working conditions survey: a comparison between South Korea and EU countries." *Ind Health.* 2009;47:50–4.
11. International Labor Office. *International Standard Classification of Occupations*, 2012. Available at: http://www.ilo.org/public/english/bureau/stat/isco/isco08/index.htm. Accessed 29 February 2017.
12. Kasch FW, Boyer JL, Van Camp SP, Verity LS, Wallace JP. "The effect of physical activity and inactivity on aerobic power in older men." *Phys Sportsmed.* 1990;18:73–83.
13. Smith EL, Gilligan C. "Physical activity for the older adult." *Fam Pract Recertif.* 1984;6(12):89–107.

14. Miyamoto M, Shirai Y, Nakayama Y, Gembun Y, Kaneda K. "An epidemiologic study of occupational low back pain in truck drivers." *J Nippon Med Sch.* 2000;67:186–90.
15. Hoy J, Mubarak N, Nelson S, Sweerts de Landas M, Magnusson M, Okunribido O, et al. "Whole body vibration and posture as risk factors for low back pain among forklift truck drivers." *J Sound Vib.* 2005;284:933–46.
16. Bovenzi M. "A longitudinal study of low back pain and daily vibration exposure in professional drivers." *Ind Health.* 2010;48:584–95.
17. Chang V, Hiller C, Keast E, Nicholas P, Su M, Hale L. "Musculoskeletal disorders in support workers in the aged care sector." *Phys Ther Rev.* 2013;18:185–206.
18. Haukka E, Leino-Arjas P, Solovieva S, Ranta R, Viikari-Juntura E, Riihimäki H. "Co-occurrence of musculoskeletal pain among female kitchen workers." *Int Arch Occup Environ Health.* 2006;80:141–8.
19. Hong Kong. *Final Report on the Study of Work-Related Musculoskeletal Disorders in Catering Industry in Hong Kong.* Occupational Safety & Health Council, Hong Kong, 2011. Available at: http://www.oshc.org.hk/oshc_data/files/OSHInformation/Musculoskeletal%20Disorders_Catering_Eng.pdf. Accessed 29 March 2017.
20. Holmström E, Engholm G. "Musculoskeletal disorders in relation to age and occupation in Swedish construction workers." *Am J Ind Med.* 2003;44:377–84.
21. Okunribido O, Wynn T. *Ageing and Work-Related Musculoskeletal Disorders. A Review of the Recent Literature. Research Report.* Health and Safety Executive, 2010. Available at: http://www.hse.gov.uk/research/rrpdf/rr799.pdf. Accessed 29 March 2017.
22. Zwart D, Frings-Dresen D. "Physical workload and the aging worker: a review of the literature." *Int Arch Occup Environ Health.* 1995;68:1–12.

Chapter 10

Relation between Overall Health Status and Environmental Satisfaction of Community Elders

Seonhye Lee, Chang Heon Cheong, and Jimee Kim

THE NEED FOR THE STUDY

Elderly[1] influence on the Korean society is growing with the rapid increase of their population and is expected to grow continuously, so it is becoming more necessary to understand them in depth. According to the 2011 population projection by Statistics Korea, the size of elderly population is estimated to reach 7.12 million in 2017, or 14.0 percent of the entire population, and 10.33 million in 2025, entering the age of 10 million elders (Jung, Oh, Kang, Kim, Seon-Woo, Oh, et al., 2014). Due to the retirement from the community, role change within the family, and physical aging process, the quality of life for elderlies may decline with accumulated physical and mental problems (Kim, Lee, & Park, 2010). The life expectancy of a 65-year-old person is 18.3 years for male and 22.8 years for female per the 2014 Senior Citizen Statistical Data (Statistics Korea, 2016), identifying health as the greatest concern for elderlies since they would be spending more of their advanced age in an unhealthy state (Lee, 2014).

Since 43.7 percent of the Korean elders consider themselves unhealthy and the elderly medical expense takes up 36.8 percent of the entire national expense with the amount being 3.43 million won per capita, about three times of the national average of 1.15 million won (Statistics Korea, 2016), the concern for elderly health is the most important challenge for both the national finance and the improvement of their quality of life. The health status in particular can significantly vary depending on the region, so health education programs and such must proceed with consideration of characteristics of the local environment (Lee, Park, & Kim, 2015). Importance of environment lies in its impact on mobility, safety from dangers and crimes, health-related behaviors, and social participations of the individual residents (Jung, 2010). Accordingly, the current research trend expands on the influence of regional environment on health and diseases (Son et al., 2010), being free of the limited perspectives which used to consider the regional factor only in the social-economic stance, and taking a multiangled approach in physical, social, cultural, and institutional aspects, such as land uses (Kim & Kang, 2011) and state of local sports facilities (Kim, Lee, Lee, & Lee, 2015), with many ongoing researches in multidisciplinary fields on the relationship between environment and health in a region (Belon & Nykiforuk, 2013; Kim & Kim, 2013; Kim, 2014; Kim & Kim, 2015; Lee, Park, & Kim, 2015; Renalds, Smith, & Hale, 2010).

For elderlies, their limited activity by the weakened physical strength is one of the major factors which make the environment of their community more important. Some recent studies are making progress on the relationship between elderly health and environment (Jung & Lee, 2015; Yi & Kim, 2015), yet there still lacks one that considers characteristics of elderly health.

Therefore, this study has been conducted to verify the relationship between health and environmental satisfaction of community elders, so that it can be utilized as a baseline study for development of community environment to help elders spend their remaining years healthier.

RESEARCH GOALS

The purpose of this study is to verify the relationship between overall health status and satisfaction on surrounding environment of community elders. The detailed goals are as follows:

1. To analyze the differences in overall health status, environment satisfaction, and health level by general characteristics.
2. To analyze the difference in overall health status by level of environment satisfaction.
3. To analyze the influence factors on overall health status.

METHODS

Research Design

This study is a descriptive correlation study to comprehend the relationship between overall health status and level of environment satisfaction of elder residents in communities.

Databases

The population data for this study was a total of 228,781 that consisted of 900 adults selected from each of the 254 public health centers in cities, districts, and boroughs for a community health study by Korea Centers for Disease Control (KCDC), and the 61,552 elders of over 65 were chosen for the data analysis. The data used in this study was provided, after the personal information was deleted, through an electrical counter of KCDC after a review and an approval for data use according to the raw data use protocol of "2013 Community Health Study."

Measurement

Overall Health Status

Overall health status was taken from the EuroGoL Visual Analogue Scale (EQ-VAS), designed to record on a scale the subjective and general health status of an individual on the day of measuring the health-related quality of life. The range is between 0 and 100, with the higher number indicating the better health (Kim, 2012).

Environment Satisfaction

Environment satisfaction is level of environment satisfaction regarding the overall level of safety, natural environment, living environment, traffic condition, and medical service in one's neighborhood. The score was summed up for the five questions with a "satisfactory" answer receiving 1 point each. The higher number indicated the higher level of environment satisfaction.

Health Level

Health level was taken as both the mental and the physical health problems experienced by an elder.

- Mental health problem

Mental health problem section consisted of four questions related to mental health, regarding stress, sadness, suicidal thoughts, and depression diagnosed by a doctor, and the answer score was summed up with "yes" receiving 1 point for each. The higher number indicated the worse mental health.

- Physical health problem

Physical health problem is on five diseases: high blood pressure, diabetes, hyperlipidemia, arthritis, and osteoporosis, which were the most frequent chronic diseases in elderlies over sixty according to the 2012 National Health and Nutritions Survey (2013). The answer score was summed up with "yes" receiving 1 point for each disease diagnosis by a doctor. The higher number indicated the worse physical health.

General Characteristics

General characteristics consisted of age, sex, marital status, education level, residential area, and residential periods. The residential area was categorized by the administration division, with the metropolitan and the rest as "rural areas," and the residential periods were categorized into "less than fifteen years" and "more than fifteen years," based on the fact that an average residential period of a rural resident is over fifteen years (Son et al., 2010).

Statistical Analysis

The data was translated to a SPSS file, which was then analyzed using IBM SPSS statistical software program (ver.22, IBM, Armonk, NY) for the general conditions, descriptive statistics for the level of health and environment satisfaction, *t*-test or ANOVA for the differences in level of health and environment satisfaction by general characteristics, Pearson's correlation for the correlation between the major factors, and multiple regression for the analysis of influence factors on overall health status. The significance level was <0.05.

RESULTS

General Characteristics, Health Level, Environment Satisfaction, and Overall Health Status of Subjects

The general characteristics of the subjects in this study were elders between sixty-five and seventy-four at 59.6 percent, 58.9 percent female, 69.1 percent of less than elementary education, 63.5 percent married, 76.6 percent of living in rural areas, and 86.1 percent of less than fifteen years of residence. The health score was 1.01 for mental health problem and 1.41 for physical health problem, whereas the average total score of environment satisfaction was 3.98 out of 5, in the order of 0.88 for natural environment, 0.87 for level of safety, 0.86 for living environment, 0.69 for medical service, and 0.68 for traffic condition. EQ-VAS, or the point for overall health status, was 62.63 (table 10.1).

Table 10.1 General Characteristics, Health Level, Environment Satisfaction, and Overall Health Status of Subjects (n = 61,552)

Variables			N (%)	M (SD)	Min-Max
General characteristics	Age (years)				
		65–74	36,678(59.6)		
		≥75	24,874(40.4)		
	Sex				
		Male	25,300(41.1)		
		Female	36,252(58.9)		
	Educational level				
		≤Primary	42,551(69.1)		
		Middle	8,008(13.0)		
		≥High	10,993(17.9)		
	Marital status				
		With spouse	39,072(63.5)		
		Without spouse	22,480(36.5)		
	Residential areas				
		Metropolitan	14,373(23.4)		
		Rural areas	47,179(76.6)		
	Residential period(years)†				
		<15	53,015(86.1)		
		≥15	8,530(13.9)		
Health level	Mental health problem†			1.01(0.53)	0.00–3.00
	Physical health problem†			1.41(1.15)	0.00–5.00
Environment satisfaction				3.98(1.20)	0.00–5.00
	Level of safety			0.87(0.34)	0.00–1.00
	Natural environment			0.88(0.32)	0.00–1.00
	Living environment			0.86(0.35)	0.00–1.00
	Traffic condition			0.68(0.47)	0.00–1.00
	Medical health service			0.69(0.46)	0.00–1.00
Overall health status†				62.63(21.33)	0.00–100.00

†Missing value involved.

Overall Health Status, Environment Satisfaction, and Health Level according to General Characteristics

The differences in the overall health status, environment satisfaction, and health level were as shown on table 10.2. The overall health status showed significant differences across all the general characteristics, whereas the environment showed significant differences for every factor except sex and

Table 10.2 Overall Health Status, Environment Satisfaction and Health Level According to General Characteristics (n = 61,552)

General Characteristics		*Overall Health Status*		*Environment Satisfaction*		*Mental Health Problem*		*Physical Health Problem*	
Variables	*Categories*	*M(SD)*	*t or F value*	*M(SD)*	*t or F value*	*M(SD)*	*t or F value*	*M(SD)*	*t or F value*
Age (years)	65–74	65.21 (20.48)	36.753*	3.96 (1.21)	–4.365*	0.98 (0.52)	–15.217*	1.41 (1.16)	–1.568
	≥75	58.82 (21.99)		4.00 (1.19)		1.05 (0.55)		1.42 (1.13)	
Sex	Male	67.13 (20.16)	44.317*	3.98 (1.21)	–0.196	1.00 (0.47)	–4.214*	0.97 (0.93)	–84.477*
	Female	59.49 (21.57)		3.98 (1.20)		1.01 (0.57)		1.72 (1.18)	
Educational level	≤Primary	59.52 (21.69)	1634.075*	3.97 (1.21)	4.591*	0.97 (0.50)	–21.806*	1.29 (1.11)	–35.413*
	Middle	67.05 (19.37)		3.97 (1.22)		1.07 (0.57)		1.63 (1.18)	
	≥High	71.41 (18.04)		3.96 (1.22)		1.00 (0.53)		1.45 (1.17)	
Marital status	With spouse	64.94 (20.83)	35.715*	3.99 (1.19)	4.591*	0.97 (0.50)	–21.806*	1.29 (1.11)	–35.413*
	Without spouse	58.60 (21.61)		3.95 (1.22)		1.07 (0.57)		1.63 (1.18)	
Residential area	Metropolitan	65.60 (20.29)	19.065*	4.05 (1.22)	8.039*	1.00 (0.53)	–2.794*	1.45 (1.17)	4.062*
	Rural areas	61.73 (21.56)		3.96 (1.20)		1.01 (0.54)		1.40 (1.14)	
Residential periods (years)	<15	66.47 (20.44)	17.918*	3.78 (1.32)	–16.460*	1.03 (0.54)	4.191*	1.46 (1.19)	3.915*
	≥15	62.01 (21.41)		4.01 (1.18)		1.00 (0.53)		1.41 (1.14)	

education level. The group of elders between sixty-four and seventy-four, male, more than high school education, married, living in metropolitan, and less than fifteen years of residence showed a significantly high overall health status. As for the environment satisfaction, the group of over seventy-five, married, living in metropolitan, for more than fifteen years showed a significantly high satisfaction level (table 10.2).

In the health level, the mental health problem showed significant differences across all the general characteristics, whereas the physical health problem showed significant differences for all factors except age. The mental health problem was significantly greater in the group of over seventy-five, female, less than elementary education, not married, living in rural areas, and less than fifteen years of residence. The physical health problem was significantly greater in the group of female, less than elementary education, not married, living in metropolitan, and less than fifteen years of residence. Both the mental and physical health problems were greater in the group of female, less than elementary education, not married, and less than fifteen years of residence (table 10.2).

Overall Health Status and Health Level according to Environment Satisfaction

The overall health status showed significant differences in all items by environment satisfaction, whereas the mental and physical health problem showed significant differences for level of safety, natural environment, and traffic condition (table 10.3). The group with the higher overall satisfaction on level of safety, natural environment, and traffic condition showed a low level of mental and physical health problem and a high overall health status. The group with the higher satisfaction on living environment and medical service showed only a high overall health status score.

Correlation between Major Variables

The correlation between major variables is shown in table 10.4. The overall health status represents a positive correlation between environment satisfaction (r = 0.103, $p < 0.05$), and mental health problem ($r = -0.048$, $p < 0.05$) and physical health problem ($r = -0.181$, $p < 0.05$) indicates a negative relationship.

Effects Variables on the Overall Health Status

The effects of analyzing the effects of the overall health status are shown in table 10.5. Overall health status (Adj. $R^2 = 0.101$ $F = 762.537$, $p < 0.05$) was

Table 10.3 Overall Health Status and Health Level According to Environment Satisfaction ($n = 61,552$)

				Health level			
		Overall Health Status		*Mental Health Problem*		*Physical Health Problem*	
Variables	*Characteristics*	*M(SD)*	*t-value*	*M(SD)*	*t-value*	*M(SD)*	*t-value*
Level of safety	Satisfaction	64.00(21.27)	10.952*	1.00(0.52)	–4.791*	1.40(1.14)	–5.851*
	Dissatisfaction	60.23(21.60)		1.03(0.60)		1.49(1.18)	
Natural environment	Satisfaction	62.76(21.30)	4.127*	1.01(0.53)	–2.427*	1.41(1.14)	–3.176*
	Dissatisfaction	61.66(21.57)		1.02(0.57)		1.45(0.18)	
Living environment	Satisfaction	62.99(21.25)	10.145*	1.01(0.53)	–0.397	1.41(1.15)	–1.173
	Dissatisfaction	60.51(21.67)		1.01(0.57)		1.43(1.15)	
Traffic condition	Satisfaction	64.14(20.86)	25.730*	1.00(0.52)	–4.430*	1.40(1.15)	–4.439*
	Dissatisfaction	59.40(21.97)		1.02(0.56)		1.44(1.15)	
Medical health service	Satisfaction	63.88(21.02)	21.763*	1.01(0.52)	–1.177	1.41(1.15)	–0.161
	Dissatisfaction	59.82(21.76)		1.01(0.56)		1.41(1.14)	

*$p < 0.05$.

Table 10.4 Correlation between Major Variables (n = 61,552)

Variables	*Overall Health Status*	*Environment Satisfaction*	*Mental Health Problem*	*Physical Problem*
Overall health status	1.00			
Environment satisfaction	0.103*	1.00		
Mental health problem	–0.048*	–0.017*	1.00	
Physical health problem	–0.181*	–0.019*	0.034*	1.00

$^{*}p < 0.05$.

Table 10.5 Effects Variables on the Overall Health Status (n = 61,552)

	ß	*t-value*
Constant(B)	(56.840)	12.744*
Age	–0.112	27.845*
Sex	0.065	13.850*
Educational level	0.125	29.769*
Marital status	0.036	8.072*
Residential area	0.044	-11.225*
Residential periods	–0.046	-11.730*
Mental health problem	–0.030	-7.756*
Physical health problem	–0.142	-34.956*
Environment satisfaction	0.103	26.677*
Adj. R^2 : .101 F : 762.537* Durbin Watson : 1.660		

$^{*}p < 0.05$, ‡Referent group: age (≥75 = 1), sex (male = 1), educational level (≥high school = 1), marital status (with spouse = 1), residential areas (metropolitan = 1), length of living (≥15 = 1).

explained as 10.1 percent through age (β = –0.112), sex (β = 0.065), educational level(β = 0.125), marital status (β = 0.036), residential area (β = 0.044), residential periods (β = –0.046), mental health problem (β = –0.030), physical health problem (β = –0.142) and environment satisfaction (β = 0.103) (table 10.5).

DISCUSSION

This study was done to comprehend the relationship between health and environment satisfaction of community elders using data from the Korean Community Health Study conducted in 2013.

Community elders had an average of 1.01 mental health problems and 1.41 physical health problems, indicating that a Korean elder suffers about one mental problem among stress, sadness, suicidal thought, and depression, and more than one physical problem among high blood pressure, diabetes, hyperlipidemia, arthritis, and osteoporosis. The mental physical health problems were significantly more in the group of female elders, less than elementary education, not married, living in rural areas, and less than fifteen years of residence. A factual survey on elders revealed that 90.4 percent of the entire elderly population had at least one chronic illness, and 72.2 percent suffered multiple. In the case of depression, a common mental health problem, the likeliness of elderlies over eighty-five to suffer it was more than twice of that of ones between sixty-five and sixty-nine, and was also high in unmarried cases (Jung et al., 2014). This study also showed a high occurrence of mental health problems in elders over seventy-five with statistical significance. According to a 2015 study by Statistics Korea on mortality due to intentional self-injury (e.g., suicide) in elders over 65, 58.6 suicides per 100,000 was reported with the highest suicide rate among ones over eighty. The rapid increase of super-aged population indicates the same increase of demand for mental care service for community elders, and since most elders suffer chronic illnesses, they require more active management solution for integrated mental physical health problems.

The overall health status for elders in this study was 62.63 in average. The EQ-VAS for elders over sixty-five according to the 2010–2012 National Health and Nutrition Survey data (Lee, 2014) was 70.0 for male, and 63.7 for female, and the value in the study on elders with arthritis (Yang & An, 2011) was 64.03, so the even lower score of the subjects in this study indicates a lack of improvement in elderly health. The group of elders over seventy-five, female, less than high school education, unmarried, living in rural areas, and more than fifteen years of residence showed a significantly lower overall health status. Korea in particular have more physical laborers living in farming and fishing rural areas than in large cities (MOHW·KCDC, 2010), and the lower score for females agrees with the result by Lee (2014) in which the female elders also had the lower scores than the males, the result of which Kim (2013) viewed as the dispositional difference in men taking physical illness or damage less seriously than women. Such individual characteristics seem to result from the reality of an abundance of less-educated female elders living alone in a rural area for an extensive time.

Environment satisfaction was 3.98 out of 5 which was a relatively higher level of satisfaction, with natural environment, level of safety, and living environment scoring higher than 80 when converted to a percentage value, but medical service and traffic condition scored only 68–69 revealing a large disparity. During the elderly ages with diminished physiologic functions, the resulting limited mobility and frequent visits to medical facilities seemed to lead to the lower satisfaction level than other environmental factors. Lopez (2012) also pointed out that many elders who no longer drove could have problems living in non-walkable environment or place without appropriate transportation options. Medical service as a part of social service infrastructure is a basic requirement important in personal well-being, and traffic condition as a public infrastructure is closely related to environmental well-being. Such factors are basic needs for residents, and must be resolved before creating a livable city (Cho & Hwang, 2014). Traffic and medical services in particular are among the requirements for Age-Friendly Cities according to WHO, so there must be an establishment of age-friendly policies and development of environment for elders with the limited activity and various health problems.

Considering that environment satisfaction is an influence factor for elderly health and that residents of metropolitan have a significantly high level of environment satisfaction, clearly the health and environment conditions for the elderly rural residents are relatively poorer. Kim's study (2014) suggested a need to improve medical care accessibility and spatial equity, as a minute increase of hospital arrival time for an elderly in rural areas would reduce the chance to receive a necessary medical care by about 0.92 percent. The study by Kim & An (2011) also showed that a good physical environment in neighborhood has a role in promoting physical activities for elders and has a positive impact on their mental health, since places with fine pedestrian environment and well-made public transportation system have active senior welfare centers, senior citizen centers, and clan gatherings, leading to improved physical health and reduced depression. Kim & Kim (2013) stressed that an individual in an inadequate neighborhood shows a poor health status stemming from the negative perception of the surroundings, so it is important not just for a local government to improve the environment but also for the residents to have a positive perception of it. Jung and Cho (2005) also said that a subjective evaluation by the individuals should be included in residential characteristics. However, they noted that in Korea, unlike in the western world, people of high and low socioeconomical status coexist within a single administration division. According to them, how to conceptualize the regional units is an important factor when studying the regional impact on individual health status.

Therefore, an improvement of localized medical service for elderlies must be done through its subdivision into the smaller administration division and their analysis to understand the regional factor of environment in elderly health. Additionally, to understand and improve factors influencing the subjective perception of elders on their environment satisfaction, there must be a network of experts with various academic backgrounds in important factors of daily lives for elderlies, such as housing, traffic, food, medical, public health, and others, aided by attention of the local governments in support of its operation and collaboration.

While this study is a secondary analysis using the raw data in 2013 Community Health Survey and thus is limited in understanding of characteristics of each concepts, its significance lies in the consideration of physical environment for study of elderly health. Future studies need to establish the empirical evidence for the relation with health and environment and the strategies development for the elderly well-being through repeated studies of living environment and health outcome.

CONCLUSION

This study was conducted to confirm the relationship between health of elders over sixty-five in all parts of the country and their environment through a secondary analysis of the raw data in 2013 Community Health Survey.

The result showed that age, sex, education level, marital status, residential area, residential periods, mental health problem, physical health problem, and environment satisfaction accounted for 10.1 percent in the overall health status value of the Korean elderly. Female and unmarried residents living in rural areas scored worse in all health level, such as the mental, physical health problems, and overall health status, so specialized policies and services for them must be offered to minimize the inequality of available health services.

In summary of the results, the elders over seventy-five scored worse in both mental health problem and overall health status, indicating a need for an improved mental care service specialized for the elders in later years. For evaluation of health services for elders, the overall health status value summarized in one visual item appears to be a useful evaluation tool for elders and caregivers, as it can reduce inconveniences and excessive time consumption which can arise during application of various evaluation tools to elders. Therefore, any later study must conduct a comparison study with other comprehensive evaluation tools for its validity verification. Also, improving the health status of elderly rural residents would require cares for physical mental health problems on an individual level, attention for improving environment satisfaction on an environmental level, and preparation of measures with multidisciplinary and integral approaches. As such, a later study requires a repetition study of impact by environment satisfaction on health, and a classification study with a multilevel statistical analysis to understand impact level of each regional characteristic.

NOTE

1. This chapter was previously published as Lee, Seonhye, Chang Heon Cheong, and Jimee Kim. "Relation between Overall Health Status and Environmental Satisfaction of Community Elders." *Journal of Korean Living Environment System* 24, no. 4 (2017): 517–525.

REFERENCES

Belon, A. P. & Nykiforuk, C. (2013). "Possibilities and challenges for physical and social environment research in Brazil: a systematic literature review on health behaviors," *Cadernos de saúde pública*, 29(10), 1955–73. doi:10.1590/0102-311X00044513.

Cho, N. S. & Hwang, E. J. (2014). "A Comparative study on conditions of a livable city," *Collection of Social Science Research*, 30(2), 235–267.

Jung, K. H., Oh, K. H., Kang, E. N., Kim, J. H., Seonwoo, D., Oh, M. A., et al. (2014). *2014 Survey of Senior Citizens*. Ministry of Health and Welfare & Korea Institute for Health and Social Affairs.

Jung, K. H. (2010). "International trends in the establishment of age-friendly cities: background and significance," *Health and Welfare Forum*, 10, 102–112.

Jung, Y. J. & Lee, S. G. (2015). "The study on the causality among built environment, social relationship, and health of the elderly," *Journal of the Korean Regional Development Association*, 27(2), 75–94.

Jung, S. W. & Cho, Y. T. (2005). "Neighborhood characteristics and individual health under Korean context," *Journal of Preventive Medicine Public Health*, 38(3), 259–266.

Kim, E. J. & Kang, M. G. (2011). "Effects of built environment and individual characteristics on health condition," *Journal of the Korean Regional Science Association*, 27(3), 27–42.

Kim, E. J. & Kim, T. H. (2014). "Healthy-friendly environmental correlates of population health," *The Korea Spatial Planning Review*, 81, 185–200.

Kim, H. K., Lee, H. J., & Park, M. (2010). "Factors influencing quality of life in elderly women living alone," *Journal of Korean Gerontological Society*, 30(2), 279–292.

Kim, H. R. (2014). "Predicting factors of health related quality of life among older adults at senior centers in Korea," *Journal of Korean Gerontological Nursing*, 16(2), 95–106.

Kim, J. I. (2013). "Level of health-related quality of life(EQ-5D) and its related factors among variable elders receiving home visiting health care services in some rural areas," *Journal of Korean Academy Community Health Nursing*, 24(1), 99–109.

Kim, J. M., Lee, S. H., Lee, E. Y., & Lee, H. Y. (2015). "Community-based environment and walking among adults," *Journal of the Korean Society of Living Environment System*, 22(1), 75–86.

Kim, S. N. (2014). "The effect of the physical environment on walking behavior, medical service utilization, and EQ-5D results of the elderly in rural areas: a multilevel path analysis with complex survey data," *Statistics Research*, 19(2), 99–126.

Kim, T. H. (2012). *Validity and Reliability Evaluation for EQ-5D in the General Population of South Korea*. Unpublished Doctoral Dissertation, The University of Ulsan, Ulsan.

Kim, Y. J. & An, K. H. (2011). "Influences of neighborhood's physical environments on physical and mental health to the elderly," *Journal of Urban Design Institute of Korea*, 12(6), 89–99.

Kim, W. J. & Kim, T. Y. (2013). "A study on the neighborhood physical and social environment and health: the mediating role of perceived environments," *Journal of Community Welfare*, 46, 23–47.

Lee, H. S. (2014). "The factors influencing health-related quality of life in the elderly-focused on the general characteristics, health habits, mental health, chronic disease, and nutrient intake status: data from the fifth Korea National Health and Nutrition Examination Survey(KNHANES V), 2010–2012," *Korea Journal of Community Nutrition*, 19(5), 479–489. doi:10.5720/kjen.2014.19.5.479.

Lee, J. A., Park, J. H., & Kim, M. (2015). "Social and physical environments and self-rated health in urban and rural communities in Korea," *International Journal of Environmental Research and Public Health*, 12, 14329–14341. doi:10.3390/ijerph121114329.

Lopez, R. P. (2012). *The Built Environment and Public Health* (1st ed.). San Francisco, CA: Wiley.

Ministry of Health and Welfare Korea Centers for Disease Control and Prevention. (2010). *2009 National Health Statistics: Korea National Health and Nutrition Examination Survey IV-3.* Seoul: Ministry of Health and Welfare Korea Centers for Disease Control and Prevention.

Ministry of Health and Welfare Korea Centers for Disease Control and Prevention. (2013). *National Health Statistics National Health and Nutrition Survey 5th Year 3rd Year*, 2012.

Renalds, A., Smith, T. H., & Hale, P. J. (2010). "A systematic review of built environment and health," *Family & Community Health*, 33(1), 68–78. doi:10.1097/FCH.0b013e3181c4e2e5.

Son, K. Y., Kim, M. K., Kim, J. Y., Na, S. W., Wi, J. Y., Lee, Y. R., et al. (2010). "Investigation of association between social capital and health-related quality of life among residents in a rural area," *Korean Journal of Health Promotion*, 10, 113–122.

Statistics Korea. (2016). *2016 Statistics of the Aged.* http://kostat.go.kr/portal/korea/kor_nw/2/6/5/index.board?bmode=read&aSeq=356426.

Yang, S. J. & An, J. S. (2010). "Health status, health behavior and quality of life in the elderly with osteoarthritis," *Nursing Science*, 23(2), 23–33.

Yi, Y. J. & Kim, E. J. (2015). "The effects of accessibility to medical facilities and public transportation on perceived health of urban and rural elderly: using generalized ordered logic model," *Journal of Korea Regional Development Association*, 27(1), 65–88.

Chapter 11

The Effect of Health and Functional Limitation on Sexual Life Satisfaction

Evidence from Elderly Korean Couples

Jaeeon Yoo

Sexual[1] life encompasses vaginal intercourse for reproduction and various sexual activities including petting, oral sex, and masturbation (DeLamater & Karraker, 2009). Sexual life provides a variety of meanings to elderly couples including power, the vitality of life, pleasure, the flower of life, the necessities of life, the expression of love between couples, the passage of sympathy, emotional satisfaction, seasoning and flavoring life, and usefulness as a woman (Lee, 2014, 2016). The sexual life satisfaction of the elderly is closely related to ego-integrity (Choi, 2008), depression (Ganong & Larson, 2011), couple relations (DeLamater, Hyde, & Fong, 2008; Lodge & Umberson, 2012), life satisfaction (Hwang & Shin, 2012), and successful aging and happiness (Karraker, DeLamater, & Schwartz, 2011). Although there is no official statistical data on the sexual life of the Korean elderly, previous studies using in-depth interviews and surveys with convenience sampling consistently reported that many Korean elderly people had active sexual lives (Shin & Park, 2014). A study conducted on American elderly couples showed that approximately 70.1 percent had engaged in sexual activities within the past 12 months (Karraker & DeLamater, 2013). The results of these studies revealed that although sexual functioning had deteriorated and physical health had declined with age, libido was maintained (DeLamater & Sil, 2005), and the elderly could continue various types of sexual activities into their seventies, eighties, and nineties (DeLamater & Moorman, 2007; Lodge & Umberson, 2012) with the help of sexual enhancers (e.g., erectile-dysfunction medicine and vaginal lubricants) (Kingsberg, 2002).

Sexual life is an important part of the life of the elderly and many elderly people have an active sexual life. However, a previous report (Kim & Lee,

2013) showed that only 30.3 percent of South Korean elderly were satisfied with their sex lives. Although the majority of elderly people are dissatisfied with their sex lives, there is little social support to improve the sexual satisfaction of the elderly, and it is not easy to publicize the topic in the fields of academia, media, or politics (Gott & Hinchliff, 2003). Biological age in itself is not a direct obstacle to having a sexual life (Gott & Hinchliff, 2003). However, the cognitive, psychological, and social schemes that a sex life symbolizes, such as vitality, pleasure, beauty, and youth, have become popularized by the mass media. Consequently, the wrinkled face of the elderly individual or the no longer trim body is mistakenly perceived as having little sexual attraction (Montemurro & Gillen, 2013; Montemurro & Siefken, 2014). The sexual activities of the elderly have been suppressed in South Korea because ageism and a male-oriented sexual regime have dominated society (Laumann et al., 2006). Our objective in this study was to pose the necessity of developing counseling and education, nursing, and long-term care services for improving the elderly's satisfaction with their sexual lives.

This is a starting point for developing sexual counseling and sex education programs that raise awareness of the theme of a sexual life in elderly individuals, and ultimately lead them to experiencing a pleasant and satisfying sexual life. Our intention was to evaluate how physical and cognitive health and the limitations in living independently as a husband and a wife mutually affected the sexual satisfaction of elderly couples. The uniqueness of this study was to analyze survey data representing the elderly living in South Korea according to the couple as a unit, and to simultaneously estimate the effects on each party; by focusing on the physical and cognitive problems and the mediating effects of the limitations in independent living caused by those problems it is possible to highlight the gender differences in these relationships.

LITERATURE REVIEW

Theories: The Linked Lives Perspective and Intersectionality

The linked lives perspective is one of the core principles of life-course theory, and it is useful for explaining the relationship between the health of elderly couples and their satisfaction with their sex lives (Angela, 1996; Lodge & Umberson, 2012). According to this perspective, the couples' health is closely related, and the results of their interactions are accumulated over the life course because the members of a family share daily life and exchange care (Elder, 1994). This perspective suggests that physical and cognitive health, and the sexual life of couples are closely related, and the pattern is more distinctive for elderly couples who have shared their daily life and sexual life for decades (Biddle & Yap, 2010; Elder, 1998; Franks, Lucas,

Stephens, Rook, & Gonzalez, 2010). When one half of an elderly couple has restrictions on the activities of daily living (ADL) or the instrumental activities of daily living (IADL), the spouse becomes a primary caregiver (Wolff & Kasper, 2006), and it becomes harder to maintain a sexual life in the same way as before (Lee, 2014). Consequently, deterioration in physical or cognitive health and the restrictions of independent living can hinder both husband and wife's satisfaction in their sexual life (Kim & Hong, 2016; Lee, 2014; Yoo, 2017).

It is possible to understand the sexual life of the elderly couples better by integrating the linked lives perspective and the perspective of intersectionality (Lodge & Umberson, 2012). The concept of intersectionality is primarily used in women's studies; however, the main idea of this perspective is to respect the diversity of subgroups that are subgroups whose identities may be suppressed by belonging to a wider group. From this perspective, a husband and a wife may give different meanings and values to their sex life (Hirayama & Walker, 2011; Karraker & DeLamater, 2013; Karraker, DeLamater, & Schwartz, 2011) owing to the gender ideologies of masculinity and femininity, which have been constructed in their contemporary manner for several decades (Lodge & Umberson, 2012; Waite, Laumann, Das, & Schumm, 2009). Although this relationship between exogenous and endogenous variables can be explained logically according to the two theories (i.e., linked lives and intersectionality), there is no empirical study that evaluates how the limitations in physical and cognitive health affect a couple's satisfaction in their sexual life in Korea. Our aim is to provide empirical evidence for this relationship in an East Asian context.

Physical and Cognitive Health, Independent Living, and Sexual Life Satisfaction in Elderly Couples

This section will examine what is known about this topic by reviewing previous studies on the physical and cognitive health problems, limitations in independent living, and sexual life satisfaction of elderly couples. Moreover, it will identify the issues to be evaluated further in this study. Some studies have argued that sexual life satisfaction varies according to the age, gender, and household income of the elderly husbands and wives (Kim, 2018; Kim & Lee, 2013; Yoo, 2017). However, other studies have reported contradictory results, namely that sexual life satisfaction can be maintained at a high level, although the pattern of sexual relations changes and frequency decreases as the couple ages (Kim & Lee, 2013; Lee, 2014; Lindau et al., 2007; Lodge & Umberson, 2012). Some research has claimed that deteriorating health rather than biological age influences the sexual life directly and negatively (Karraker, DeLamater, & Schwartz, 2011; Shin & Park, 2014). However, there are arguments that take an opposing perspective. For example, Waite et al. (2009) reported that mental health is more closely related to dissatisfaction with sexual life than physical health. Previous studies have also revealed that the prescribed medicine for chronic diseases causes a loss of libido only in female patients and that diagnosed chronic diseases do not affect various sexual activities including petting, oral sex, and masturbation (DeLamater & Moorman, 2007). Moreover, physical sexual dysfunctions can be overcome by using sexual function enhancers (Kingsberg, 2002). Overall, many researchers agree that the elderly individual's gender is related to their sexual functioning, libido, and sexual life satisfaction. However, different opinions exist on whether the main factor hindering sexual life satisfaction is biological age, physical health, or mental health. It is difficult to find a dyadic-structure study that evaluates the effects of the husband or wife's health on their own sexual life satisfaction in elderly Korean couples.

The results of previous studies did not agree on the relationships among age, physical health, cognitive functioning, and the sexual life satisfaction of the elderly. It is possible that the limitations in independent living, which occur when age, physical health issues, or deteriorated cognitive functions exceed a certain level, may affect the sexual life satisfaction of a partner. This is because the limitations in independent living due to a physical health issue or worsened cognitive functions can have adverse effects on the marital relationship between an elderly person with a health problem and a spouse providing care. The elderly, who have health issues due to chronic illness or who use long-term care services, also have a desire for a sexual life (Doll, 2013). An elderly person, who needs long-term care, and his or her spouse have more severe difficulties in engaging in a sexual life than those who live independently, thus their sexuality is neglected and excluded from the subject of sexual life support (Doll, 2013; Harris, Adams, Zubatsky, & White, 2011). Studying the sexual lives of the elderly who have limitations in independent living and identifying measures to support them is therefore particularly a timely issue (Bentrott & Margrett, 2011; Frankowski & Clark, 2009).

The Current Study

We examined whether the linked life perspective actually explained the relationship between the health of the elderly couple and sexual life satisfaction; our aim was to complement and develop several tasks identified by previous studies conducted on the sexual life satisfaction of the elderly. First, most previous studies conducted surveys or in-depth interviews with the elderly using a specific facility in a specific area and adopting convenience sampling; these studies recommended that follow-up studies should use data representing the whole population (Hwang & Shin, 2012; Yoo, 2017). Therefore, our intention was to verify the results of previous studies by using the Survey on Elderly Life Conditions (SELC) in 2011, which is representative of the elderly in South Korea.

Second, the sexual life and satisfaction of a married person should be considered as a bilateral relationship, but previous studies analyzed data at the individual level and could not adequately reflect the characteristics of the spouse (Kim & Lee, 2013). Therefore, we analyzed the physical and cognitive health of the husband and the wife, their limitations in independent living, and how their individual sexual life satisfaction influenced their partner by using the Actor-Partner Interdependence Model (APIM) (Cook & Kenny, 2005).

Third, sexual life satisfaction in the later period of life is not solely determined by biological age or the level of physical and cognitive functioning, and it may differ because of the occurrence of limitations in independent living. However, it is difficult to identify previous studies examining the effects of the limitations caused by the deteriorated physical and cognitive health of a husband or a wife and how they affect sexual life satisfaction. Therefore, we evaluated how the limitations in the couple's independent living affected each other's sexual life satisfaction by focusing on the mediating effects.

Lastly, our aim was to conduct analyses emphasizing intersectionality whereby the elderly were divided into various subgroups having diverse and different attributes, because it was not clear how the factors affecting their sexual life satisfaction differed specifically according to physical health, cognitive function, actor, partner, and gender.

Objectives and Research Questions

Our objective was both to seek ways to improve the sexual life satisfaction of the elderly and guarantee the sexual rights of those who had poor physical and cognitive health conditions and limitations in independent living. To accomplish this objective, we analyzed the data of 1,930 couples over sixty-five years old from the SELC in 2011, which represented the elderly of South Korea, and conducted an extended version of the APIM analysis.

The specific research questions were as follows:

- Question 1: How do the physical health problems and worse cognitive functions of elderly couples directly affect the sexual life satisfaction of the husband and the wife?
- Question 2: What are the mediating effects of the limitations in independent living due to physical health problems and the worsened cognitive functions on the individuals' sexual life satisfaction?

- Question 3: Are there direct effects of the physical health problems and worsened cognitive function on sexual life satisfaction and do the indirect effects mediated by independent living differ by actor, partner, or gender?

METHOD

Data and Subjects

The subjects in this study were 1,930 couples representative of elderly couples older than 65 years living in South Korea. We used the SELC (2011) conducted by the Ministry of Health and Welfare and the Korea Institute for Health and Social Affairs to analyze information regarding sexual life satisfaction, cognitive functioning, independent living, age, and household income. The SELC in 2011 was carried out according to Article 5 of the Welfare of the Aged Act; it targeted 10,674 elderly people (65 years old or older) residing in 3,142 survey districts created by applying a stratified two-stage cluster sampling method to cities and provinces. Sixty-eight professionally trained investigators visited the houses and interviewed subjects; the information obtained was subsequently verified by phone interviews with over 91 percent of respondents. We obtained consent from participants before collecting sensitive information on sexual life satisfaction and informed participants that they could voluntarily refuse to answer an uncomfortable question or end their participation in the study at any time. Furthermore, investigators were trained on these issues before conducting the interviews. We also received Institutional Review Board (IRB) approval from our institution so as to comply with established research ethics before conducting the study and analyzing the data obtained. The SELC data collected through this process in 2011 are not only representative and credible but also include a variety of material about the sexual life satisfaction, physical and cognitive health, independent living, and social and demographic characteristics of the couples thus it provided data suitable for the analytic purposes of this study.

The elderly couple in a dyadic structure (rather than an individual elderly person) was used as a unit of analysis because we examined the bilateral relationship between a husband and a wife. To analyze the couple unit, we excluded 2,508 subjects who did not have a spouse, who had a spouse but one member of the couple was younger than 65, or those where only one member participated in the SELC in 2011. Most of the subjects excluded from the study had either had their spouses die or had spouses who were too under sixty-five. Moreover, sixty-eight subjects were excluded from the study because their spouses were very ill (e.g., dementia and long-term hospitalization), and they could not answer the SELC questions directly. An additional seventy-seven subjects were excluded from the analysis because they denied answering questions related to sexual life satisfaction, a dependent variable of this study. Finally, we used 1,930 couples (total 3,860 individual persons: 1,930 husbands and 1,930 wives), who were over sixty-five years old and responded to the survey as study subjects.

MEASURES

Endogenous Variables

Sexual Life Satisfaction of a Husband and a Wife

Sexual life satisfaction was evaluated by one item ("Overall, how satisfied are you with your current sexual life?") and each husband and wife selected one of very satisfied, satisfied, average, unsatisfied, and very unsatisfied. These responses were coded as 5, 4, 3, 2, and 1, respectively; a higher score meant higher satisfaction with their sexual life.

Mediators: Limitations in the Independent Living of a Husband and a Wife

When a respondent indicated that the person needed the other's help for any of the seven ADL items or any of the ten IADL items, ADL or IADL was scored as 1. When a respondent could do all seven ADL items or all ten IADL items, ADL or IADL was scored as 0. The seven ADL items are (1) dressing; (2) washing face, teeth cleaning, and shampooing; (3) bathing or showering; (4) eating; (5) lying down, getting up, and moving; (6) using the bathroom, cleaning after using a toilet, and dressing; and (7) controlling bladder and bowel movements. The ten IADL items are (1) dressing; (2) household chores; (3) preparing meals; (4) laundry; (5) taking prescribed medicine on time; (6) financial management; (7) going out to nearby areas; (8) making purchasing decisions, paying money, and receiving change; (9) making and receiving telephone calls; and (10) using transportation.

Exogenous Variables

Physical Health Problems

The latent variable of physical health problems consisted of the number of chronic diseases diagnosed by a medical doctor that had persisted over three months, and the number of prescribed medications that the subject had been taking for more than three months. Chronic disease, the first observation variable, included thirty-four diseases (possible range: 0–34) encompassing circulatory, endocrine, musculoskeletal, respiratory, sensory, cancer, digestive, genitourinary, and other disease categories. In this study, subjects had a minimum of zero and a maximum of six diseases. Medication, the second observation variable, ranged from 0 to 10. The latent variables of physical health problems consisted of chronic diseases and medication. Greater value indicated that there were more physical health problems.

Worse Cognitive Function

The cognitive functions of the elderly were measured using the Mini-Mental State Examination-Korean Version (MMSE-KC) scale (range: 0–30). This was coded by multiplying the raw score of the cognitive function by −1 to make it easy to interpret the results according to the physical health score (higher score = poorer health). In other words, a higher cognitive function score meant a more severe decline of cognitive function.

Control Variables: Husband Age, Wife Age, and Household Income

We included age and household income as control variables in the analytic model of this study because previous studies reported that they were closely related to physical and cognitive health, and to sexual life satisfaction (Kim & Lee, 2013; Yoo, 2017). The age of the study subjects ranged between 65 and 101. The first, second, third, fourth, and fifth quintiles of annual gross household income were below 7.63, 764–11.93, 11.94–18.49, 18.50–31.70, and over 31.71 KRW million, respectively.

Data Analysis

Figure 11.1 shows the conceptual framework of the study. This conceptual framework assumed that a decrease in the physical and cognitive health of a husband or a wife would cause limitations in independent living and these factors could affect the sexual life satisfaction of either the husband or wife. We used an extended version of APIM for this analysis. The strength of APIM is that it can quantify the effects of an actor's attributes on a partner and vice versa by using multiple people having close interactions as a group (Cook & Kenny, 2005). The application of APIM, which considers the characteristics of both people, is appropriate because the sexual life of elderly couples involves the physical and emotional interaction between a husband and a wife; a spouse becomes a primary caregiver

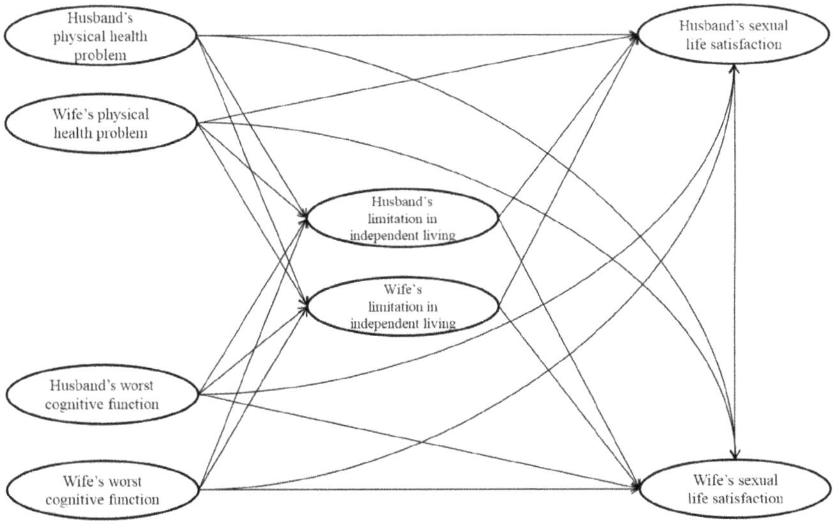

Figure 11.1 The Analytical Framework for the Study.

when the other person has physical and cognitive limitations in independent living. The extended version of APIM was used to reflect the mediating effects in the interdependent relationship between the husband and the wife because the physical health problem and the decline in cognitive function could induce limitations to independent living, and these factors could, at the same time, influence the sexual life satisfaction of the couple. It also has several advantages as it is based on full information maximum likelihood method (FIML), which includes missing cases of exogenous variables, minimizes measurement error by using the latent variables of physical health problems, and can consider multiple endogenous variables, including parameters, at the same time (Duncan, Duncan, & Strycker, 2013; Enders & Bandalos, 2001).

We conducted the following intensified process according to the research questions. To evaluate the first research question, we estimated the direct path actor-partner effect of the physical health problem and the worse cognitive functions of the couple on the sexual life satisfaction for each partner and compared the estimated values. To address the second research question, we evaluated the mediating effects of the limitations in independent living on the path from worse physical health problems and cognitive functions of the couple to sexual life satisfaction. Lastly, the third research question constrained each path of the direct and the indirect effects of the limitations in independent living that were estimated for previous questions, and compared the differences in model fitness x^2 between the free model, which set all paths

Table 11.1 Descriptive Statistics and Pearson Correlations among Variables (N = 1,930)

Variables	*1)*	*2)*	*3)*	*4)*	*5)*	*6)*	*7)*	*8)*	*9)*	*10)*	*11)*	*12)*	*13)*
1)	1.00												
2)	0.53	1.00											
3)	–0.10	–0.05	1.00										
4)	–0.06	–0.06	0.29	1.00									
5)	–0.13	–0.07	0.89	0.24	1.00								
6)	–0.08	–0.08	0.27	0.83	0.28	1.00							
Variables	*1)*	*2)*	*3)*	*4)*	*5)*	*6)*	*7)*	*8)*	*9)*	*10)*	*11)*	*12)*	*13)*
7)	–0.14	–0.10	0.21	0.07	0.21	0.06	1.00						
8)	–0.13	–0.10	0.10	0.24	0.07	0.24	0.11	1.00					
9)	–0.15	–0.11	0.10	0.06	0.11	0.07	0.35	0.03	1.00				
10)	–0.11	–0.13	0.01	0.10	–0.01	0.12	0.05	0.31	0.29	1.00			
11)	–0.08	–0.04	0.09	0.11	0.07	0.11	0.20	0.10	0.27	0.23	1.00		
12)	–0.08	–0.04	0.08	0.12	0.07	0.13	0.17	0.15	0.21	0.30	0.78	1.00	
13)	0.05	0.05	0.04	–0.10	–0.02	–0.09	–0.06	–0.06	–0.18	–0.18	–0.20	–0.18	1.00
M	3.04	3.05	2.17	2.80	1.82	2.25	0.11	0.13	25.2	23.8	75.5	72.1	3.10
SD	0.91	0.87	1.53	1.62	1.44	1.53	0.31	0.34	3.92	3.99	5.13	4.67	1.25
Range	1–5	1–5	0–6	0–6	0–9	0–10	0–1	0–1	0–30	5–30	65–101	65–90	1–5

Note. (1) Husband's sexual life satisfaction; (2) Wife's sexual life satisfaction; (3) The number of chronic diseases of husband; (4) The number of chronic diseases of wife; (5) The number of medications of husband; (6) The number of medications of wife; (7) Husband's limitations in independent living; (8) Wife's limitations in independent living; (9) Husband's worse cognitive function; (10) Wife's worse cognitive function; (11) Husband's age; (12) Wife's age; and (13) Annual household income.

free, and the other models. We conducted identity verification and compared the specific differences in physical health, cognitive function, actor, partner, and gender.

RESULTS

Descriptive Statistics

Table 11.1 shows the results of the descriptive statistics and the correlation analysis of the variables. The mean sexual life satisfaction of the husband and that of the wife were similar to each other at approximately 3.0. The mean number of chronic diseases was 2.2 and 2.8 for the husband and wife, and the mean number of medications taken was 1.8 and 2.3, respectively. The results showed that the wife had more physical health problems. Approximately 10 percent of subjects had limitations in ADL and IADL: the percentage was higher for the wife (husband = 11 percent and wife = 13.0 percent). The mean cognitive function scores were 25 for the husband and 24 for the wife. When the cognitive functions of the subjects were determined based on the MMSE-KC scores, 20 percent of the elderly showed deteriorated cognitive functions. However, people who are admitted to a hospital or a nursing home owing to severely deteriorated cognitive function are excluded from the SELC, which examines the elderly living in local communities. Therefore, only 3 percent of the total subjects were confirmed by doctors as having dementia. The mean age of the husband was 75.5 years and that of the wife was 72.1 years. The results of the correlation analysis between variables showed that the sexual life satisfaction of the husband and that of the wife were closely related ($r = 0.53$, $p < 0.001$). The correlations between chronic diseases and taking medication were also very high ($r = 0.83$ for wife, $r = -0.89$ for husband, $p < 0.001$), and the results revealed that they were appropriately used as observational variables to constitute the latent variables of physical health problems. The results indicated that the age of the couple, the worse cognitive function, and the limitations in independent living were highly correlated ($p < 0.001$).

Results of APIM Analysis

Table 11.2 and figure 11.2 show the results of the structural equation modeling of the physical health problem of each subject, the direct effects of the worse cognitive function, and the indirect effects of limitations in independent living, affecting sexual life satisfaction. The root mean squared error of approximation (RMSEA) for the model fit was 0.06, comparative fit index (CFI) was 0.98, Tucker-Lewis Index (TLI) was 0.93, and standardized root mean square residual (SRMR) was 0.01, which were all excellent.

Table 11.2 Actor-Partner Interdependence Model Result on Sexual Life Satisfaction among Korean Elderly Couples (*N* = 1,930)

	Husband			*Wife*		
Paths	*b*	*SE*	*β*	*b*	*SE*	*β*
SS← Husband's PHP	–0.06***	0.02	–0.09	–0.02	0.02	–0.04
SS ← Wife's PHP	–0.00	0.00	–0.00	–0.02	0.02	–0.04
SS ← Husband's WCF	–0.08***	0.03	–0.09	–0.05*	0.03	–0.06
SS ← Wife's WCF	–0.05	0.03	–0.05	–0.08**	0.03	–0.10
SS ← Husband's LIL	–0.21**	0.07	–0.07	–0.15*	0.07	–0.06
SS ← Wife's LIL	–0.26***	0.07	–0.10	–0.14*	0.07	–0.05
LIL ← Husband's PHP	0.04***	0.01	0.17	0.01	0.01	.02
LIL ← Wife's PHP	–0.00	0.01	–0.01	0.05***	0.01	.22
LIL ← Husband's WCF	0.10***	0.01	0.32	–0.03**	0.01	–0.07
LIL ← Wife's WCF	–0.02**	0.01	–0.07	0.10***	0.01	0.29
SS ← Husband's age	–0.00	0.01	–0.02	0.00	0.01	0.01
SS ← Wife's age	0.00	0.01	0.01	0.00	0.01	0.02
SS ←Household income	0.01	0.02	0.01	0.01	0.02	0.02
DCF ← Husband's age	0.01*	0.00	0.07	–0.00	0.00	–0.02
LIL ← Wife's age	0.00	0.00	0.05	0.00	0.00	0.06
LIL←Household income	0.00	0.01	0.01	0.00	0.01	0.01
X^2 (*df*)	174.72 (22)***					
RMSEA	0.06					
CFI	0.98					
TLI	0.93					
SRMR	0.01					

Note. CFI = Comparative fit index; WCF = Worse cognitive function; LIL = Limitation in independent living; PHP = Physical health problem; RMSEA = Root mean squared error of approximation; SRMR = Standardized root square residual; SS = Sexual life satisfaction; TLI = Tucker–Lewis Index.
*$p < 0.05$. **$p < 0.01$. ***$p < 0.001$.

The Effects of Physical Health Problems and Worse Cognitive Function on Sexual Life Satisfaction

As a first research question, we evaluated the results of actor-partner effects of pathways that directly connected sexual life satisfaction with physical health problems and worse cognitive function. First, having more physical health problems decreased the sexual life satisfaction of the husband, and showed significant direct actor effects ($\beta = -0.09$, $p < 0.001$), but the sexual life satisfaction of the wife was not significantly influenced by own physical health problems. Second, the sexual life satisfaction of the husband and of the wife did not show significant differences because of the direct physical health problems of the partner. Third, a more severe decline in the cognitive function of the husband lowered his sexual life satisfaction and revealed significant and direct actor effects ($\beta = -0.09$, $p < 0.01$), while the more

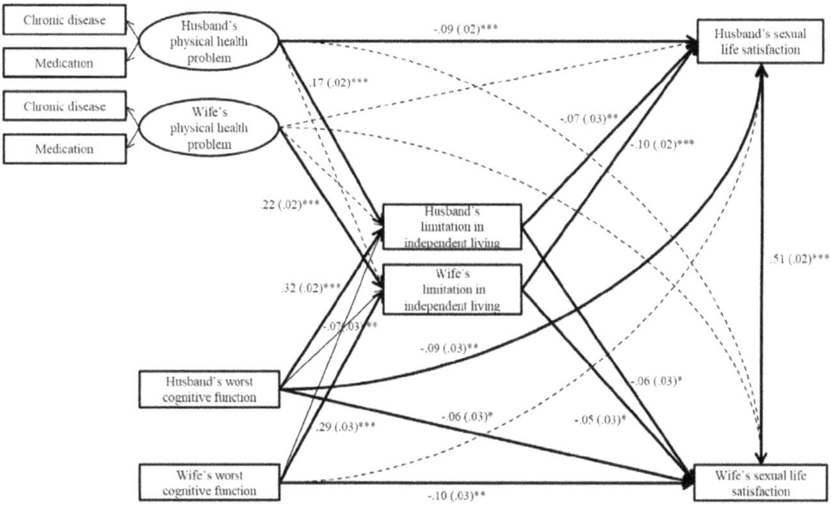

Figure 11.2 Actor-Partner Interdependence Model Results on Sexual Life Satisfaction among Korean Elderly Couples. Note: Significant paths are solid lines, and nonsignificant pathways are dotted lines. Husband's age, wife's age, and household income are controlled in these results. Path coefficients in this figure are standardized values. *$p < 0.05$. **$p < 0.01$. ***$p < 0.001$.

severe decline in the cognitive function of the wife decreased her sexual life satisfaction and indicated significant and direct actor effects ($\beta = -0.10$, $p < 0.01$). Fourth, the sexual life satisfaction of the husband was not significantly affected by the worse cognitive function of the wife directly but that of the wife significantly decreased with the worse cognitive function of the husband, and showed direct partner effects ($\beta = -0.06$, $p < 0.05$). The age of the husband, the age of the wife, and the household income, which were used as control variables, did not have significant effects on sexual life satisfaction for either actor effects or partner effects.

Indirect Actor-Partner Effects Influencing Sexual Life Satisfaction Mediated by Limitations in Independent Living

The second research question examined the results of actor-partner effects in the pathway indirectly connecting worse cognitive function to sexual life satisfaction mediated by the limitations of independent living. First, the husband's physical health problems ($\beta = 0.17$, $p < 0.001$) and worse cognitive function ($\beta = 0.32$, $p < 0.001$) began to limit his independent living. The limitations in the husband's independent living had significant negative effects on both husbands' sexual life satisfaction ($\beta = -0.07$, $p < 0.01$) and wives' sexual life satisfaction

(β = – 0.06, $p < 0.05$). Like the husband, the wife's physical health problems (β = 0.22, $p < 0.001$) and worse cognitive function (β = 0.29, $p < 0.001$) also led to limitations in her independent living, and the limitations in independent living negatively influenced her husband's sexual life satisfaction (β = –0.10, $p < 0.001$) and her sexual life satisfaction (β = –0.05, $p < 0.05$). Although the husband's old age mediated the limitation in independent living of the husband, and indirectly affected the sexual life satisfaction of the husband and the wife negatively, other control variables did not have even indirect significant effects.

Intersectionality: Differences in Actor, Partner, and Gender Effects

In addition, we conducted identity verification for each pathway to evaluate if the directs effects of the physical health problem, the worse cognitive function on sexual life satisfaction, and the mediating effects of the limitations in independent living differed by actor, partner, and gender. First, the husband's sexual life satisfaction was similarly influenced by his physical health problem and worse cognitive function ($\triangle x^2$ (1) = 0.62), but it was not significantly affected by the wife's physical health problem and worse cognitive function. Therefore, there was no direct partner effect. Second, the wife's sexual life satisfaction was similarly affected by her own worse cognitive function and the husband's worse cognitive function ($\triangle x^2$ (1) = 0.58), but there was no significant difference between actor and partner effects because neither party was significantly affected by own or partner's physical health problems. In summary, the husband's sexual life satisfaction was directly affected more by his own health condition than by his partner's health condition regardless of physical health and worse cognitive function. By contrast, the wife's sexual life satisfaction was only influenced directly by her own worse cognitive function and that of her spouse.

The results of identity verification on mediator effects revealed that both husband and wife showed significantly larger effects of worse cognitive function than of physical health problems on the limitations in independent living [$\triangle x^2$ (2) = 57.73, $p < 0.001$], and the actor effects were significantly larger than the partner effects [$\triangle x^2$ (4) = 246.42, p < 0.001]. However, the effects of the limitations on independent living, a parameter, or on the husband's and the wife's sexual life satisfaction were not significantly different for actor, partner, or gender. The results indicated that worse cognitive function rather than physical health problems, and own rather than partner's physical and cognitive levels induced the limitations in independent living. However, after occurring, the limitations in independent living had a negative effect on sexual life satisfaction regardless of actor, partner, or gender.

DISCUSSION

Using a structural equation model, we analyzed how physical health problems and worse cognitive functions directly affected the sexual life satisfaction of elderly couples, and how the interdependent relationship indirectly influenced it by mediating the limitations in independent living.

The most important finding of this study was that physical health problems and worse cognitive functions mediated the limitations in independent living to hinder own and his/her partner's sexual life satisfaction. As it has been considered natural that people have more physical health problems and that their cognitive functions decline with age, people may have accepted decreased sexual life satisfaction as part of the natural aging process. Although aging is an inescapable developmental process, the results of this study showed that biological age had little effect on sexual life satisfaction. In particular, the factors found in this study that hinder sexual life satisfaction could be delayed or eliminated, so sexual dissatisfaction among the elderly should not be assumed as a matter of course. For example, physical health problems and worse cognitive function can be prevented, delayed, or treated, and the limitations in independent living can be addressed by the society. It is urgently necessary to prevent and delay physical health problems and worse cognitive functions through intervention programs in order to improve sexual life satisfaction (Karraker & DeLamater, 2013; Waite et al., 2009). Moreover, it is necessary to expand nursing, long-term care, family education, and family counseling services to elderly couples suffering from physical health problems and worse cognitive functions, and provide sexual counseling and sexual education programs for couples with limited capacity for independent living (Bentrott & Margrett, 2011).

Although a wife's worse cognitive function led to limitations in independent living and lowered the husband's sexual life satisfaction, the husband's sexual life satisfaction was not directly affected by the physical and cognitive health level of his wife but was mainly determined by his own physical and cognitive health levels. The results may suggest that elderly Korean males still have a self-centered unilateral sexuality that emphasizes sexual function and that they do not understand their spouse sufficiently (Kim & Hong, 2016).

Unlike the husband who had few partner effects but large actor effects, the wife's sexual life satisfaction was directly or indirectly affected by the husband's worse cognitive function as well as her own worse cognitive function. In other words, the results showed that the wife's sexual life satisfaction was influenced by both her husband's and her cognitive function level and limitations in independent living. The results can be understood according to the results of Lee (2014), who showed that an elderly male enjoyed sexual life in various ways including sexual intercourse with a spouse, watching an adult video, and masturbation, while an elderly female mainly had a sexual relationship with a spouse, and valued the emotional and relational aspects of that relationship. It is interesting that the partner effects influenced wife's sexual life satisfaction as much as the actor effects. In addition, it is noteworthy that the physical health problems of the husband and the wife did not directly affect the wife's sexual life satisfaction. The results of the study revealed that the sexual life satisfaction of the elderly female is not solely determined by her physical health status (DeLamater, Hyde, & Fong, 2008) and that cognitive functions are important in sexual life satisfaction. The results were also consistent with the results of Waite et al. (2009), who emphasized the effects of mental health over those of physical health. Therefore, maintaining the husband's cognitive functions and independent living should be supported to effectively enhance the wife's sexual life satisfaction.

We can make some suggestions for future research based on the results of this study. First, we excluded the elderly who did not have spouses for various reasons such as being widowed, divorced, or single because the objective of this study was to examine the interdependent relationship of elderly couples. However, while the elderly can maintain a sexual life without a spouse (Lindau et al., 2007), they may experience greater difficulties in having a sexual life than the elderly person living with a spouse (DeLamater & Karraker, 2009; Jeon, Oh, & Kim, 2017; Kim & Lee, 2013). Therefore, follow-up studies are expected to study the sexual life of the elderly without spouses in detail and seek ways to improve their sexual life satisfaction.

Second, the data need to be updated by repeating the primary survey. Moreover, the new survey and analysis should use more advanced measurement tools and the analysis should be more sophisticated. Since the original data were collected in 2011, the results may be different from the contemporary situation of elderly Koreans in 2018. However, it was necessary to use the data before 2011 because the SELC measured sexual life satisfaction only until that date. Therefore, it is necessary to conduct a further survey that examines the sex life of elderly Korean people and compares that with the past results. In addition, future studies should measure sexual life satisfaction more elaborately by using more advanced scales than were used here. Physical health can be measured by taking into account not only the number but also the types of medicine taken. These limitations should be considered when interpreting and generalizing the results of this study.

Lastly, we could not discuss the policy support measures for enhancing the sexual life of elderly couples with limited independent living ability. The results, however, showed that wives' limitations in independent living lowered husbands' sexual life satisfaction as well as their own sexual life satisfaction. Consequently, we expect that future studies will develop nursing, recuperation, counseling, and education services to enhance the sexual life satisfaction of elderly couples having limitations in independent living; effective measures to address these should be introduced based on the scientific evidence.

CONCLUSION

It is necessary to prepare for specific nursing, long-term care, family education, and family counseling services that can enable the elderly to maintain a satisfactory sexual life. However, this study is meaningful insofar as its results provide the basis for necessary policy interventions to improve the sexual life of the elderly by evaluating the direct, indirect, and mediating effects of own and partner's physical and cognitive functions on sexual life satisfaction. We expect that this topic will be discussed more actively in women's studies and family studies to raise awareness that the elderly can enjoy a sexual life and maintain sexual life satisfaction despite limitations in independent living due to deterioration in the physical and cognitive health of the husband or wife.

NOTE

1. This chapter was previously published as Yoo, Jaeeon. "The Effect of Health and Functional Limitation on Sexual Life Satisfaction: Evidence from Elderly Korean Couples." *Asian Women* 34, no. 4 (2018).

REFERENCES

Angela, M. O. (1996). "The precious and the precocious: Understanding cumulative disadvantage and cumulative advantage over the life course." *The Gerontologist*, 36(2), 230–238.

Bentrott, M. D., & Margrett, J. A. (2011). "Taking a person-centered approach to understanding sexual expression among long-term care residents: Theoretical perspectives and research challenges." *Ageing International*, 36(3), 401–417. doi:10.1007/s12126-011-9110-7.

Biddle, N., & Yap, M. (2010). *Demographic and Socioeconomic Outcomes Across the Indigenous Australian Lifecourse: Evidence from the 2006 Census*. Canberra: ANU Press.

Choi, K. (2008). "Sexual life and ego-integrity among elderly people." *Journal of Korean Gerontological Nursing*, 10(2), 109–102 (In Korean).

Cook, W. L., & Kenny, D. A. (2005). "The actor-partner independence model: A model of bidirectional effects in developmental studies." *International Journal of Behavioral Development*, 29(2), 101–109.

DeLamater, J., Hyde, J., & Fong, M. C. (2008). "Sexual satisfaction in the seventh decade of life." *Journal of Sex and Marital Therapy*, 34, 439–454.

DeLamater, J., & Karraker, A. (2009). "Sexual functioning in older adults." *Current Psychiatry Reports*, 11(1), 6–11.

DeLamater, J., & Moorman S. (2007). "Sexual behavior in later life." *Journal of Aging and Health*, 19, 921–945.

DeLamater, J., & Sil, M. (2005). "Sexual desire in later life." *Journal of Sex Research*, 42, 138–149.

Doll, G. M. (2013). "Sexuality in nursing homes: Practice and policy." *Journal of Gerontological Nursing*, 39(7), 30–37. doi:10.3928/00989134-20130418-01.

Duncan, T. E., Duncan, S. C., & Strycker, L. A. (2013). *An Introduction to Latent Variable Growth Curve Modeling: Concepts, Issues, and Application.* New York, NY: Routledge Academic.

Elder, G. H. (1998). "The life course as developmental theory." *Child Development*, 69(1), 1–12.

Elder, G. H. (1994). "Time, human agency, and social change: Perspectives on the life course." *Social Psychology Quarterly*, 57(1), 4–15.

Enders, C. K., & Bandalos, D. L. (2001). "The relative performance of full information maximum likelihood estimation for missing data in structural equation models." *Structural Equation Modeling*, 8(3), 430–457.

Frankowski, A. C., & Clark, L. J. (2009). "Sexuality and intimacy in assisted living: Residents' perspectives and experience." *Sexuality Research and Social Policy*, 6(4), 25–37.

Franks, M. M., Lucas, T., Stephens, M. A. P., Rook, K. S., & Gonzalez, R. (2010). "Diabetes distress and depressive symptoms: A dyadic investigation of older patients and their spouses." *Family Relations*, 59(5), 599–610.

Ganong, K., & Larson, E. (2011). "Intimacy and belongings: The association between sexual activity and depression among older adults." *Society and Mental Health*, 1(3), 153–172. doi:10.1177/2156869311431612.

Gott, M., & Hinchliff, S. (2003). "How important is sex in later life? The views of older people." *Social Science & Medicine*, 56(8), 1617–1628.

Harris, S. M., Adams, M. S., Zubatsky, M., & White, M. (2011). "A caregiver's perspective of how Alzheimer's disease and related disorders affect couple intimacy." *Aging & Mental Health*, 15(8), 950–960. doi:10.1080/13607863.2011.583629.

Hirayama, R., & Walker, A. J. (2011). "When a partner has a sexual problem: Gendered implications for psychological well-being in later life." *Journal of Gerontology, Series B: Psychological Sciences and Social Sciences*, 66(6), 804–813. doi:10.1093/geronb/gbr102.

Hwang, E., & Shin, S. (2012). "Relationship between life satisfaction and sexuality among community-dwelling elderly." *The Korean Academic Society of Adult Nursing*, 24(2), 183–190. doi:10.7475/kjan.2012.24.2.183 (In Korean).

Jeon, K., Oh, H., & Kim, J. (2017). "A study on the types of the experiences of sexual life of elderly men living alone." *Asia-Pacific Journal of Multimedia Services Convergent with Art, Humanities, and Sociology*, 7(8), 853–862. doi:10.14257/ajmahs.2017.08.51 (In Korean).

Karraker, A., & DeLamater, J. (2013). "Past-year sexual inactivity among older married persons and their partners." *Journal of Marriage and Family*, 75(1), 142–163. doi:10.1111/j.1741-3737.2012.01034.x.

Karraker, A., DeLamater, J., & Schwartz, C. R. (2011). "Sexual frequency decline from midlife to later life." *Journal of Gerontology, Series B: Psychological Sciences and Social Sciences*, 66(4), 502–512. doi:10.1093/geronb/gbr058.

Kim, D., & Hong, G. (2016). "Sexuality and sexual life experience of community dwelling older adults." *Journal of Korean Gerontological Nursing*, 18(3), 128–137. doi:10.17079/jkgn.2016.18.3.128 (In Korean).

Kim, H. (2018). "Male elderly's sexual life and it's [sic] satisfaction in Daegu area." *The Journal of the Korea Contents Association*, 18(6), 314–323. doi:10.5392/JKCA.2018.18.06.314 (In Korean).

Kim, H., & Lee, H. (2013). "Factors related to the elderly's sexual satisfaction." *The Journal of the Humanities*, 69, 579–604 (In Korean).

Kingsberg, S. A. (2002). "The impact of aging on sexual function in women and their partners." *Archives of Sexual Behavior*, 31, 431–437.

Laumann, E. O., Paik, A., Glasser, D., Kang, J. H., Wang, T., Levinson, B., . . . Gingell, C. (2006). "A cross-national study of subjective sexual well-being among older women and men: Findings from the global study of sexual attitudes and behaviors." *Archives of Sexual Behavior*, 35(2), 143–159.

Lee, M. (2016). "Study on the sex recognition of male elderly." *Journal of Digital Convergence*, 14(5), 433–443. doi:10.14400/JDC.2016.14.5.433 (In Korean).

Lee, H. (2014). "The old man's sexual partner about the phenomenon compared." *Journal of Community Welfar*e, 51, 103–125. doi:10.15300/jcw.2014.51.4.103 (In Korean).

Lindau, S. T., Schumm, L. P., Laumann, E. O., Levinson, W., O'Muircheartaigh, C. A., & Waite, L. J. (2007). "A study of sexuality and health among older adults in the United States." *New England Journal of Medicine*, 357, 762–774. doi:10.1056/NEJMoa067423.

Lodge, A. C., & Umberson, D. (2012). "All shook up: Sexuality of mid-to later life married couples." *Journal of Marriage and Family*, 74(3), 428–443. doi:10.1111/j.1741-3737.2012.00969.x.

Montemurro, B., & Gillen, M. M. (2013). "Wrinkles and sagging flesh: Exploring transformations in women's sexual body image." *Journal of Women & Aging*, 25(1), 3–23. doi:10.1080/08952841.2012.720179.

Montemurro, B., & Siefken, J. M. (2014). "Cougars on the prowl? New perceptions of older women's sexuality." *Journal of Aging Studies*, 28, 35–43. doi:10.1016/j.jaging.2 013.11.004.

Shin, S., & Park, H. (2014). "Effect of sexual attitude of aged people on sexual life: Moderating effect of general characteristics." *Korean Journal of Adult Nursing*, 26(3), 320–329. doi:10.7475/kjan.2014.26.3.320 (In Korean).

Waite, L. J., Laumann, E. O., Das, A., & Schumm, L. P. (2009). "Sexuality: Measures of partnerships, practices, attitudes, and problems in the national social life, health, and aging study." *The Journal of Gerontology, Series B: Psychological Sciences and Social Sciences*, 64(Suppl. 1), i56–i66.

Wolff, J. L., & Kasper, J. D. (2006). "Caregivers of frail elders: Updating a national profile." *The Gerontologist*, 46(3), 344–356.

Yoo, Y. (2017). "The effects of sexual knowledge and attitudes on sexual satisfaction in the aged." *Journal of the Korea Entertainment Industry Association*, 11(6), 237–245. doi:10.21184/jkeia.2017.08.11.6.237 (In Korean). *11) 12) 13)*

Chapter 12

Mothers' Working Hours and Children's Obesity

Data from the Korean National Health and Nutrition Examination Survey, 2008–2010

Goeun Lee and Hyoung-Ryoul Kim

Obesity[1] in childhood and adolescence can lead to obesity in adulthood, and it is well known that obesity causes several diseases, such as hypertension, dyslipidemia, diabetes, cardiovascular disease, and colon cancer [1,2]. In particular, this issue emerged as a social problem that exacerbates the burden of future medical problems and costs [3]. One study estimated the social and economic cost of adolescent obesity in Korea was 1,363,800 million Won [4]. Obesity prevalence in children and adolescent aged two to eighteen increased from 5.8 percent in 1995 to 9.7 percent in 2007 in Korea (6.1 percent to 11.3 percent, and 5.5 percent to 8.0 percent in boys and girls, respectively) [5].

Childhood and adolescent obesity is affected by home and society which he or she belongs to and genetic factors. One study reported that childhood and adolescent obesity is more related to parents' socioeconomic position (SEP) [6]. As parents' occupation is an important factor determining the household's SEP, children's obesity can be associated with their parent's job.

With the rapid industrialization for decades in Korea, the number of married women who has occupation is getting higher. Since 2001, the employment rate of married women has been maintained above 50 percent [7]. In the past, even if a woman before marriage participated in economic activities, she had to quit the job after marriage due to having a baby, housework, and parenting at home. But, in recent years, many married women with children are working outside. However, married working women still do a lot of household chores such as taking care of their children, making foods, and cleaning. Married woman who has children works both in her workplace and home [8,9]. With regard to the association between mothers' work and their children's obesity, many researches were performed in developed countries [10–13]. There is a study that mothers' working long hours have positively related to child's obesity [14]. This result explained that working mothers spend less time with their children at home, and they do not have enough time to prepare good and slow foods and to guide child's recreational activities [14,15].

There was no study showing the relevance of the mothers' work hours and children's obesity in Korea. In addition, most studies dealing with this issue did not consider children's age and gender. Therefore, we intended to find out the association between mother's working hours and children's obesity according to children's gender and age, using the data of the Korea National Health and Nutrition Examination Survey (KNHANES).

MATERIALS AND METHODS

Subjects

This study used the data of KNHANES in 2008, 2009, and 2010, which are the second and third year of KNHANES IV and the first year in KNHANES V, respectively. The KNHANES is a stratified multistage clustered probability design for selecting representative samples. In total, 29,235 people were involved in this survey. We chose households consisting of "children of a couple" or "children of a single mother." Among them, by selecting only children and adolescents of the age from 6 to 18 years and their mothers who have jobs, 2,016 children and 1,220 mothers were selected in this study.

Methods

All information about household income, children's age, gender, and BMI and mother's job, working hours per week, work schedule, education, and BMI were included in the KNHANES raw data. BMI was calculated by directly measured height and weight. Other information was based on the health questionnaire survey.

The height was measured up to 1 cm, and the weight was measured up to 0.1 kg. BMI was divided by the weight (kilogram) by the square of the height (meter) and the second decimal point was permitted. Obesity of children and adolescents abided by the BMI cut-off point considering gender- and age-based growth curve. Depending on the 2007 Korea Childhood and Youth Standard Growth Chart percentiles, by up to the age of eighteen, overweight was defined as BMI at 85th percentile or above 85th percentile. Obesity was defined as 95th percentile or above 95th percentile considering gender and age in month. If BMI is 25.0 or over 25, it is also obesity even though he or she was under 95th percentile for age in month [16].

The 2007 Korea Childhood and Youth Standard Growth Chart provided weight, height and BMI according to gender and age in month. We estimated odds ratio in two groups, which are comparing obese children (BMI ≥ 95 percent for gender and age or BMI ≥ 25) with normal weight children (BMI < 95 percent) and comparing overweight children including obese children (BMI ≥ 85 percent for gender and age) with normal weight children (BMI < 85 percent for gender and age). On two groups, "normal" has two different meanings. The first "normal weight" included overweight, but the second "normal weight" excluded overweight. For convenience and avoiding confusion, we distinguished "overweight" and "overweight (including obesity)."

Mothers' working hours in a week are classified as under forty hours, forty to forty-eight hours, forty-nine to sixty hours, and over sixty hours, respectively.

Household income was categorized into quartiles such as low, middle low, middle high, and high. Mother's education was classified into elementary school, middle school, high school, and college or more. Mother's BMI divided into two groups; < 25 was normal and ≥25 was obese. Mother's occupational classification in KNHANES followed the major groups of the Korean Standard Classification of Occupations (KSCO). We reclassified them into three categories, which are white collars (managers, professionals and related workers, and office clerks), pink collars (service and sales workers), and blue collars (skilled agricultural, forestry and fishery workers, crafts and related workers, equipment, machine operating and assembling workers, elementary workers and military officers). Status of shift work was classified into day work and shift work (all types of shift work, except day work).

This study received an exemption from screening by the Institutional Review Board of Songeui Medical Campus, the Catholic University of Korea, Seoul, Korea (ID: MC12EASI0158).

Statistical Analysis

KNHANES IV and V data were made of stratified multistage clustered probability design and all statistical analyses incorporated into survey weights. First, we carried out frequency analysis for mothers' and children's general characteristics and prevalence. Children and adolescents were stratified by age (six to twelve years old and thirteen to eighteen years old) and gender. Survey logistic regression was used to calculate odds ratio (OR) and 95 percent confidence interval (CI) to assess the association of mother's working hours with overweight or obesity of her children. We adjusted household income, mothers' education and obesity, mothers' job characteristics—occupational classification and shift work. All statistical analyses were performed using IBM SPSS STATISTICS version 20.0, and we considered $P < 0.05$ to be statistically significant.

RESULTS

The general characteristics of subjects are shown in tables 12.1 and 12.2. Among children, obesity prevalences were 12.8 percent in boys and 7.7 percent in girls, respectively (table 12.1). In mothers, mothers who work less than forty hours per week was 38.8 percent and mothers working forty-nine hours or more per week were 27.1 percent (table 12.2).

Mostly, obesity and overweight (including obesity) prevalence in children whose mothers worked forty to forty-eight hours was low, while obesity or overweight (including obesity) prevalence was higher in children whose mothers worked over forty-nine hours or under forty hours (table 12.3).

Table 12.4 shows ORs of children's obesity and overweight (including obesity) according to mothers' working hours per week. Among six- to twelve-year-old boys, overweight (including obesity) decreased in children whose mother worked over sixty hours per week. OR was 0.24 (95 percent CI: 0.06–0.89). Thirteen- to eighteen-year-old boys whose mothers worked under forty hours per week were higher risk for obesity and overweight (including obesity) than thirteen- to eighteen-year-old boys whose mothers worked forty to forty-eight hours. OR was 4.23 (95 percent CI: 1.79–10.00)

Table 12.1 General Characteristic of the Children (*n* = 2,016)

	Total N (%+)	*Male* N (%+)	*Female* N (%+)	P-*value*
Total	2,016(100.0)	1,058(100.0)	958(100.0)	
Age (years)				0.774
6–12	1,051(44.0)	549(43.6)	502(44.4)	
13–18	965(56.0)	509(56.4)	456(55.6)	
Body Mass Index (kg/m^2)				0.008
Underweight	121(6.3)	54(5.5)	67(7.4)	
Normal weight	1,534(76.1)	799(75.6)	735(76.8)	
Overweight	167(7.1)	81(6.1)	86(8.1)	
Obese	194(10.4)	124(12.8)	70(7.7)	
Household income				0.477
Low	145(8.2)	79(7.8)	66(8.6)	
Middle low	480(26.1)	236(25.4)	244(27.0)	
Middle high	719(35.7)	367(35.2)	352(36.3)	
High	662(30.0)	371(31.7)	291(28.2)	
Missing	10(0.0)	5(0.0)	5(0.0)	

+ Column and estimated percentage.

Table 12.2 General Characteristic of the Mothers (*n* = 1,220)

		Mothers *N (%¶)*
Age (years)	Mean ± S.E.†	41.21(±0.158)
Body Mass Index (kg/m2)	< 25	907(75.5)
	≥25	289(24.5)
Education	Elementary school	48(4.5)
	Middle school	103(9.2)
	High school	694(56.7)
	Some college or more	375(29.6)
Job ‖	Managers	9(0.8)
	Professionals and related workers	272(21.5)
	Office clerks	188(15.0)
	Service workers	190(15.8)
	Sales workers	230(19.5)
	Skilled agricultural, forestry, and fishery workers	38(2.4)
	Crafts and related workers	54(4.5)
	Equipments, machine operating, and assembling workers	33(2.3)
	Elementary workers	206(18.1)
	Military officer	0(< 0.1)
Working hours per week	<40	459(38.8)
	40–48	422(33.9)
	49–60	193(15.7)
	>60	145(11.6)
Work schedule	Day work	991(86.5)
	Shift work	156(13.5)

† standard error, ¶ estimated percentage, ‖by Korean Standard Classification of Occupations, 6th version.

in obesity and 3.83 (95 percent CI: 1.76–8.31) in overweight (including obesity). Six- to twelve-year-old girls whose mothers worked forty-nine to sixty hours per week were more overweight (including obesity) than girls whose mothers worked forty to forty-eight hours per week. OR was 2.51 (95 percent CI: 1.03–6.10). Thirteen- to eighteen-year-old girls whose mothers worked over sixty hours were more overweight (including obesity) than the reference. OR was 2.62 (95 percent CI: 1.04–6.62).

DISCUSSION

In this study, children's overweight (including obesity) increased among girls whose mothers worked longer and boys whose mothers worked shorter. Researchers in North America and Europe showed that longer working hours of mothers increased BMI of their children [11,12,17–19].

Table 12.3 Prevalence of Children's Obesity and Overweight in Their Mothers' Working Hours Per Week According to Age and Gender

Age	*Gender*	*Mothers' Working Hours*	*Total N(%++)*	*Obese N(%++)*	P-*value*	*Overweight and Obese N(%++)*	P-*value*
6–12	Male				0.692		0.362
	(*N* = 548)	< 40	244(100.0)	25(10.0)		47(19.8)	
		40–48	172(100.0)	12(8.2)		40(23.4)	
		49–60	76(100.0)	6(11.8)		15(22.9)	
		>60	56(100.0)	4(5.7)		9(11.1)	
	Female				0.078		0.192
	(*N* = 502)	< 40	222(100.0)	12(5.4)		38(18.3)	
		40–48	174(100.0)	6(3.8)		25(13.6)	
		49–60	67(100.0)	9(12.7)		20(26.2)	
		>60	39(100.0)	5(11.2)		8(17.8)	
13-18	Male				0.006*		0.008*
	(*N* = 509)	< 40	152(100.0)	33(24.0)		39(26.5)	
		40–48	185(100.0)	19(9.8)		25(12.1)	
		49–60	94(100.0)	11(9.8)		13(11.8)	
		>60	78(100.0)	14(20.4)		17(22.4)	
	Female				0.588		0.356
	(*N* = 456)	< 40	145(100.0)	11(11.1)		19(16.7)	
		40–48	165(100.0)	12(5.9)		18(9.6)	
		49–60	80(100.0)	8(9.3)		13(15.2)	
		>60	66(100.0)	7(10.6)		15(19.6)	

++ row and estimated percentage.
*p-value < 0.05.

The reason for such results was analyzed as the following: long working hours of mothers made lack of time for taking care of their children. So their children spend more time to watch TV, do less physical activity, and eat unbalanced diet [18]. Compared with nonworking or part-time working mothers, full-time working mothers are likely to have their children with overweight and obesity [20].

In our study, we found three interesting results. First, obese and overweight boys whose mothers work under forty hours per week were more prevalent among thirteen- to eighteen-year-old boys. These patterns are shown similarly in other age and gender groups (not significant statistically). Employment rate of Korean married women was very low if they had children under six [7,9,17]. Raising small children interrupted mother's occupations, while mother's employment rate increased when their children became school-aged or adolescent for their children's education cost. However, married women whose career was disconnected are usually hired as part-time or nonregular employees. It makes them working under forty hours in a week [17,21]. It is possible to assume that social economic position of mothers who work under forty hours can be relatively low in Korea. In Korean studies, married women

Table 12.4 Odds Ratios of Children's Obesity and Overweight in Their Mothers' Working Hours Per Week Stratified by Age and Gender

Childrens'		Mothers'	*Obese Odds Ratio (95% CI)§*		*Overweight and Obese Odds Ratio(95% CI)§*	
Age	*Gender*	*Working Hours*	*Crude OR*	*Adjusted OR†*	*Crude OR*	*Adjusted OR†*
6–12	Male	< 40	1.25 (0.51–3.05)	1.40 (0.54–3.64)	0.81 (0.48–1.36)	0.73 (0.40–1.33)
		40 ~ 48	1	1	1	1
		49–60	1.50 (0.42–5.40)	1.59 (0.44–5.74)	0.97 (0.44–2.16)	0.94 (0.39–2.27)
		> 60	0.68 (0.15–2.99)	0.37 (0.06–2.35)	0.41 (0.15–1.10)	0.24 (0.06–0.89)
	Female	< 40	1.42 (0.54–3.70)	1.51 (0.51–4.41)	1.42 (0.77–2.62)	1.14 (0.57–2.30)
		40–48	1	1	1	1
		49–60	3.65 (1.09–12.22)	3.40 (0.86–13.54)	2.26 (1.06–4.85)	2.51 (1.03–6.10)
		> 60	3.17 (0.75–13.37)	3.24 (0.63–16.82)	1.38 (0.52–3.67)	1.35 (0.43–4.28)
13–18	Male	< 40	2.89 (1.36–6.15)	4.23 (1.79–10.00)	2.62 (1.31–5.25)	3.83 (1.76–8.31)
		40–48	1	1	1	1
		49–60	0.99 (0.40–2.45)	1.15 (0.42–3.11)	0.97 (0.44–2.14)	1.14 (0.48–2.72)
		> 60	2.34 (0.97–5.66)	2.39 (0.90–6.39)	2.10 (0.92–4.78)	2.09 (0.82–5.32)
	Female	< 40	1.97 (0.65–5.94)	2.20 (0.73–6.65)	1.89 (0.80–4.47)	2.02 (0.84–4.89)
		40–48	1	1	1	1
		49–60	1.62 (0.57–4.57)	1.22 (0.36–4.22)	1.69 (0.67–4.29)	1.35 (0.47–3.92)
		> 60	1.87 (0.64–5.50)	1.90 (0.65–5.52)	2.30 (0.94–5.65)	2.62 (1.04–6.62)

§ confidence interval (CI).
† adjusted with children's age, household income and mothers' education, mothers' BMI, occupational classification and shift work.

who worked as part-time or nonregular employment were much more prevalent than unmarried women or married men. Such women were relatively low-educated and service-sales workers. The women in the case of highly educated-college are more engaged in education service, mostly [9,22,23]. Part-time working married women in service-sales were hired in order to respond to changes in seasonal workload and worked low level of difficulty and simple tasks, while part-time working married women in education service were hired in order to cut down labor costs or substitute regular worker. One study reported their average contract periods were 6.8 months. So, in any cases, part-time working married women were employed as day laborer or temporary workers, and their jobs were unstable and paid low wages [23]. Low SEP of mothers can be associated with their children's obesity. In developed countries, childhood and adolescents of high SEP groups usually consume more vegetables and fruits, which are low calories, than low SEP group [24]. Additionally, children of low-income households do eating higher cholesterol intake, binge eating, and more TV watching [25,26]. Also, SEP of household is associated with physical activity of adolescence. High parental education was related with increased physical activity of adolescents and decreased TV watching time [27,28].

The second interesting result was decreasing obesity and overweight of six- to twelve-year-old boys whose mothers worked over sixty hours, differed from other age and girls. Working over sixty hours a week is very long time. Mothers may go to work very early before their children finish breakfast or return home very late time past supper. Young boys' meals can be neglected, not being taken care of by mothers for a long time. Adolescents can solve meals without mothers' help, and young girls can take care of themselves relatively compared to boys of same ages. So we thought that young boys eat very irregular meals or skip meals. But more researches about this issue will be needed.

Finally, in six- to twelve-year-old girls whose mothers work forty-nine hours or more per week, prevalence of obesity and overweight was much higher. Girls are usually more influenced by their mothers than boys. So girls whose mothers spend less time with them possibly do less physical activity and watch TV longer. However, boys are usually more outgoing and do more physical activities without their mothers' control, when their mothers work longer, and adolescent girls, compared to adolescent boys, usually do not participate in moderate- to high-intensity exercise and spend more time watching TV and have less physical activity as grade increases [29,30]. This can be an explanation for this difference according to gender.

The risk for obesity increases in the children and adolescents with using computer and watching TV longer, short sleeping time, and fewer intakes of fruit [31–33]. Working mothers spend less time for cooking, eating with their children, playing, and having leisure time with their children [15,18,34]. It is possible for them to supervise the daily activities of children less [14]. Full-time working mothers who work harder usually may buy instant foods, processed foods, and high-calorie food for their families. Furthermore, they rarely serve fruits and vegetables, while they eat high caloric foods [35–37]. In the case of many working mothers, whose working hours are long or who do shift work, it is more frequent that family members tend to eat out and often skip meals and overeat later [38,39]. In the UK, eight- to thirteen-year-old children whose mothers are employed full-time spend more time watching TV than the same aged children whose mothers are nonemployed or are part-time employed [40].

In this study, we examined the relevance of children's obesity and mothers' working hours according to developmental stages—childhood and adolescence—and gender. Through using these stratifications, we intended to find the different effects of mothers' working hours on their children's obesity according to gender and age. So we found the gender difference in this association. This study also used reliable and representative data of Korea. This is the strength of our study unlike other studies dealing with this issue.

This study has some limitations. First, we did not consider fathers' factors such as occupation and BMI. As we know, father's occupation can represent SEP of his family. However, information about fathers with growing children in the KNHANES IV and V data is somewhat limited, and especially in single mothers' households. So we excluded fathers' variables—BMI and employment. We considered household incomes instead of fathers' occupation. Second, we used cross-sectional and secondary data for analysis. We did not consider mothers' working period. Results may vary depending on child's developmental stage when the mother has a job. A study showed that mothers' full-time employment around the age of eleven affected probability of overweight at the age of sixteen [41]. And another study reported that the duration of mothers' employment was associated with higher BMI of their children cumulatively [42]. Additionally, there was no information about mother's work schedules—whether on weekdays or weekends. There will be a difference in children's lives depending on whether their mothers work on weekend.

Future studies should consider the working period of mothers, calorie intake, routine diet, physical activity, time of using computer, watching TV, study time of children and adolescents, and food selection at home in order to clarify the cause of children's obesity according to the mothers' working hours.

NOTE

1. This chapter was previously published as Lee, Goeun, and Hyoung-Ryoul Kim. "Mothers' working hours and children's obesity: Data from the Korean National Health and Nutrition Examination Survey, 2008–2010." *Annals of Occupational and Environmental Medicine* 25, no. 1 (2013): 28.

REFERENCES

1. Rolland-Cachera MF, Deheeger M, Maillot M, Bellisle F. "Early adiposity rebound: causes and consequences for obesity in children and adults." *Int J Obes* (2005) 2006, 30 (Suppl. 4):S11–S17.

2. Dietz WH. “Childhood weight affects adult morbidity and mortality.” *J Nutri* 1998, 128:411S–414S.
3. Ebbeling CB, Pawlak DB, Ludwig DS. “Childhood obesity: public-health crisis, common sense cure.” *Lancet* 2002, 360:473–482.
4. Jung YH, Ko S, Lim HJ. “The socioeconomic cost of adolescent obesity.” *Health Soc Welfare Rev* 2010, 30:195–219. Korean.
5. Oh KW, Jang MJ, Lee NY, Moon JS, Lee CG, Yoo MH, Kim YT. “Prevalence and trends in obesity among Korean children and adolescents in 1997 and 2005.” *Korean J Pediatr* 2008, 51:950–955. Korean.
6. Gnavi R, Spagnoli TD, Galotto C, Pugliese E, Carta A, Cesari L. “Socioeconomic status, overweight and obesity in prepuberal children: a study in an area of Northern Italy.” *Eur J Epidemiol* 2000, 16:797–803.
7. Kim YO. “A dynamic study of women’s labour market transitions: career interruptions and its determinants.” *Korean J Popul Stud* 2002, 25:5–40. Korean.
8. Kim JW. “An empirical study on the dual burden of married working women: testifying the adaptive partnership, dual burden and lagged adaptation hypotheses.” *Korean J Soc Welfare* 2005, 57:51–72. Korean.
9. Park SM, Sun BY, Kim JW. *A Study on the Life-World of Women in Korea*. Seoul: Korean Women’s Development Institute, 2005. Korean.
10. Takahashi E, Yoshida K, Sugimori H, Miyakawa M, Izuno T, Yamagami T, Kagamimori S. “Influence factors on the development of obesity in 3-year-old children based on the Toyama study.” *Prev Med* 1999, 28:293–296.
11. Anderson PM, Butcher KF, Levine PB. “Maternal employment and overweight children.” *J Health Econ* 2003, 22:477–504.
12. Phipps SA, Lethbridge L, Burton P. “Long-run consequences of parental paid work hours for child overweight status in Canada.” *Soc Sci Med* (1982) 2006, 62:977–986.
13. Hesketh K, Crawford D, Salmon J, Jackson M, Campbell K. “Associations between family circumstance and weight status of Australian children.” *Int J Pediatr Obes* 2007, 2:86–96.
14. Brown JE, Broom DH, Nicholson JM, Bittman M. “Do working mothers raise couch potato kids? Maternal employment and children’s lifestyle behaviours and weight in early childhood.” *Soc Sci Med* 2010, 70:1816–1824.
15. Cawley J, Liu F. “Maternal employment and childhood obesity: a search for mechanisms in time use data.” *Econ Human Biol* 2012, 10:352–364.
16. Korea Center for Disease Control and Prevention, The Korean Pediatric Society. *The Committee for the Development of Growth Standard for Korean Children and Adolescents. Korean Children and Adolescents Growth Standard (Commentary for the Development of 2007 Growth Chart).* [Government Report Online]. Seoul: Division of Chronic Disease Surveillance, 2007 November. Available from: http://www.cdc.go.kr/CDC/info/CdcKrInfo0201.jsp?menuIds=HOME001-MNU0004-MNU0007-MNU0025&fid=28&q_type=&q_value=&cid=1235&pageNum=1. Korean.
17. Hong J-L. “Decomposition of changes in labor force participation of married women: 1998–2007.” *Women’s Stud* 2011, 80:143–180. Korean.

18. Ziol-Guest KM, Dunifon RE, Kalil A. "Parental employment and children's body weight: mothers, others, and mechanisms." *Soc Sci Med* 2013, 95:52–59.
19. Miller DP. "Associations between the home and school environments and child body mass index." *Soc Sci Med* 2011, 72:677–684.
20. Pinot de Moira A, Power C, Li L. "Changing influences on childhood obesity: a study of 2 generations of the 1958 British birth cohort." *Am J Epidemiol* 2010, 171:1289–1298.
21. Keum JH. *Labor Market for Women Workers and Challenges* (translated by Lee G). Seoul: Korea Labor Institute, 2002. Korean.
22. Youn AY, Chun YM. "An analysis on women's irregular work and causal factors in its choice." *J Women Econ* 2008, 5:1–30. Korean.
23. Kim JHKD, Lee IJ, Mun MK. *The Development of High Quality Short-Time Working Models to Promote Women Employment* (translated by Lee G). Seoul: Korea Labor Institute, 2007. Korean.
24. Neumark-Sztainer D, Story M, Resnick MD, Blum RW. "Correlates of inadequate fruit and vegetable consumption among adolescents." *Prev Med* 1996, 25:497–505.
25. Casey PH, Szeto K, Lensing S, Bogle M, Weber J. "Children in food-insufficient, low-income families: prevalence, health, and nutrition status." *Arch Pediatr Adolesc Med* 2001, 155:508–514.
26. Casey PH, Simpson PM, Gossett JM, Bogle ML, Champagne CM, Connell C, Harsha D, McCabe-Sellers B, Robbins JM, Stuff JE, Weber J. "The association of child and household food insecurity with childhood overweight status." *Pediatrics* 2006, 118:e1406–e1413.
27. von Rueden U, Gosch A, Rajmil L, Bisegger C, Ravens-Sieberer U. "Socioeconomic determinants of health related quality of life in childhood and adolescence: results from a European study." *J Epidemiol Comm Health* 2006, 60:130–135.
28. Kantomaa MT, Tammelin TH, Nayha S, Taanila AM. "Adolescents' physical activity in relation to family income and parents' education." *Prev Med* 2007, 44:410–415.
29. Kim J. "Leisure-time activities associated with obesity in adolescents." *J Korean Acad Comm Health Nurs* 2008, 19:587–599. Korean.
30. Oh I-HLG, Oh CM, Choi K-S, Choe B-K, Choi J-M, Yoon T-Y. "Association between the physical activity of Korean adolescents and socioeconomic status." *J Prev Med Public Health* 2009, 42:305–314. Korean.
31. Kang HT, Ju YS, Park KH, Kwon YJ, Im HJ, Paek DM, Lee HJ. "Study on the relationship between childhood obesity and various determinants, including socioeconomic factors, in an urban area." *J Prev Med Public Health* 2006, 39:371–378. Korean.
32. Chen X, Beydoun MA, Wang Y. "Is sleep duration associated with childhood obesity? A systematic review and meta-analysis." *Obesity (Silver Spring, Md)* 2008, 16:265–274.
33. Lee HH, Park HA, Kang JH, Cho YG, Park JK, Lee R, Yoon JY, Kim OH. "Factors related to body mass index and body mass index change in korean

children: preliminary results from the obesity and metabolic disorders cohort in childhood." *Korean J Family Med* 2012, 33:134–143.

34. Angela Fertig GG, Tcherins R. "The connection between maternal employment and childhood obesity: inspecting the mechanisms." *Rev Econ Household* 2009, 7:227–255.
35. Courtemanche C. "Longer hours and larger waistlines? The relationship between work hours and obesity." *Forum Health Econ Policy* 2009, 12 (2). http://libres.uncg.edu/ir/uncg/f/C_Courtemanche_Longer_2009.pdf.
36. Blake CE, Devine CM, Wethington E, Jastran M, Farrell TJ, Bisogni CA. "Employed parents' satisfaction with food-choice coping strategies. Influence of gender and structure." *Appetite* 2009, 52:711–719.
37. Bauer KW, Hearst MO, Escoto K, Berge JM, Neumark-Sztainer D. "Parental employment and work-family stress: associations with family food environments." *Soc Sci Med* (1982) 2012, 75:496–504.
38. Devine CM, Farrell TJ, Blake CE, Jastran M, Wethington E, Bisogni CA. "Work conditions and the food choice coping strategies of employed parents." *J Nutri Ed Behav* 2009, 41:365–370.
39. Blake CE, Wethington E, Farrell TJ, Bisogni CA, Devine CM. "Behavioral contexts, food-choice coping strategies, and dietary quality of a multiethnic sample of employed parents." *J Am Diet Assoc* 2011, 111:401–407.
40. Mullan K. "Young people's time use and maternal employment in the UK." *British J Sociol* 2009, 60:741–762.
41. von Hinke Kessler Scholder S. "Maternal employment and overweight children: does timing matter?" *Health Econ* 2008, 17:889–906.
42. Morrissey TW. "Trajectories of growth in body mass index across childhood: associations with maternal and paternal employment." *Soc Sci Med* 2013, 95:60–68.

Chapter 13

Subjective and Objective Indicators of Socioeconomic Status and Self-Rated Health in Korean Adolescents

Kyungwon Choi

Socioeconomic[1] status (SES) is a multidimensional construct (Chen & Paterson, 2006) and is usually derived from information on education, occupational status, and income. In adolescence, SES is conventionally constituted by parental occupation, levels of income and education, and material deprivation. In other words, parental SES has been considered to determine adolescent SES because adolescents typically have no job and no income. However, such data can be problematic when the participants are adolescents. Previous studies have shown that not only inaccuracies but also a significant amount of data remain absent in adolescent self-reporting of the level of parental education, occupation, and income (Ensminger et al., 2000; Goodman, Huang, Schafer-Kalkhoff, & Adler, 2007; Wardle, Robb, & Johnson, 2002). Such inaccuracies and information gaps could stem from the fact that a significant proportion of adolescents might not know the actual SES of their parents, or simply that they do not wish to accurately report on these indicators. Therefore, these SES may not be appropriate for adolescents' SES (Wardle et al., 2002). To overcome these flaws and assess the SES of adolescents, the family affluence scale (FAS) (Currie et al., 2008) and the subjective social status (Quon & McGrath, 2014) have been proposed. FAS is composed of four questions, all easily answerable, that may reflect the level of affluence or material deprivation of adolescents (Torsheim et al., 2004; Wardle et al., 2002). FAS, therefore, may be a useful alternative approach in the study of SES in adolescent health because it is less vulnerable to nonresponses and inaccurate reporting. Some studies have measured the subjective social status of adolescents such as subjective household economic status and subjective school achievement (Goodman et al., 2007; Lemeshow et al., 2008; Piko & Fitzpatrick, 2007; Richer, Moor, & van Lenthe, 2012). Subjective household economic status was used to measure the perceived SES of the family in society by simply asking them their perceived family wealth using a five-point scale (Piko & Fitzpatrick, 2007; Richer et al., 2012) or by using a ten-point self-anchoring scale (Goodman et al., 2007). The ten-point self-anchoring scale is presented as a ladder representing American society; adolescents are asked to choose the rung on the ladder that they think best represents their family's position in American society. Subjective school achievement was used to measure the personal social position in school (Koivusilta, Rimpelä, & Kautiainenk, 2006; Lemeshow et al., 2008). Different SES indicators may have different implications for health (Chen, Matthews, & Boyce, 2002), and there is no single best indicator of SES that can be applied equally across all health outcomes and age groups (Iversen & Holsen, 2008). Understanding which SES indicators are associated with adolescents' health is critical for introducing effective interventions that can reduce health disparities. Thus, different types of SES indicators should be used to understand the broader impact of SES (Chen & Paterson, 2006).

While many studies have investigated the relationship between SES and the health outcomes of adolescents (Barros et al., 2009; Chen & Paterson, 2006; Koivusilta et al., 2006; Vingilis, Wade, & Silly, 2002), studies of Korean adolescents in this regard are generally problematic since they have depended on unrepresentative samples (An & Kim, 2013), or limited samples (examining only certain age groups) (Khang, Cho, Yang, & Lee, 2005), and/or include only a few conventional SES indicators in their analyses (An & Kim, 2013). Therefore, the aim of this study is to assess the relative contribution of various SES to adolescents' health (as measured by self-rated health (SRH)) of adolescents utilizing a nationally representative sample dataset.

METHODS

The Korea Youth Risk Behavior Web-Based Survey

The present study drew on data from the Korea Youth Risk Behavior Web-based Survey (KYRBWS)-VII conducted by the Korean Centers for Disease Control and Prevention (KCDCP). KYRBWS has been carried every year by the Korean Center for Disease Control with the purpose of calculating representative and confidential public health index information related to the health-related behavior of Korea's adolescents. KYRBWS includes questions related to the following: tobacco, alcohol, and drug use; eating habits, obesity, and weight control; physical activity; injury prevention; sexual behavior;

mental health; dental health; and individual hygiene. KYRBWS is an anonymous, Internet-based, self-administered, structured questionnaire that uses a stratified three-stage clustering design on the basis of geographic area, school size, and grade level. The KCDCP have reported all data collection procedures utilized for the KYRBWS-VII. After determining the sampling, participants were randomly assigned identification numbers. Upon accessing the survey webpage using their ID numbers, the participants were asked to respond to a question about their willingness to participate. If they chose not to participate by "disagreeing," they did not progress any further. A total of 79,202 students in grade seven to twelve from 400 middle schools and 400 high schools completed the web-based survey with guidance from trained teachers, the response rate was 95.5 percent (N = 75,643). However, those students who did not answer important questions such as whether they lived together with their parents, the level of parental education were excluded from the present study. Accordingly, data from 74,936 students aged twelve to eighteen years were analyzed. The characteristics of the participating students are shown in Table 13.1.

Instruments

SES in this study included FAS, level of parental education, subjective household economic status, and subjective academic achievement. To adjust the effects of other associated factors, health-related behavioral (smoking, alcohol consumption, physical activity, consumption of breakfast), and psychological factors (depression, perceived stress, body weight perception) were included (Boardman, 2006; Breidablik, Meland, & Lydersen, 2008; Heshmat et al., 2015; Moor et al., 2014; Page & Suwanteerangkul, 2009; Piko, 2007; Vingilis et al., 2002).

Data Analysis

Analyses were separately conducted for male and female adolescents. Sampling weights which have been described in detail by the KCDCP (KCDCP, 2011) were used to report on estimates representative of the Korean adolescent population and the complex sampling design of the survey. The complex sampling design took into account stratification, clustering, and multistage sampling to obtain the variances. Multivariate logistic regression analysis was carried out in order to evaluate the relationship between various SES and SRH after adjusting for covariates such as health-related behavioral and psychological factors. In model 1, the level of parental education was included as a SES indicator. In model 2, FAS was included. subjective household economic status comprised model 3, and subjective academic

Table 13.1 Overview of Instruments

Variables	*Operationalization*
Socioeconomic	
Family structure	Possible responses were having both parents, having father or mother, having father or mother, having father or mother with step-parent, having no parents (orphaned or living with other relatives).
The level of parental education	The level of parental education was categorized as (1) college or higher, (2) high school, (3) middle school or less, and (4) do not know.
Family Affluence Scale (FAS)	FAS consists of four items: family car ownership, whether the student shared a bedroom, the number of computers at home, and time spent on holiday in the past twelve months. The composite FAS score was calculated by summing the responses to these four questions, the results of which were categorized of low (0–3), middle (4–5), or high (6–7) group.
Subjective family economic status	Participants were asked of their perception of their household's economic status. Possible responses from low to high.
Subjective academic achievement	Participants were asked of their perception of the grades' at school over the past twelve months. Possible responses from low to high.
Psychological	
Perceived stress	Participants were asked how much stress they usually felt using a 5-item scale. Adolescents who felt stressed were placed in the perceived stress group.
Experience of depression	This was measured with a question if they had ever experienced sadness or despair to the extent that it had interrupted their everyday life for more than two weeks at a time over the past twelve months (dichotomized: yes/no).
Body weight perception	Participants were asked of subjective evaluation of their own body weight. The responses were classified of very underweight, normal, and overweight.
Behavioral	
Lifetime smoking experience Lifetime drinking experience	This was measured using dichotomized (yes/no) questions inquiring into lifetime smoking experience, lifetime drinking experience.
Frequency of Breakfast consumption	This was assessed with a question inquiring into the frequency of having breakfast during the previous week (less than two times a week/three to four times a week/more than five times a week).
Level of physical activity	Activity was assessed by a single question pertaining to the number of days on which they engaged in vigorous physical activity during the previous week ($\geq$5 days, 1–4 days, or 0 days).
Self-rated health	Adolescents' perception of their health. The responses were then dichotomized into unhealthy (Very poor, poor, fair) and healthy (good, very good) for the analysis.

achievement model 4, while all SES indicators were included model 5 in sequence. All models were adjusted for school grade, health-related behavioral and psychological factors. All data were analyzed using SPSS 18.0.

RESULTS

General Characteristics of the Participants

Table 13.2 details the characteristics of the participants in this study. A total of 74,936 students participated of which 49.9 percent were male adolescents. The overall percentage of participants who rated their health as poor was 34.6 percent. Specifically, 40.2 percent of female adolescents and 28.3 percent of male adolescents rated themselves as having poor health. Compared to male adolescents, female adolescents were more likely to evaluate their health negatively. 50.7 percent of the participants were middle-school students, and 92.1 percent of adolescents lived with both parents. 44.5 percent of the participants had middle FAS grade. Approximately 47.4 percent of the students rated their own socioeconomic status as being in the middle. With regard to the level of parental education, more than one-third of respondents reported that their father had graduated from college or higher, while a smaller proportion (32.8 percent) had mothers with that level of education. About 37.8 percent of the adolescents reported that their school achievement was low, while 35.2 percent rated their school achievement as high. Nearly 83.9 percent of participants reported they were stressed, and 32.7 percent reported they experienced depression. 26.1 percent said they smoked, 51.0 percent said they consumed alcohol, while 41.2 percent reported they did no physical activity. More than half of participants had breakfast more than five times a week, and 33.5 percent stated that their weight was normal.

Associations of Socioeconomic Status with Self-Rated Health among Male Adolescents

The calculated odds ratios (ORs) that show the relationship between SES and SRH in male adolescents are presented in table 13.3. In all models except for the full model, when school grade, psychological, and health-related behavioral factors were adjusted for, all SES were significantly associated with the reported fair/poor perceptions of health. Parent(s) with high school or less educational attainment, lower FAS scores, lower subjective academic achievement, and household economic status were significantly correlated with a higher prevalence of poor self-rated health in each model. In model 5, the full model, subjective household economic status (middle, OR; 1.31,

Table 13.2. Self-Rated Health According to Selected Socioeconomic Characteristics by Sex

		Total Population		*Male (N=37,414)*		*Female (N=37,522)*	
Characteristics	*Categories*	*N*	*EV %*	*Poor/fair (N/EV %)*	*SE*	*Poor/fair (NEV /%)*	*SE*
Grade of school	Middle school	38,025	50.7	5,224 (46.4)	1.1	7,060 (46.1)	1.1
	High school	36,911	49.3	5,397 (53.6)	1.1	8,230 (53.9)	1.1
Family structure	Having both parents	68,493	92.1	34,113 (91.7)	0.2	34,380 (92.5)	0.1
	Having father or mother	4,225	5.2	2,175 (5.6)	0.1	2,050 (4.9)	0.1
	Having father or mother with new spouse	1,133	1.4	462 (1.2)	0.1	671 (1.6)	0.1
	No parents	1,085	1.3	664 (1.6)	0.1	421 (1.0)	0.1
FAS	High	20,724	27.7	2,545 (24.1)	0.5	3,700 (25.3)	0.5
	Middle	33,371	44.5	4,740 (45.1)	0.5	6,866 (45.5)	0.4
	Low	20,841	27.8	3,336 (30.8)	0.5	4,724 (29.2)	0.5
Subjective household economic status	High	22,197	29.6	12,391 (33.1)	0.2	9,806 (26.1)	0.2
	Middle	35,490	47.4	16,757 (44.8)	0.5	18,733 (49.9)	0.5
	Low	17,249	23.0	8,266 (22.1)	0.3	8,983 (23.9)	0.2
Paternal education	College or higher	32,298	43.1	4,278 (42.2)	0.7	6,003 (42.8)	0.8
	High school	26,355	35.2	3,552 (32.8)	0.6	5,802 (36.2)	0.6
	Middle school or less	3,733	5.0	599 (5.3)	0.2	878 (4.9)	0.2
	Unknown	12,550	16.7	2,192 (19.7)	0.5	2,607 (16.1)	0.4
Maternal education	College or higher	24,565	32.8	3,238 (31.6)	0.7	4,513 (32.1)	0.7
	High school	34,359	45.8	4,523 (42.9)	0.6	7,555 (48.6)	0.6
	Middle school or less	3,737	5.0	547 (4.7)	0.2	919 (5.3)	0.2
	Unknown	12,275	16.4	2,313 (20.8)	0.5	2,303 (14.0)	0.4
Subjective academic achievement	High	13,459	35.2	13,459 (36.0)	0.2	12,920 (34.4)	0.2

	Middle	20,202	27.0	9,941 (26.6)	0.3	10,261 (27.3)	0.3
	Low	28,355	37.8	14,014 (37.5)	0.2	14,341(38.2)	0.3
Perceived stress	Stressed	63,037	83.9	29,854 (79.9)	0.2	33,183(88.4)	0.2
	Unstressed	11,899	16.1	7,560 (20.1)	0.2	4,339 (11.6)	0.2
Experience of depression	No	50,056	67.3	26,956 (72.1)	0.3	23,100 (61.9)	0.3
	Yes	24,880	32.7	10,458 (27.9)	0.3	14,422 (38.1)	0.3
Experiences of lifetime	No	55,511	73.9	24,715 (65.8)	0.4	30,796 (82.8)	0.3
Smoking	Yes	19,425	26.1	12,699 (34.2)	0.4	6,726 (17.2)	0.3
Experiences of lifetime	No	36,655	49.0	17,446 (46.2)	0.4	19,209 (52.1)	0.4
Alcohol consumption	Yes	38,281	51.0	19,968 (53.8)	0.4	18,313 (47.9)	0.4
Level of physical activity	None	31,636	41.2	11,030 (29.3)	0.3	20,606 (54.6)	0.4
	One to four days/a week	36,058	48.0	20,861 (55.0)	0.3	15,197 (40.1)	0.4
	Five days over/a week	7,949	10.8	5,982 (15.7)	0.3	1,967 (5.3)	0.1
Frequency of breakfast consumption	More than five times a week	46,802	62.6	23,445 (62.4)	0.4	23,357 (62.9)	0.4
	Three to four times a week	9,896	13.1	4,628 (12.5)	0.2	5,268 (13.8)	0.2
	Less than two times a week	18,238	24.3	9,341 (25.2)	0.3	8,897 (23.3)	0.3
Body weight perception	Standard weight	25,206	33.5	11,640 (31.0)	0.3	13,566 (36.2)	0.3
	Overweight	28,592	37.6	12,429 (33.0)	0.3	16,163 (42.7)	0.3
	Underweight	21,138	28.9	13,345 (36.0)	0.2	7,793 (21.1)	0.2

EV; estimated value, SE; standard error, To reflect the stratified cluster sampling design of the 2011 Korea Youth Risk Behavior Web-based Survey, frequencies were calculated by using the "survey frequency procedure" of SPSS.

Table 13.3 Estimated Odds Ratios of the Association of SES on the Likelihood of Poor/Fair Self-rated Health among Korean Male Adolescents (n = 37,414)

Characteristics	*Model 1*[a] *OR (95%CI)*	*Model*[b] *OR (95%CI)*	*Model*[c] *OR (95%CI)*	*Model*[d] *OR (95%CI)*	*Model*[e] *OR (95%CI)*
Paternal education					
College or higher	1				1
High school	1.08 (1.01–1.15)				0.99 (0.93–1.07)
Middle school or less	1.27 (1.11–1.45)				1.13 (0.98–1.29)
Unknown	1.11 (1.11–1.33)				1.07 (0.97–1.17)
Maternal education					
College or higher	1				1
High school	1.09 (1.03–1.17)				1.02 (0.96–1.09)
Middle school or less	1.08 (0.95–1.23)				0.95 (0.84–1.09)
Unknown	1.29 (1.18–1.41)				1.10 (0.99–1.29)
FAS					
High		1			1
Middle		1.21 (1.32–1.51)			1.14 (0.99–1.13)
Low		1.14 (1.16–1.32)			1.2 (0.89–1.19)
Subjective family economic status					
High			1		1
Middle			1.41 (1.33–1.50)		1.31 (1.12–1.39)
Low			1.84 (1.71–1.97)		1.59 (1.47–1.72)
Subjective academic achievement					
High				1	1
Middle				1.12 (1.05–1.19)	1.04 (0.97–1.11)
Low				1.44 (1.35–1.19)	1.24 (1.17–1.32)

OR: odds ratio, CI: confidence interval.

* All models were adjusted for other covariates (family structure, grade of school, perceived stress, experience of depression, experiences of lifetime smoking/drinking, breakfast consumption, level of physical activity, body weight perception).

a Including paternal and maternal education as a SES variable.

[b] FAS (family affluence scale) as a SES variable.

c Including subjective family economic status as a SES variable.

[d] subjective academic achievement as a SES variable.

e Including all SES variables.

95% CI; 1.23–1.39; low, OR; 1.59, 95% CI; 1.47–1.72), as well as subjective academic achievement (low, OR 1.24, 1.17–1.32) remained significant.

Associations of Socioeconomic Status with Self-Rated Health among Female Adolescents

Table 13.4 shows the calculated ORs for the relationship between SES and SRH in female adolescents with respect to grade of school, psychological and behavioral factors. In female adolescents, like male adolescents, having parent with high school or less educational attainment, lower FAS scores, lower subjective academic achievement, and household economic status were significantly correlated with a higher prevalence of poor self-rated health in each model. In the full model (model 5), subjective household economic status (middle, OR; 1.30, 95% CI; 1.23–1.39; low, OR; 1.49, 95% CI; 1.39–1.60), and subjective academic achievement (middle, OR; 1.07, 95% CI; 1.01–1.13; low, OR; 1.13, 95% CI; 1.07–1.20) remained significant.

DISCUSSION

The aim of this study was to explore the relationship between various SES indicators and SRH among Korean adolescents. Based on previous research, the hypothesis in this study was that FAS and subjective social status indicators including subjective household economic status and subjective academic achievement would be significantly associated with SRH, even after controlling for covariates. In this study, all SES was associated with the odds ratio of poor SRH in separate multivariate logistic models adjusted for behavioral and psychological factors. However, in the full models that combined subjective and objective indicators of SES, only subjective social status indicators maintained their independent association to SRH. These results support previous research that showed higher subjective household economic status as being protective against a poor perception of health as compared with objective indicators, and adolescent's social position as indicated by school achievement is closely related with SRH (Hagquist, 2006; Koivusilta et al., 2006; Piko & Fitzpatrick, 2001). This is also in agreement with the assumption that as young people increasingly gain independence, the influence of parental SES is reduced, and peers become a more important reference group (Torsheim et al., 2004). Adolescents' perception of SRH may contribute to the relationship between school achievement and SRH. Whereas SRH among adults is characterized as both an enduring self-concept and a spontaneous health assessment, SRH among adolescents is deemed to be an enduring self-concept (Bailis, Segall, & Chipperfield, 2003). This is because adolescents

Table 13.4 Estimated Odds Ratios of the Association of SES on the Likelihood of Poor/Fair Self-Rated Health among Korean Female Adolescents (n = 37,414)

Characteristics	*Model 1*[a] *OR (95%CI)*	*Model*[b] *OR (95%CI)*	*Model*[c] *OR (95%CI)*	*Model*[d] *OR (95%CI)*	*Model*[e] *OR (95%CI)*
Paternal education					
College or higher	1				1
High school	1.05 (0.99–1.11)				0.99 (0.93–1.06)
Middle school or less	1.18 (1.05–1.33)				1.07 (0.95–1.21)
Unknown	1.19 (1.10–1.29)				1.08 (0.99–1.18)
Maternal education					
College or higher	1				1
High school	1.04 (0.98–1.09)				0.98 (0.92–1.04)
Middle school or less	1.15 (1.03–1.29)				1.05 (0.93–1.18)
Unknown	1.12 (1.02–1.23)				1.04 (0.94–1.14)
FAS					
High		1			1
Middle		1.26 (1.19–1.33)			1.04 (0.98–1.10)
Low		1.12 (1.06–1.18)			1.06 (0.99–1.13)
Subjective family economic status					
High			1		1
Middle			1.36 (1.28–1.44)		1.30 (1.23–1.39)
Low			1.60 (1.50–1.71)		1.49 (1.39–1.60)
Subjective Academic Achievement					
High				1	1
Middle				1.13 (1.07–1.19)	1.07(1.01–1.13)
Low				1.25 (1.19–1.33)	1.13 (1.07–1.20)

OR: odds ratio, CI: confidence interval.

* All models were adjusted for other covariates (family structure, grade of school, perceived stress, experience of depression, experiences of lifetime smoking/drinking, breakfast consumption, level of physical activity, body weight perception).

a Including paternal and maternal education as a SES variable.

[b] FAS (family affluence scale) as a SES variable.

c Including subjective family economic status as a SES variable.

[d] subjective academic achievement as a SES variable.

e Including all SES variables.

do not usually have serious illnesses or consequent symptoms. For this reason, adolescents are more likely than adults to assess their health in terms of competence (Mechanic & Hansell, 1987). The self-identities of adolescents are less stable and require more external corroboration. Accordingly, social feedback reflecting consensually based norms and expectations may influence the self-rated health of adolescents (Mechanic & Hansell, 1987). School achievement is a good indicator of competence in adolescents in that it mirrors strong parent-oriented norms and expectations.

In previous studies, adolescents with low FAS scores had a higher risk of reporting poor SRH (Moor et al., 2014; Torsheim et al., 2004; Richer et al., 2012). In this study, FAS was significantly associated with boys and girls' SRH in separate multivariate logistic regression models, but showed no association in full models that combine all SES indicators. One plausible reason for this result is that items of FAS may not be sensitive when measuring family affluence in Korean adolescents. The rate of computer possession in this study was 96.8 percent, and 75.5 percent of adolescents reported they had their own room. It is worth remembering that Korea has one of the highest rates of computer possession at home (Korea National Statistical Office, 2012), and Korea's declining birthrates over the past two decades have meant that most families have only child or two children (Korea National Statistical Office, 2013). The items that reflect family vary across countries and culture, more specific items are needed to improve the sensitivity of FAS.

In this study, the level of parental education was not significantly correlated with SRH in both boys and girls. The evidence for correspondence between levels of parental education and SRH in adolescence is somewhat inconsistent (Duarte-Salles et al., 2011; Hagquist, 2006; West, 1997). Given the literature review, the level of parental education has both direct and indirect effects on adolescents' SRH (Duarte-Salles et al., 2011; Hagquist, 2006; West, 1997). The findings in this study may be partially influenced by high expectations among parents for good grades for their children. The pressure for academic achievement may cause adolescents' psychological discomfort including stress and depression, which are reported to be associated with adolescents' poor SRH (Piko, 2007; Tremblay, Dahinten, & Kohen, 2003; Vingilis et al., 2002). Adolescents' psychological discomfort may accentuate the effect of level of parental education on adolescents' SRH.

Several limitations should be considered when interpreting these findings. First, this study used a cross-sectional design, which makes it impossible to make conclusive statements about causality. Longitudinal studies must be performed to confirm such statements. Another limitation is that this study excluded those students who did not answer the question as to whether they lived together with their parents (0.9 percent). This shortcoming could be attributed to the KYRBWS. A 2008 Korean society index showed a school enrollment rate of 95.5 percent. Therefore, the relationship between SRH and SES for excluded or unenrolled students could not be determined. Lastly, some variables such as depressed mood and stress perception were measured by only one question for each, neither of which was standardized or validated. As a result, there may be concerns as to whether confounding factors were adequately and correctly considered.

CONCLUSION

The results of the present study indicate that subjective indicators of SES are significantly associated with SRH, while objective indicators such as FAS and levels of parental education show no such association. To assess family affluence more precisely and prevent exclusion of adolescents who fail to correlate with conventional SES, the specific items of FAS need to be replaced with more country-specific elements. Moreover, subjective social status indicators proved to be reliable indicators that can be used to assess adolescents' SES and link it to SRH as a health outcome. Findings in this study underline the fact that adolescent-specific indicators should be used when assessing adolescents' SES. Identifying vulnerable adolescent populations could make for effective health promotion and preventive interventions and reduce health disparities.

NOTE

1. This chapter was previously published as Choi, Kyungwon. "Subjective and objective indicators of socioeconomic status and self-rated health in Korean adolescents." *Korean Society for Health Education and Promotion* 32, no. 5 (2015): 53–62.

REFERENCES

Adler, N. E., Epel, E. S., Castellazzo, G., & Ickovics, J. R. (2000). "Relationship of subjective and objective social status with psychological and physiological functioning: preliminary data in healthy white women." *Health Psychology*, 19(6), 586–592.

An, J. S., & Kim, H. J. (2013). "A study on the determinants of children and adolescents' health inequality in Korea." *Studies on Korean Youth*, 24, 205–231.

Bailis, D. S., Segall, A., & Chipperfield, J. G. (2003). "Two views of self-rated general health status." *Social Science & Medicine*, 56, 203–217.

Barros, M. B., Zanchetta, L. M., de Moura, E. C., & Malta, D. C. (2009). "Self rated health and associated factors, Brazil, 2006." *Revista de Saude Publica*, 43(Suppl. 2), 27–37.

Boardman, J. D. (2006). "Self-rated health among U.S. adolescents." *Journal of Adolescent Health*, 38(4), 401–408.

Breidablik, H. J., Meland, E., & Lydersen, S. (2008). "Self-rated health in adolescence: a multifactorial composite." *Scandinavian Journal of Public Health*, 43, 246–252.

Chen, E., & Paterson, L. Q. (2006). "Neighborhood, family and subjective socioeconomic status: how do they relate to adolescent health?" *Health Psychology*, 25(6), 704–714.

Chen, E., Matthews, K. A., & Boyce, W. T. (2002). "Socioeconomic differences in children's health: how and why do these relationships change with age?" *Psychological Bulletin*, 128(2), 295–329.

Currie, C., Molcho, M., Boyce, W., Holstein, B., Torsheim, T., & Richter, M. (2008). "Researching health inequalities in adolescents: the development of the health behavior in school-aged children (HBSC) Family Affluence Scale." *Social Science & Medicine*, 66(6), 1429–1436.

Duarte-Salles, T., Pasarin, M. I., Borrell, C., Rodriguez-Sanz, M., Rajmil, L., Ferrer, M., Pellise, F., & Balague, F. (2011). "Social inequalities in health among adolescents in a large southern European city." *Journal of Epidemiology and Community Health*, 65, 166–173.

Ensminger, M. E., Forrest, C. B., Riley, A. W., Kang, M., Green, B. F., Satrfield, B., & Ryan, S. A. (2000). "The validity of measures of socioeconomic status of adolescents." *Journal of Adolescent Research*, 15(3), 392–419.

Fismen, A. S., Samdal, O., & Torsheim, T. (2012). "Family affluence and cultural capital as indicators of social inequalities in adolescent's eating behaviors: a population-based survey." *BMC Public Health*, 12, 1036–1044.

Goodman, E., Huang, B., Schafer-Kalkhoff, T., & Adler, A. E. (2007). "Perceived socioeconomic status: a new type of identity which influence adolescents' self-rated health." *Journal of Adolescent Health*, 41, 479–487.

Hagquist, C. E. (2006). "Health inequalities among adolescents-the impact of academic orientation and parents' education." *European Journal of Public Health*, 17(1), 21–26.

Heshmat, R., Kelishadi, R., Motamed-Gorji, N., Motlagh, M. E., Ardalan, G., Arifirad, T., Rastad, H., Asayesh, H., Djalalinia, S., Larijani, B., & Qorbani, M. (2015). "Association between body mass index and perceived weight status with self-rated health and life satisfaction in Iranian children and adolscents: the CASPIAN-III study." *Quality life Research*, 24(1), 263–272.

Iversen, A. C., & Holsen, I. (2008). "Inequality in health, psychosocial resources and health behavior in early adolescence: the influence of different indicators of socioeconomic position." *Child Indicators Research*, 1, 291–302.

Jung, S. H., Tsakos, G., Sheiham, A., Ryu, J. I., & Watt, R. G. (2010). "Socioeconomic status and oral health-related behaviors in Korean adolescents." *Social Science & Medicine*, 70(11), 1780–1788.

Khang, Y. H., Cho, S. I., Yang, S., & Lee, M. S. (2005). "Socioeconomic differentials in health and health related behaviors: finding from the Korea Youth Panel Survey." *Journal of Preventive Medicine and Public Health*, 38, 391–400.

Kent, E. E., Sender, L. S., Morris, R. A., Grigsby, T. J., Montoya, M. J., Ziogas, A., et al. (2013). "Multilevel socioeconomic effects on quality of life in adolescent and young adult survivors of leukemia and lymphoma." *Quality of Life Research*, 22(6), 1339–1351.

Koivusilta, L. K., Rimpelä, A. H., & Kautiainenk, S. M. (2006). "Health inequality in adolescence. Does stratification occur by familial social background, family affluence, or personal social position?" *BMC Public Health*, 6, 110–118.

Korea Centers for Disease Control and Prevention. (2011). *Instructions for the Statistics of 7th Korea Youth Risk Behavior Web-based Survey (KYRBWS) in 2011.* Korea Centers for Disease Control and Prevention.

Korea National Statistical Office. (2012). *International Statistics Yearbook.* Seoul: Korea National Statistical Office.

Korea National Statistical Office. (2013). *Major Features and Analysis of Change across the Life-Cycle.* Seoul: Korea National Statistical Office.

Lee, H., Harris, K. M., & Lee, J. (2013). "Multiple levels of social disadvantage and links to obesity in adolescence and young adulthood." *Journal of School Health*, 83(3), 139–149.

Lemeshow, A. R., Fisher, L., Goodman, E., Kawachi, I., Berkey, C. S., & Colditz, G. A. (2008). "Subjective social status in the school and change in adiposity in female adolescents: findings from a prospective cohort study." *Archives of Pediatrics and Adolescent Medicine*, 162(1), 23–28.

Mariu, K. R., Merry, S. N., Robinson, E. M., & Wason, P. D. (2012). "Seeking professional help for mental health problems, among New Zealand secondary school students." *Clinical Child Psychology and Psychiatry*, 17(2), 284–297.

Mazzuco, S., & Meggiolaro, S. (2014). "Family structures and health behaviors in adolescents." *Child Indicators Research*, 7, 155–175.

Mechanic, D., & Hansell, S. (1987). "Adolescent competence, psychological well-being, and self-assessed physical health." *Journal of Health and Social Behavior*, 28, 364–374.

Moor, I., Rathmann, K., Stronks, K., Levin, K., Spallek, J., & Richiter, M. (2014). "Psychosocial and behavioral factors in the explanation of socioeconomic inequalities in adolescent health: a multilevel analysis in 28 European and North American countries." *Journal of Epidemiology and Community Health*, 68, 912–921.

O' Farrell, A., Flanagan, E., Bedford, D., James, D., & Howell, F. (2005). "Factors associated with self-reported depression and self-esteem among school-going adolescents from a geographically defined region in Ireland." *Irish Journal of Medical Science*, 174(4), 17–22.

Page, R. M., & Suwanteerangkul, J. (2009). "Self-rated health, psychosocial functioning, and health-rated behavior among Thai adolescents." *Pediatrics International*, 51, 120–125.

Piko, B. (2007). "Self-perceived health among adolescents: the role of gender and psychosocial factors." *European Journal of Pediatrics*, 166, 701–708.

Piko, B. F., & Fitzpatrick, K. M. (2001). "Does class matter? SES and psychosocial health among Hungarian adolescents." *Social Sciences & Medicine*, 53, 817–830.

Piko, B. F., & Fitzpatrick, K. M. (2007). Socioeconomic status, psychosocial health and health behaviors among Hungarian adolescents." *European Journal of Public Health*, 17(4), 353–360.

Quon, E. C., & McGrath, J. J. (2014). "Subjective socioeconomic status and adolescent health: a meta-analysis." *Health Psychology*, 33(5), 433–447.

Richer, M., Moor, I., & van Lenthe, F. J. (2012). "Explaining socioeconomic differences in adolescent self-rated health: the contribution in material, psychosocial and behavioral factors." *Journal of Epidemiology & Community Health*, 66, 691–697.

Rueden, U. V., Gosch, A., Rajmil, L., Bisegger, C., Ravens-Sieberer, U., & European KIDSCREEN Group. (2006). "Socioeconomic determinants of health related quality of life in childhood and adolescence: results from a European study." *Journal of Epidemiology & Community Health*, 60, 130–135.

Torsheim, T., Currie, C., Boyce, W., Kalnins, I., Overpeck, M., & Haugland, S. (2004). "Material deprivation and self-rated health: a multilevel study of adolescents from 22 European and North American countries." *Social Sciences & Medicine*, 59, 1–12.

Tremblay, S., Dahinten, S., & Kohen, D. (2003). "Factors related to adolescents' self-perceived health." *Health Reports*, 14(Suppl.), 7–16.

Vingilis, E. R., Wade, T. J., & Seeley, J. S. (2002). "Predictors of adolescent self-rated health. Analysis of the National Population Health Survey." *Canadian Journal of Public Health*, 93, 193–197.

Wardle, J., Robb, K., & Johnson, F. (2002). "Assessing socioeconomic status in adolescents: the validity of a home affluence scale." *Journal of Epidemiology & Community Health*, 56, 595–599.

West, P. (1997). "Health inequalities in the early years: is there equalisation in youth?" *Social Science and Medicine*, 44, 833–858.

Xu, Z., Su, H., Chen, J., Wu, J., & Chang, W. (2011). "Self-rated health of Chinese adolescents: distribution and its associated factors." *Scandinavian Journal of Caring Sciences*, 25, 780–786.

Chapter 14

Health Status and Associated Health Risks among Female Marriage Immigrants in Korea

Hyekyeong Kim, Seunghyun Yoo, Seon Cho, Eun-Joo Kwon, Suyoung Kim, and Ji-Youn Park

Marriages[1] between foreign women and Korean men have notably increased in the past twenty years. In fact, the marriages between foreign women and Korean men increased from 2.4 percent of all marriages in Korea in 1997 to 8.4 percent in 2007 (Statistics Korea, 2007). Among over 122,000 international marriages in Korea in 2008, 87 percent were between foreign female and Korean men. Of those women, 29.1 percent were ethnic Koreans from China, 26.2 percent were Chinese, and 22.1 percent were Vietnamese (MPAS, 2008).

As the life adjustment and quality of life issues of multicultural families deserve attention, health of the immigrant wives plays a central part in the adjustment of immigrant wives and mothers after life-changing events such as immigration, marriage, childbirth, and employment. Health examination results of migrant wives show that they had higher prevalence of obesity, hypertension, anemia, and cervical cancer risks than Korean women (KAHP, 2008).

Migrant wives also face financial difficulties: A half of households with migrant wives fall below poverty line, and only 1.7 percent of the households receive National Basic Livelihood Security support (KIHASA, 2010). Almost a quarter of the migrant wives (23.5 percent) are often left out of the National Health Insurance (NHI) and Medicaid programs despite they experience the burden of health-care costs and low accessibility to health-care services, and subsequently give up getting health care (KIHASA, 2010).

Despite the need and importance, immigrant wives have limited access to health-care services and support due to language barriers, financial difficulties, lack of adequate information, and/or insurance coverage. For many of the immigrant wives are younger than forty years, they are not eligible for the national health examination program which is offered free-of-charge by the NHI Cooperation.

In this respect, this study reports the results of recent health examination for migrant wives with the aims of (1) describing health status of those women; (2) identifying their health risks; and (3) providing a basis for public health strategies to address health issues among female marriage immigrants to Korea.

METHODS

Study Participants

The participants of this study were 3,069 immigrant wives who were registered at district offices and public health centers nationally and had taken free-of-charge health examination opportunities supported by the Ministry of Health and Welfare in 2008.

These health examination opportunities were promoted mainly through fliers. Immigrant wives and their spouses were eligible for the health examination regardless of the citizenship status of the women. The promotion fliers were made in four languages (Korean, Chinese, English, and Vietnamese) to be more accessible to immigrant wives.

Data Collection

Health Examination

The health examination was conducted by the Korea Association of Health Promotion (KAHP) from July to November 2008 using mobile health examination equipment and services. For those who wanted the health examination but could not participate on the day of the KAHP visit were scheduled to come to KAHP branch facilities in fifteen cities and towns throughout Korea.

The health examination program consisted of twenty-one medical tests to detect chronic and acute health conditions. It includes diabetes, hyperlipidemia, anemia, hepatitis B, and other conditions and abnormalities in liver functions, sexually transmitted diseases such as syphilis and HIV/AIDS, and so on (table 14.1).

Once completed, health examination results were mailed to the participants within ten days. Additional tests were arranged for those who needed further examination and confirmation of the test results. Those needed follow-up care were referred to district public health centers, local clinics,

Table 14.1 Health Examination Contents

Categories	*Test Items*	*Standard for Normal*
Basic	Height	
	Weight	
	BMI	<23 (kg/m^2)
	Systolic blood pressure	<120 mmHg
	Diastolic blood pressure	< 80 mmHg
ECG	ECG	Normal reading
Urine	PH	5–8 ph
	Pro	Negative
	Glu	Negative
	O_Blood	Negative
Anemia	Hb	Women: 12.0–16.0 g/dL
Liver	AST	≤40 IU/L
	ALT	≤45 IU/L
	γ-GTP	Women: 0–51 IU/L
Hyperlipidemia	TC	110–230 mg/dL
Diabetes	GLU	70–110 mg/dL
Hepatitis B	S-Ag	Negative
	S-Ab	Positive
	Interpretation	Immunity Present
STD	RPR(Qualitative)	Negative
AIDS	HIV(EIA)	Negative
Uterine cancer	Brush	Normal reading
Chest x-ray	Chest-Ray(100 mm)	Normal reading

and hospitals. Detected cases of tuberculosis and sexually transmitted diseases were reported to district public health centers in accordance with the Infectious Disease Prevention Act.

Health Survey

At the beginning of the health examination, the participants completed a health survey on demographic characteristics, family and disease history, health-related behaviors such as eating behavior, smoking, alcohol drinking, physical activity, and mental health. The surveys were developed in aforementioned four languages.

Data Analysis

Baseline characteristics of the participants, health survey items, and health examination results are compared across five groups categorized by country of origin using chi-square tests or analysis of variance. Multivariable logistic regression analysis was performed on models with health status and health behavior practices as outcomes. All analyses were conducted by using SPSS 17.0 software.

RESULTS

Demographic Characteristics of Participants

A total of 3,069 immigrant wives completed the health examination and surveys. An average age of the women was 30.3 years (52.0 percent in the twenties and 28.9 percent in the thirties). About 50 percent of the women (51.3 percent) were recent immigrants who had spent less than three years in Korea at the time of this health examination, 20.2 percent had lived in Korea for three to five years, and 28.5 percent had spent more than five years. One-third of the women were Vietnamese (34.3 percent), and another third was Chinese (30.4 percent). The next largest group was Filipina (11.8 percent), followed by Japanese (10.5 percent) and Cambodian women (5.4 percent). More than a half of the women (58.4 percent) were full-time housewives (table 14.2).

Health Status and Health Behaviors

For comparison by countries where immigrant wives originally came from, results were pulled for women from the following five countries in the order of group size: Vietnam, China, Philippines, Japan, and Cambodia ($n = 2,658$) (table 14.3). Japanese women were older, and lived in Korea for longer than

Table 14.2 Demographic Characteristics

Characteristics		*Percent (%)*
Age (30.6±9.1, SE=0.2)	15–19 years	3.5
	20–29 years	52.0
	30–39 years	28.9
	40–49 years	11.8
	50 and older	3.7
Country of origin	Vietnam	34.3
	China	30.4
	Philippines	11.8
	Japan	10.5
	Cambodia	5.4
	Others	7.6
Years of residence	> 5 years	28.5
	3–5 years	20.2
	< 3 years	51.3
Occupation	Housewife	58.4
	Employed	6.2
	Self-owned business	1.7
	Farming/Fishing	4.2

other women, while women from Vietnam and Cambodia were younger and relatively recent immigrants.

Generally Vietnamese women fell in lower ranges of disease prevalence and health risk factors in the participant group. Although the mean BMI of the immigrated women did not vary much by their countries of origin, obesity prevalence was the highest among Filipina women (22.3 percent) when 7.8 percent of the Vietnamese women were obese ($p < 0.01$). Immigrant wives from the Philippines showed highest proportions of high blood pressure (10.9 percent, $p < 0.01$), and needing hepatitis B vaccination (64.1 percent, $p < 0.01$). Cambodian women had the highest proportion of ECG abnormal readings (7.2 percent, $p < 0.01$), and Japanese women were most anemic (4.9 percent, $p < 0.01$).

Differences found among the women by country of origin in the prevalence of urine abnormalities, liver function results, total cholesterol levels, diabetes, sexually transmitted diseases, abnormal chest X-ray reading, and uterine cancer were insignificant.

More women from Vietnam and the Philippines reported cooking salty food ($p < 0.01$) and preferring meat ($p < 0.01$), while Chinese wives cooked spicy food ($p < 0.01$), and ate irregularly ($p < 0.01$). Half of Chinese, Filipina, and Cambodian wives, respectively, responded that they cooked meals mainly by frying food ($p < 0.01$). Japanese women practiced most desirable eating behavior by eating both meat and vegetables ($p < 0.01$), eating regularly ($p < 0.01$), broiling or steaming food than frying ($p < 0.01$), not eating salty and spicy food ($p < 0.01$), and not drinking ($p < 0.01$).

Although great majorities of these women neither smoke nor drink, Chinese women present the highest proportions of current smokers (4.2 percent) and alcohol drinking (17.9 percent, $p < 0.01$). Women from the Philippines were the most physically active (39.1 percent, $p < 0.01$), while Cambodian and Japanese women were the least active. Chinese wives were most stressed (43.7 percent, $p < 0.01$).

Comparison of Health Characteristics by Age and by Years of Residence

Immigrant women who were younger than thirty-four were more likely to eat meat than older women (age$\geq$40), and this tendency was weaker as the age progressed (table 14.4). Women in their late twenties reported that they cooked food mainly by frying more than women in their forties and older (OR = 1.315, $p < 0.05$). Meanwhile, younger women were less likely to eat regularly, except for those in the late twenties.

Exercise and physical activity levels did not differ by age groups, and those younger than twenty-four were significantly not stressed than those over 40 (OR = 0.752, $p < 0.05$).

Table 14.3 Health Status and Health Behavior Practices by Country of Origin

		All Immigrants	Country of Origin					
			Vietnam	China	Philippines	Japan	Cambodia	p-value
Cases (%)		2,658 (100.0)	991 (37.3)	872 (32.8)	336 (12.6)	303 (11.4)	156 (5.9)	
Age, mean, year			24.7	34.1	32.0	40.2	24.1	<0.001
Years of residence in Korea (%)			7.8	30.4	50.3	83.6	3.2	<0.001
≥5 years			21.4	24.2	17.4	8.9	9.6	
3–4.99 years			70.8	45.4	32.4	7.6	87.2	
< 3 years								
Health status	BMI	21.9	20.9	22.7	22.8	22.3	21.2	<0.01
	Mean Overweight (%)	16.4	11.0	20.6	18.5	19.1	16.0	
	Obese (%)	15.6	7.8	21.0	22.3	14.9	10.9	
	BP abnormal (%)	5.4	4.6	6.0	10.9	7.9	4.5	<0.01
	ECG abnormal (%)	6.0	4.1	5.1	4.2	4.3	7.2	<0.01
	Urine abnormal (%)	10.8	9.6	10.8	13.3	6.8	8.6	
	Anemia (%)	2.3	1.6	1.7	4.1	4.9	3.8	<0.01
	Liver abnormal (%)	2.0	1.4	1.8	2.9	1.6	2.6	
	Total cholesterol	2.7	2.3	3.1	2.9	4.3	3.8	
	Borderline (%) Abnormal (%)	2.1	2.2	2.2	3.5	2.3	0.6	
	Mean	170.3	167.3	170.8	173.2	179.0	167.1	
	Diabetes	0.9	1.0	1.3	0.3	0.3	–	
	Borderline (%) Abnormal (%)	0.7	0.6	0.8	0.6	0.3	1.3	
	Mean	85.2	83.8	86.9	84.8	85.1	83.6	
	Hepatitis B vulnerable (%)	44.1	43.4	37.2	64.1	44.5	56.9	<0.01
	Syphilis + (%)	0.6	0.1	1.4	0.3	0.3	—	
	HIV+ (%)	1 case	1 case	—	—	—	—	
	Chest x-ray Abnormal (%)	4.1	0.3	0.1	—	0.3	—	
	Uterine cancer (%)	0.7	0.4	1.3	0.5	—	—	

Health behaviors and mental health	Food seasoning (%)							<0.01
	Average Salty Spicy	77.9	78.6	71.5	80.7	90.1	83.9	
	Salty and spicy	10.1	11.4	9.3	11.8	6.1	8.1	
		5.6	4.2	10.0	2.2	1.0	4.7	
		6.3	5.8	9.1	5.3	2.7	3.4	
	Food preference (%)							<0.01
	Vegetables	22.5	20.0	28.5	18.0	18.5	22.4	
	Mixed Meat	66.5	63.9	66.6	67.8	78.8	60.5	
		11.0	16.1	4.9	14.1	2.7	17.0	
	Eating regularly (%)							<0.01
	Always Sometimes Irregular	46.1	46.9	37.5	57.2	61.0	44.1	
		38.5	36.7	43.8	30.0	32.5	44.1	
		15.4	16.3	18.8	12.8	6.5	11.7	
	Cooking style (%)							<0.01
	Fry Broil, Steam Uncooked	46.8	45.6	50.9	52.9	34.1	53.6	
		42.2	45.7	35.1	35.9	58.9	33.3	
		11.0	8.7	13.9	11.1	7.0	13.0	
	Drinking (%)							<0.01
	0	88.7	95.2	82.1	91.1	95.8	95.0	
	2–3 times/month	8.0	3.4	13.5	5.8	2.8	4.3	
	> Once a week	3.3	1.4	4.4	3.2	1.4	0.7	
	Not smoking (%)	96.9	99.5	95.8	97.7	99.0	100.0	
	Exercise (%)							<0.01
	0/week 1–2/week 3+/week	72.3	73.8	72.3	65.8	75.3	76.4	
		18.5	18.5	16.8	27.0	18.5	19.4	
		9.2	7.7	10.9	12.1	6.2	4.2	
	Stressed (%)	37.1	29.3	43.7	40.6	41.0	22.3	<0.01

Table 14.4 Adjusted Odds Ratios of Health Behavior Practice and Conditions, by Age and Years of Residence

	Age (Ref: 40 and older)				Years of Residence (Ref: >5 years)	
	≤24	25–29	30–34	35–39	<3 years	3–5 years
Eating more meat	2.246***	2.324***	1.893*	0.981	1.357	1.056
Cooking fried foods	1.258	1.315*	1.076	0.925	1.280*	1.364*
Eating regularly	0.708*	0.779	0.539***	0.658**	0.850	0.693**
Exercise regularly	0.825	0.915	1.050	0.968	0.974	0.771*
More physical activity	0.852	0.896	0.772	1.044	0.792*	1.043
Stressed a lot	0.752*	1.043	1.005	1.201	0.744**	0.767*
BMI	0.196***	0.442***	0.585**	0.756	0.896	0.980
BP	0.392***	0.281***	0.426***	0.443**	0.791	0.916
ECG	1.193	1.239	0.915	1.170	0.562*	0.606
Anemia	0.344*	0.170***	0.624	0.696	1.019	0.555
Total cholesterol	0.622	0.332*	0.358*	0.441	1.483	1.488

Note: $p < 0.05$*, $p < 0.01$**, $p < 0.001$***

Younger women were significantly less likely to be obese (age≤34) and to have hypertension (age≤39), anemia (age≤29), and hyperlipidemia (age twenty-five to thirty-four) that older women (age≥40). Age difference was not observed for diabetes and liver diseases.

Compared to the women who had lived in Korea for longer than five years, those who immigrated rather recently were more likely to have fried food and were less stressed. Those who had lived in Korea for less than three years were less physically active (OR = 0.792, p<0.05). Those who had lived in Korea for three to five years were less likely to eat (OR = 0.693, p<0.01) and—exercise regularly (OR = 0.771, p<0.05) than more seasoned immigrants.

There were not significant differences by years of residence in Korea among the immigrants in obesity, hypertension, anemia, hyperlipidemia, liver diseases, and diabetes except for abnormal ECG readings, which was significantly lower among recent immigrants (< 3 years, OR = 0.562, p<0.05).

Association between Health Behavior and Health Conditions

Adjusted odds ratios were computed for elevated BMI, blood pressure, total cholesterol, and glucose level, ECG abnormal reading, anemia, and liver

Table 14.5 Adjusted Odds Ratios of Health Conditions, by Age, Years of Residence and Health Behaviors

Variables		*BMI*	*BP*	*ECG*	*Anemia*	*Total Cholesterol*
Age	Ref 40 & older					
	≤24	0.196***	0.392***	1.193	0.344 *	0.622
	25–29	0.442***	0.281***	1.239	0.170 **	0.332*
Years of residence	30–34	0.585**	0.426**	0.915	0.624	0.358*
	35–39	0.756	0.443**	1.170	0.696	0.441
	Ref: >5 years					
Food preference	<3 years	0.896	0.791	0.562*	1.019	1.483
	3–5 years	0.980	0.916	0.606	0.555	1.488
	Ref: Meat					
Eating regularly	Vegetables	0.992	1.124	1.896	0.591	1.068
	Mixed	1.199	1.237	1.177	0.864	1.623
	Ref: Irregular	1.049	1.066	0.717	0.913	1.127
Cooking style	Ref: Fry					
	Broil, steam	0.974	1.080	0.970	1.062	0.983
	Uncooked	1.158	0.691	1.447	1.014	1.216
Regular exercise	Ref: 0/week	1.457**	1.216	1.468	1.170	1.878*
Lifetime physical activity	Ref: physically inactive	0.786*	1.774**	0.852	1.061	0.422**
Stressed	Ref: not stressed	1.027	0.907	0.837	1.066	1.844*

Note: $p < 0.05$*, $p < 0.01$**, $p < 0.001$***

diseases in association with health behaviors of eating (i.e., preferring meat or vegetables, eating regularly, and cooking food mainly by frying, broiling/steaming, and eating raw), exercising regularly, and being stressed (table 14.5). None of these behaviors was significantly associated with abnormal ECG readings, anemia, liver diseases, and glucose level. While eating behavior was not associated with BMI and blood pressure, those who exercised regularly were more likely to have elevated levels of BMI (OR = 1.457, $p = 0.002$) and total cholesterol (OR = 1.878, $p = 0.033$). Women at higher level of physical activity were less likely to have elevated levels of BMI (OR = 0.786, $p = 0.042$) and total cholesterol (OR = 0.422, $p = 0.006$) but more likely to have higher level of blood pressure (OR = 1.774, $p = 0.001$). Those stressed were more likely to have higher level of total cholesterol (OR = 1.844, $p = 0.034$).

DISCUSSION

The overall prevalence of obesity was 15.6 percent in this study. Compared to the 2008 health examination results by KAHP, the prevalence of obesity among immigrant women (9.9 percent) in their twenties in this study was slightly higher than that of Korean women (8.7 percent). Among those in their thirties, however, the difference in obesity prevalence between immigrant wives (20.1 percent) and Korean women (13.1 percent) became greater. A number of factors are thought to contribute to the obesity problem: adverse eating and physical activity patterns (Kumanyika et al., 2010); and social contexts for obesity development including types of foods and retail food outlets available, accessibility of healthy food, opportunity for physical activity, and exposure to targeted marketing of less healthful foods (Taylor et al., 2006; Powell et al., 2004; Henderson and Kelly, 2005). Yen and Kaplan (1998) suggest that low-SES areas negatively influence physical activity as physical activity-friendly environments are less common in low-SES areas. In this study, Japanese women were found to perform desirable eating behaviors comparably. However, a majority of women (72.3 percent) in this study reported that they do not exercise at all. Anyhow, those who exercised regularly were more likely to have elevated levels of BMI and total cholesterol than those who did not exercise at all. It may have to do with the fact that this was a cross-sectional study and that those who exercised regularly because they were overweight or obese and had higher total cholesterol level. On the other hand, those who were physically active, compared to those inactive, were more likely to have high blood pressure but less likely to have high BMI and total cholesterol. However, this cross-sectional study cannot explain such associations.

Anemia has been one of the most commonly found diseases among marriage immigrant women with 12.1 percent (Seol, 2006) and the prevalence of heart diseases and apoplexy is five to six times higher than that of the general public. This study reports the prevalence of anemia at 2.3 percent and ECG abnormal rate at 6.0 percent among immigrant wives, which is not as high as reported in a previous study but still requires consistent monitoring and close management. Within the immigrant women in the study, patterns of health problems differ by age and country of origin. Filipina women showed relatively high disease prevalence than any other group and had many health risk factors, whereas Vietnamese women were found to have lower disease prevalence. Cultural and behavioral background of the immigrant women are supposed to be associated with varying prevalence of health problems by heritage. Such background, therefore, should be considered importantly in developing and implementing interventions and services. Grouping immigrants together into a small number of large categories may mask important heterogeneity with regard to specific health conditions (WHO, 2008).

Immigrant women in this study were estimated two times more likely to be diagnosed with syphilis (0.6 percent, $n = 22$) than Korean women (0.3 percent) in Korea (KAHP, 2009). In addition, one case of HIV positive was reported in this study. Bacterial sexually transmitted diseases, which themselves are dangerous, are also known to increase vulnerability to HIV because they can enhance the efficacy of transmission from one person to another (Carballo and Mboup, 2005). It has also been reported that 66 percent of all heterosexually transmitted HIV infections in EU between 1997 and 2001 were diagnosed in people from countries with high HIV prevalence (Eurosurveillance Weekly, 2002). There is a sufficient need for health education on the prevention of sexually transmitted diseases with multicultural couples.

In the present study, behavior patterns differ by their heritage, age, and years of residence in Korea, which can be attributed to cultural background and experience. As the duration of residence in Korea increased, the stress level was increased. Thirty-seven percent of immigrant wives reported experience of severe stress during the last thirty days. Furthermore, the stressed women were estimated 1.8 times more likely to have high total cholesterol. These facts mean managing stress would be the priority topics of health education for immigrant wives. In so doing, psychosocial factors besides stress levels should be included in research and practice, such as isolation, social support, homesickness, and acculturation levels. It is likely that migrant wives come to marry economically challenged, rural, older Korean men from poorer places. Some of them may be expected to carry health profiles associated with poverty (Carballo and Mboup, 2005); thereafter, acculturation will occur as they spend more time in Korea. Acculturation may play a significant role in the association of health problems with increased duration of residence. In studies with Asian and Hispanic adolescents, acculturation to a U.S. lifestyle was shown to be associated with the adoption of unhealthy behaviors, such as sedentary behavior and poor dietary habits (Unger et al., 2004; Gordon-Larsen et al., 2003). Immigrant wives experience daily challenges in their new environment and roles predominantly responsible for the health of the entire family. Their health status and health behavior practices are also challenged in the adjustment process.

Most research including the present study has focused on individual indicators and their effect on health. However, extensive literature indicates that community and contextual factors (e.g., accessibility to healthcare facilities and heart-healthy foods) are associated with health outcomes in minority populations beyond the impact of individual influences (Morenoff and Lynch, 2004; Papas et al., 2007). Consideration of contextual factors may provide a more complete picture of the relationship between acculturation and health outcomes.

As for limitations of study, the present study is based on information provided by self-report, which may lead to bias from language barrier. Although the survey instrument was translated into four different languages and staff members provided assistance throughout the entire survey, the possibility of bias remains. Since this is a cross-sectional study, causal relationship cannot be established between significant variables.

Immigration to Korea by marriage is relatively a new phenomenon, thus continuing surveillance and research are needed to identify health risks, behavior patterns, and their relationships in order to unveil unique characteristics that might contribute to their health and potential influences of acculturation. Interventions and policies for the health of migrant wives, their children and families are required to strengthen cultural competence beyond language translation and adequacy. Empowerment of migrant wives and their families so that they could be competent of recognizing and addressing their health concerns should be one of core areas of health promotion approaches.

CONCLUSION

The health conditions of migrants have elicited concern from both human rights and public health points of view. Present study has identified some health issues of recent female marriage immigrants to Korea. Patterns of immigrant women's health problems differed by age and country of origin. Behavior patterns also differed by their heritage, age, and years of residence in Korea. Immigrant wives from the Philippines had the highest prevalence of obesity and high blood pressure. Vietnamese and Chinese women were less anemic, and immigrant wives from the Philippines had the largest proportion of hepatitis B unvaccinated.

In terms of dietary behaviors, Chinese women eat salty and/or spicy food, Cambodian and Vietnamese women eat more meat than vegetables. Japanese women eat regularly, and Filipina and Cambodian women cook their food mostly by frying, more so than women from other countries. Although great majorities of these women neither smoke nor drink, Chinese women present the highest proportions of current smokers and alcohol drinking. Less than a third of the immigrant wives exercise once a week or more frequently except for women from the Philippines. The proportion of women who are stressed often was the highest among Chinese women.

Immigration to Korea by marriage is relatively a new phenomenon, thus continuing surveillance and research are needed to identify health risks, behavior patterns, and their relationships in order to unveil unique characteristics that might contribute to their health and potential influences of acculturation. Interventions and policies for the health of migrant wives, their children and families are required to strengthen cultural competence beyond language translation and adequacy. Empowerment of migrant wives and their families so that they could be competent of recognizing and addressing their health concerns should be one of core areas of health promotion approaches.

NOTE

1. This chapter was previously published as Kim, Hye-Kyeong, Seungkyun Yoo, Seon Cho, Eun-Joo Kwon, Suyoung Kim, and Ji-Youn Park. "Health status and associated health risks among female marriage immigrants in Korea." *Korean Journal of Health Education and Promotion* 27, no. 5 (2010): 79–89.

REFERENCES

Eurosurveillance Weekly. 2002. "Substantial impact of the HIV pandemic on migrant populations in Europe." July 6:29. http://www.eurosurveillance.org/ViewArticle.aspx?ArticleId=1922.

Gordon-Larsen, P., Harris, K.M., Ward, D.S., Popkin, B.M. 2003. "National Longitudinal Study of Adolescent Health. Acculturation and overweight-related behaviors among Hispanic immigrants to the US: the National Longitudinal Study of Adolescent Health." *Social Science & Medicine* 57:2023–2034.

Henderson, V.R., Kelly, B. 2005. "Food advertising in the age of obesity: content analysis of food advertising on general market and African American television." *Journal of Nutrition Education and Behavior* 37:191–196.

Jeffrey, D. M., et al. 2004. "What makes a place healthy? Neighborhood influences on racial/ethnic disparities in health over the life course: critical perspectives on racial and ethnic differences in late life." In *Critical Perspectives on Racial and Ethnic Differences in Health in Late Life*. Edited by Anderson NB, Bulatao RA, Cohen B. Washington, DC: National Academies Press (US): 406–449.

KAHP. 2008. *Analysis of 2007 Health Examination Results for Female Immigrants Women in Korea*. Korea Association of Health Promotion, Unpublished Internal Report.

KAHP. 2009. *Analysis of 2008 Health Examination Results for Female Immigrants Women in Korea*. Korea Association of Health Promotion, Unpublished Internal Report.

Korea Institute on Health and Social Affairs. 2010. *A National Survey on Multicultural Families 2009*.

Kumanyika, S.K., et al. 2010. "Population-based prevention of obesity the need for comprehensive promotion of healthful eating, physical activity, and energy balance: a scientific statement from American heart association council on epidemiology on prevention, interdisciplinary committee for prevention (formerly the expert panel on population and prevention science)." *Circulation* 118:428–464.

Manuel, C., Mourtala, M. 2005. "International migration and health." *Global Commission on International Migration*, September: 1–14.

Ministry of Public Administration and Safety. 2008. www.mopas.go.kr.

Papas, M.A., Alberg, A.J., Ewing, R., Helzlsouer, K.J., Gary, T.L., Klassen, A.C. 2007. "The built environment and obesity." *Epidemiologic Reviews* 29:129–143.

Powell, L.M., Slater, S., Chaloupka, F.J. 2004. "The relationship between community physical activity settings and race, ethnicity and socioeconomic status." *Evidence-Based Preventive Medicine* 1:135–144.

Seol, D.H. 2006. "Women marriage immigrants in Korea: immigration process and adaptation." *Asia-Pacific Forum* 33:32–59.

Statistics Korea. 2007. www.kostat.go.kr.

Taylor, W.C., Poston, W.S.C., Jones, L., Kraft, M.K. 2006. "Environmental justice: obesity, physical activity, and healthy eating." *Journal of Physical Activity and Health* 3(1):s30–s54.

Unger, J.B., Reynolds, K., Shakib, S., Spruijt-Metz, D., Sun, P., Johnson, C.A. 2004. "Acculturation, physical activity, and fast-food consumption among Asian-American and Hispanic adolescents." *Journal of Community Health* 29:467–481.

World Health Organizations. 2008. *Obesity and Overweight.* Retrieved from: http://www.who.int/mediacentre/factsheets/fs311/en/index.html.

Yen, I.H., Kaplan, G.A. 1998. "Poverty area residence and changes in physical activity level: evidence from the Alameda County Study." *American Journal Public Health* 88:1709–1712.

Chapter 15

The Mental Health of Ethnic Minority Youths in South Korea and Its Related Environmental Factors

A Literature Review

Yeeun Lee, Minji Lee, and Subin Park

Cultural[1] and ethnic diversity is a growing trend in contemporary societies due to global migration [1]. South Korea, once an ethnically homogeneous society, is also experiencing a burgeoning ethnic minority population, with an influx of foreign workers and immigrants through marriage [2]. In 2008, when the Multicultural Family Support Act was first implemented, the number of multicultural families in the national survey was 1,44,000, but this number increased to 3,30,000 in 2017, suggesting that the number of multicultural families more than doubled over the past decade [3]. Although this change can help foster positive diversity, minority groups are, at best, often underrepresented and, at worst, discriminated against or socially excluded [4]. This is particularly the case for ethnic minority youths who are faced with the challenges of multicultural identities.

According to the 2018 national census data, the highest proportion of multiethnic youths (MY) comprise children born in South Korea to a Korean and a foreign spouse (who migrated mostly from China or Southeast Asian countries [80.4 percent]), followed by children born to foreign-born parents (12.8 percent), and children born in a foreign country to foreign parent(s) who later immigrated to South Korea (6.8 percent) [2]. Therefore, most MY in South Korea are 2.5 generation Korean-born youths, with one foreign-born parent. In addition to the stress of being part of an ethnic minority, including stress due to discrimination and issues about belonging and identity [5,6], MY may experience stress as a result of contact between the distinct culture of foreign parent(s) and the culture of the majority [7]. These sociocultural adversities could make MY vulnerable to mental health problems.

With the increasing MY concerns, recent studies have examined mental health outcomes in the Korean society. However, to our knowledge, no literature review has been conducted to integrate the empirical findings of these studies. Thus, the goal of the present review was to assess the mental health of MY by comparing it to that of native-born Korean youths (NKRY) in order to monitor the mental health status of MY and to systematically summarize the effect of various contextual variables on their mental health. By employing the Bronfenbrenner's ecological system model [8], which underlines the importance and influence of the child's own contextual surroundings, we also summarized findings on the influence of multiple layers of social environments on the mental health of MY, from the most proximal familial influences to the most distal school, community, and cultural influences.

METHODS

Search and Selection

We searched for empirical research papers on mental adaptation among school-aged MY and NKRY, with a minimum sample size of twenty-five. Articles were excluded if they (1) were qualitative or reviews, (2) were irrelevant to the main topic (e.g., physical health and school adaptation), or (3) used unpublished data (e.g., thesis/dissertation).

Articles written in the English and Korean languages (published up until March 2019) were searched systematically in five online databases (International journals: PubMed, Scopus, and Web of Science; Korean journals: DBPIA and RISS). The following key search terms were used: multiethnic youths (multicultural OR bicultural OR biethnic OR multiethnic) AND (children OR adolescent OR youth OR teenage) AND mental health (psychiatr* OR psycholog* OR mental OR psycho- social OR wellbeing OR adjustment OR adaptation OR protective factor OR risk factor OR vulnerability factor OR resilience OR emotion OR behavior OR behaviour) AND Korea (Korea OR Korean). The search strategy was adjusted for each database. Initially, 507 articles were identified. After excluding duplicates and irrelevant articles by reviewing the titles and abstracts, fifty-four articles were finally included (table 15.1, figure 15.1).

RESULTS

Mental Health among Multiethnic Youths

Mental health problems can be categorized into internalizing and externalizing problems. Case-control studies that compared internalizing problems in MY,

Table 15.1 Included Studies

Author	*Population*	*N*	*Mean Age (range)*	*Outcomes (Assessment Tools)*	*Comparison Group*
Ahn et al. [10]	MY	617	14.7(13–18)	Depressive mood, suicide attempt (single-item questions adopted from the KYRBS)	Native-born Korean adolescents (n=66,302)
Bahk et al. [14]	MY	2,667	N/R(13–18)	Depressive mood, suicidal ideation, plans and attempts (a single-item question adopted from the KYRBS)	Native-born Korean adolescents (n=291,657)
Cho [31]	MY (children of a foreign-born mother and a Korean-born father)	2,811	N/R(9-15)	Depressive symptoms (a single-item author' question)	
Cho [59]	MY (children of a foreign-born mother and a Korean-born father)	121	N/R(12-18)	Externalizing problems (K-YSR)	
Choi et al. [26]	MY	115	14.4 (12-18)	Online game addiction (Lemmens et al. question) [87], juvenile delinquents (three items)	Adolescents in monocultural familes (n = 131)
Choi [50]	Korean-Japanese MY	309	14.2 (12-18)	Internalizing and externalizing problems (K-YSR)	
Chung and Lim* [47]	MY (children of a foreign-born mother and a Korean-born father)	164	12.5	Depressive symptoms (CES-D), self-esteem (RSE)	
Hwang and Heo [34]	MY	86	N/R(7-12)	Social anxiety (K-SAS)	

(*Continued*)

Table 15.1 Included Studies (Continued)

Author	*Population*	*N*	*Mean Age (range)*	*Outcomes (Assessment Tools)*	*Comparison Group*
Jang et al. [16]	MY	3,423	N/R (14-19)	Depressive symptoms Native-born Korean (a single question adopted from the KYRBS)	Native-born Korean adolescents (n=323,934)
Jeong [83]	MY (children of a foreign-born mother and a Korean-born father)	480	N/R (14-19)	Psychiatric problems (SCL-47), resilience (ER)	
Jiang and Bae [51]	MY	216	11.9 (9-20)	Psychological maladjustment (a 14-item questionnaire assessing psychological maladjustment)	
Jin [48]	MY (children of a foreign-born parent and a Korean-born parent)	201	N/R(10-12)	Internalizing (K-YSR) and externalizing problems (a six-item author's questionnaire assessing aggressiveness)	
Ju et al. [13]	MY (children of a foreign-born mother and a Korean-born father)	665	N/R (13–18)	Depressive mood, suicidal ideation, plan and attempt (single-item questions adopted from KYRBS)	Native-born Korean adolescents (*n* = 62,320)
Jwa [84]	MY (foreign-born MY)	187	16.3 (9–24)	Depression/anxiety symptoms (K-YSR)	
Kang et al. [11]	MY	243	N/R (7–12)	Teacher's ratings of internalizing and externalizing problems (K-TRF)	Native-born Korean children (*n* = 243)
Kang and Kim [41]	MY (children of a foreign-born mother and a Korean-born father)	269	N/R (9–12)	Internalizing and externalizing problems (K-YSR)	
Kim and Kim [58]	MY	206	N/R (13–15)	Internalizing and externalizing problems (K-YSR)	

Kim et al. [85]	MY (children of a foreign-born mother and a Korean-born father)	113	11.3 (10–13)	Depression and anxiety symptoms (K-YSR)	
Kim et al. [12]	MY	666	14.5 (13–18)	Depressive mood, suicidal ideation, plan and attempt (single-item questions adopted from the KYRBS)	Native-born Korean adolescents (n = 71,348)
Kim and Kim [39]	MY (children of a foreign-born mother and a Korean-born father)	179	N/R (11–18)	Depression and anxiety symptoms (KGHQ-20)	
Kim et al. [37]	MY	138	9.3 (9–11)	Self-esteem (a 7-item questionnaire derived from the PCSC)	
Kim [53]	MY (children of a foreign-born mother and a Korean-born father)	120	N/R (7–12)	Internalizing problems (K-YSR), externalizing problems (a 10-item questionnaire measuring aggressiveness and delinquency adopted from KYPS)	
Kim [55]	MY (children of a foreign-born mother and a Korean-born father)	314	N/R (7–12)	Self-esteem (a 6-item questionnaire derived from RSE)	
Kim and Hong [35]	MY	204	N/R (10–12)	Internalizing and externalizing problems (K-YSR)	
Lee [23]	MY	795	N/R (12–18)	Experience of violence, stress, depression, suicidal ideation (KYRBS)	Native-born Korean adolescents (n = 62,649)
Lee [38]	MY	191	N/R (11–12)	Internalizing and externalizing problems (each ten-item questionnaire measuring depression, anxiety, and aggressiveness derived from CBCL)	

(Continued)

Table 15.1 Included Studies (Continued)

Author	*Population*	*N*	*Mean Age (range)*	*Outcomes (Assessment Tools)*	*Comparison Group*
Lee et al. [24]	MY	378	N/R (11-13)	Iinternalizing and externalizing problems (K-YSR)	Native-born Korean adolescents (n = 382)
Lee et al. [49]	MY (children of Vietnamese mother and Korean-born father)	296	11.5 (9-18)	Self-esteem (3-item from RSE)	
Lee [46]	MY	1,597	16	Depression, social withdrawal, self-esteem (questionnaires adopted from MAPS)	
Lee [61]	MY (children of a foreign-born mother and Korean-born father)	304	N/R(13-18)	Internalizing and externalizing problems (K-YSR)	
Lee et al. [60]	MY	1,348	14	Depression, social withdrawal (questionnaires adopted from MAPS)	
Moon et al. [29]	MY	1,812	N/R(9-12)	Depressive symptoms (single question)	
Moon and An [86]	MY (children of a foreign-born mother and Korean-born father)	125	11.4	Psychiatric symptoms (SCL-90)	
Oh [36]	MY	4,775	15.3(9-24)	Depressive moods (a single-item question adopted from NSMF)	
Oh and Jwa [32]	MY (Korean-born MY and foreign- born MY)	4,775	12.6 (9-24)	Depressive moods (a single-item question adopted from NSMF)	
Paik and Yeum [28]	MY	1,343	14	Depression (questionnaires adopted from MAPS)	

Park and Nahm* [22]	MY	107	N/R(9-12)	Self-esteem (self-esteem inventory for children in Korea)	Native-born Korean children (n = 100)
Park et al. [52]	MY	4,141	N/R (9-18)	Depressive moods (a single-item question adopted from NSMF)	
Park et al. [18]	MY	3,995	14.6	Substance use, suicidality (questionnaires assessing alcohol use, smoking, drug use, suicidal ideation, plan, and attempts adopted from KYRBS)	Native-born Korean adolescents (n = 12,876) North Korean adolescents (n = 297)
Park*† [45]	MY (children of a foreign-born mother and Korean-born father)	403	11.4(13-14)	Internalizing problems (K-YSR)	
Park and Jang [40]	MY (children of a foreign-born mother and Korean-born father)	88	14.0(11-19)	Ego identity (Korean ego identity scale)	
Park and Nam [15]	MY	101	7.5 (5-12)	Teacher's rating of internalizing and externalizing problems and social relationships (KPRC-TF)	Native-born Korean children (n = 248)
Park [43]	MY (children of a foreign-born mother and Korean-born father)	121	N/R (7-15)	Self-esteem (RSE)	
Park [25]	MY	734	14.5	Substance use (questionnaires assessing alcohol use, smoking, drug use adopted from KYRBS)	Native-born Korean adolescents (n = 66,217)
Park and Lee [19]	MY (children of a foreign-born mother and Korean-born father)	727	14.9	Suicide attempt (a single question adopted from the KYRBS)	
Rhee and Lee* [44]	MY (foreign-born MY, children of foreign-born mother)	210	N/R (13-14)	Internalizing and externalizing problems (K-YSR)	

(Continued)

Table 15.1 Included Studies (Continued)

Author	*Population*	*N*	*Mean Age (range)*	*Outcomes (Assessment Tools)*	*Comparison Group*
Ryou et al. [33]	MY (children of a foreign-born mother and Korean-born father)	120	16	Depression (CES-D), anxiety (Beck's inventory for measuring clinical anxiety), suicidal ideation (SSI)	
Seol et al. [56]	MY	131	11.9(11-13)	Self-esteem (RSE)	
Song and Park [54]	MY (children of a foreign-born mother and Korean-born father)	242		Withdrawal behavior (K-CBCL)	
Yang et al.* [27]	MY (children of a foreign-born mother and Korean-born father)	305	N/R (9-15)	Depressive symptoms (CDI), self-esteem (RSE)	
Yeom and Yang* [42]	MY (children of a foreign-born mother and Korean-born father)	70	N/R (7-12)	Internalizing and externalizing problems, social competence (K-CBCL)	
Yi and Kim [9]	MY (children of foreign mother)	698	14.8	Depression, suicidal ideation, smoking (a single-item question adopted from the KYRBS)	Native-born Korean adolescents (*n* = 64,728)
Yim and Park [17]	MY	804	N/R (13-18)	Depression, suicidal ideation, substance use (single-item questionnaires adopted from the KYRBS)	Native-born Korean adolescents (*n* = 70,743)
Yun and Yang [57]	MY	136	N/R (10-19)	Delinquency (author's questionnaire)	

*Indicates that sample includes child–mother pairs, †indicates longitudinal study. CDI: Kovac's Children's Depression Inventory, CES-D: Center for Epidemiological Studies-Depression, ER: Ego Resiliency Scale, K-APQ: Korean Adolescent Risk-Taking Questionnaire, K-CBCL: Korean version of Child Behavior Checklist, KGHQ-20: Korean version of the general health questionnaire, KPRC-TF: Korean Personality Rating Scale for Children-Teacher Form, K-SAS: Korean version of Social Anxiety Scale, K-TRF: Korean Teachers' Rating Form, KYPS: Korean Youth Panel Survey, KYRBS: Korea Youth Risk Behavior Web-based Survey, K-YSR: Korean Youth Self-Report, MAPS: Multicultural Adolescents Panel Study, MY: multiethnic youths, N/R: not reported, NSMF: National Survey of Multicultural Families, PCSC: Perceived Competence Scale for Children, PQ-Y: Parentification Questionnaire-Youth, RSE: Rosenberg's Self-Esteem Scale, SCL: Symptom Checklist, SSI: Scale for Suicidal Ideation

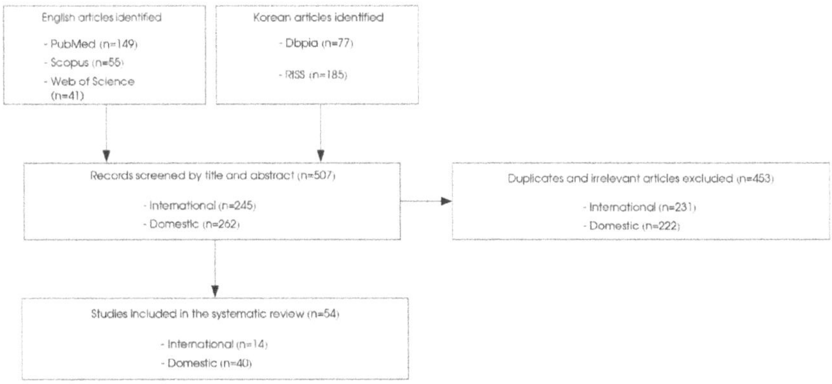

Figure 15.1 Search Strategy and Article Selection Process.

notably, depression and anxiety symptoms, with those of NKRY, showed variations in relative prevalence or severity. No significant difference was noted in reports on the prevalence and severity of internalizing symptoms including depressive and anxiety symptoms and suicidal ideation [9–12]. In other studies, however, the prevalence or severity of depressive and anxiety symptoms and suicidal behaviors among MY was high [13–16], even after adjusting for other sociodemographic variables [17,18]. Inconsistent results across studies may be attributed to varying sample characteristics. For instance, one national representative study noted that the relative risk for internalizing problems in MY differed according to sex, such that a relatively high prevalence of mood symptoms and suicidal ideation was observed only among male, but not female, youths [14]. Additionally, when compared with native-born Korean children, teacher-rated anxiety and depressive symptoms were higher only among younger (eight to ten years), but not in older, MY [15].

For more lethal symptoms, such as history of suicide attempts and hospitalization after a suicide attempt, the risk is two to three times higher among MY than among native-born adolescents, although a similar result was not obtained for suicidal ideations/plans [10,12,19]. This suggests that despite the lack of difference in the prevalence of suicidal ideations/plans between MY and NKRY, MY are more likely to attempt suicide, which warrants special attention. In addition to these clinical problems, young MY consistently report poorer self-image and higher perceived stress than do native-born children across multiple domains, including appearance, academic performance, and peer and family relationships [20–23].

Externalizing problems include diverse behavioral symptoms, such as aggressive and hyperactive behaviors and delinquencies, including smoking and drinking. One study noted that young MY, between the ages of five and twelve years, were more likely to engage in hyperactive behaviors, as rated by their teachers, in comparison to native-born peers [15]. Another study showed that young MY between the ages of eleven and thirteen years had higher scores on externalizing problems including delinquency and aggression compared to their monocultural peers [24]. For adolescent MY, studies have focused more on delinquent behaviors. In general, MY display a high rate of smoking or substance use [9,10,17,18], but behaviors differ as a function of the multicultural family type. Compared with native-born adolescents, MY with foreign-born fathers or foreign-born parents were more likely to smoke or use drugs. On the contrary, MY with foreign-born mothers were less likely to smoke or use alcohol [25]. Moreover, adolescents from multicultural families had higher game addiction factor and mood modification scores than those from monocultural families. However, there was no significant difference in juvenile delinquency between MY and NKRY adolescents [26].

Associated Environmental Factors

Sociodemographic Factors

Socioeconomic positions, such as low family income [19,27–29], nondesirable occupation of the father [30], and low parental education level [29,31] have been linked to increased mental health risks, including depressive symptoms, suicide attempts, and problematic alcohol use, among MY. Moreover, one's living arrangement was noted as a significant factor; MY who were not currently living with their parents were at a high risk of attempting suicide [19].

Family-related demographic factors are closely associated with the mental health of MY. MY with foreign-born fathers or foreign-born parents are at a greater risk of internalizing and externalizing problems, including depressive moods and suicidal behaviors, than MY with foreign-born mothers [14,19] or native Korean parents [16,18]. Moreover, foreign-born MY who migrated to South Korea experience a higher rate of social discrimination and peer victimization, and thus, report greater depressive moods as compared to Korean-born MY [32,33]. Specifically, family separation during the immigration process is a significant risk factor; the longer the separation from parents, the higher the level of depression and anxiety symptoms as well as suicidal ideation [33].

Familial Factors

Family relationship quality, which is assessed as family cohesion, support, communication, and subjective satisfaction, also plays an important role in the overall psychological adaptation of MY. It decreases mental health risks such as depression, anxiety, and suicidal ideation [28,31,33–36] and improves self-esteem [37]. In contrast, the risk for depression was high among MY who spent less time conversing with their fathers and those whose parents showed a low degree of interest in them [29]. Moreover, verbal or physical violence between parents or toward young MY predicted aggressiveness, as well as depressive and anxiety symptoms [38].

Positive parenting, which involves the adoption of an open communication style [39] and consistent and less authoritarian parenting [40], was associated with better mental health (e.g., decreased depression and anxiety and a better-developed identity) among MY. The extent of a mother's acceptance of her children's emotions was also associated with the self-esteem of young MY [22]. In addition, parentification, which is the process whereby a child is obliged to act as a parent to their own parent or sibling, was negatively correlated with both externalizing and internalizing problems among young MY, but not among monocultural family youth. This suggests that family strengths, shame, and self-differentiation are significant mediators between parentification and the mental health of young MY [24].

In addition to the influence of the mother-child relationship [41], the mother's psychosocial adaptation also affects internalizing and externalizing problems in MY [42]. Particularly, for MY with foreign mothers, the ease or difficulty with mother's sociocultural adaptation, acculturative stress, and perceived discrimination in South Korea can predict low self-esteem, depressive symptoms, and behavioral problems among MY [27,40,42–45]. One longitudinal study noted that acculturative stress and marginalization (from both host and home cultures) of foreign mothers were associated with the decreased multicultural acceptance of MYs, which also predicted greater depressive symptoms and social withdrawal three years later. Conversely, successful integration of a mother's original and host culture predicted low likelihood of the occurrence of depression and social withdrawal in children [46]. In a mediation study, a mother's perceived discrimination and acculturative stress influenced the internalizing symptoms of the MY via an increase the mother's depressive symptoms [47]. Proficiency in the Korean language was found to have a positive effect [47–49]. Given the significant association between Korean language ability and both internalizing and externalizing symptoms [29,35,36,50] and psychological maladjustment of MY [51], MY whose mothers have difficulty learning the Korean language may have poorly developed language abilities, which may indirectly influence their adaptation.

Social Relationships

The influences of other social relationships have been reported. Discrimination from friends, teachers, relatives, and even strangers, has been associated with heightened internalizing and externalizing problems [31,35,50,52,53], withdrawal behaviors [54], and decreased self-esteem among MY [55]. One mediation study suggested that experiencing social discrimination may adversely affect the self-image of MY since it leads to the internalization of stigma [56]. Another study reported that dual identity partially mediates the effect of social rejection on withdrawal behaviors [54]. Problematic relationships with peers have deleterious psychosocial impacts such as a high risk for depressive moods, suicide ideation or attempts, and delinquent behaviors [12,23,29,31,53,57]. Moreover, stress resulting from conflicts with teachers has a significant impact on suicide attempts by MY when compared to other stressors [19].

Positive aspects of social relationships can also enhance MY adaptation. In general, perceived social support is associated with decreased internalizing symptoms [53,58], delinquent behaviors [57], improved self-esteem [27], and a more developed identity in MY [40]. Specifically, support at school from peers, teachers, and after-school teachers has been independently associated with low levels of depressive symptoms [28,33]. A path analysis further noted that social support acts as a buffer against stresses from discrimination or problematic peer relationships, and attenuates the psychological impact of such distress [53].

Cultural Adjustment

Cultural adjustment can be a psychological challenge for MY when one has to navigate one's Korean culture with that of a foreign-born parent(s). The difficulty associated with cultural adaptation among MY has been linked to internalizing and externalizing problems [41,48]. A number of mediation studies noted that stress associated with cultural adaptation among MY influences internalizing problems by decreasing one's sense of identity [58]. Additionally, stress associated with cultural adaptation predicts externalizing problems (e.g., delinquency and aggressiveness) via an increase difficulty in school adaptation [59]. One moderation study showed that acculturation stress in MY affects the levels of psychological maladjustment, whereas resilience moderates the relationship between acculturation stress and the levels of psychological maladjustment [51]. While marginalization by both the Korean culture and that of foreign parents is associated with greater depressive symptoms and social withdrawal [31,60], bicultural acceptance [27,60], bicultural efficacy [48], and a well-established ethnic identity [49,50] are consistently linked to better psychological adaptation. In another study, the degree of the perception of an individual as Korean by others, rather than one's own self-perception, is associated with overall internalizing (social withdrawal, anxiety, and depression) and externalizing problems [61], highlighting the significance of the social perception of MY.

DISCUSSION

This review addressed a range of mental health risks among children from multicultural families. We aimed to, first, compare the mental health outcomes of MY with those of NKRY and, second, identify multiple layers of environmental factors that may facilitate or inhibit psychological adjustment (figure 15.2).

Ethnic minority status and relevant socioeconomic disadvantages pose mental health risks for MY [62,63]. Consistent with the results of studies on ethnic minorities in other countries [64,65], much empirical evidence supports disparities in mental health outcomes between MY, who are at a higher risk for emotional and behavioral problems, and their native-born counterparts. However, it should be noted that risks/outcomes vary across studies. Differences may be attributed to the heterogeneous outcome variables or samples examined across studies. Specifically, large-scale studies reveal more than a twofold risk for suicidal behavior among MY [14,19] compared to NKRY. This suggests the need for early preventive interventions.

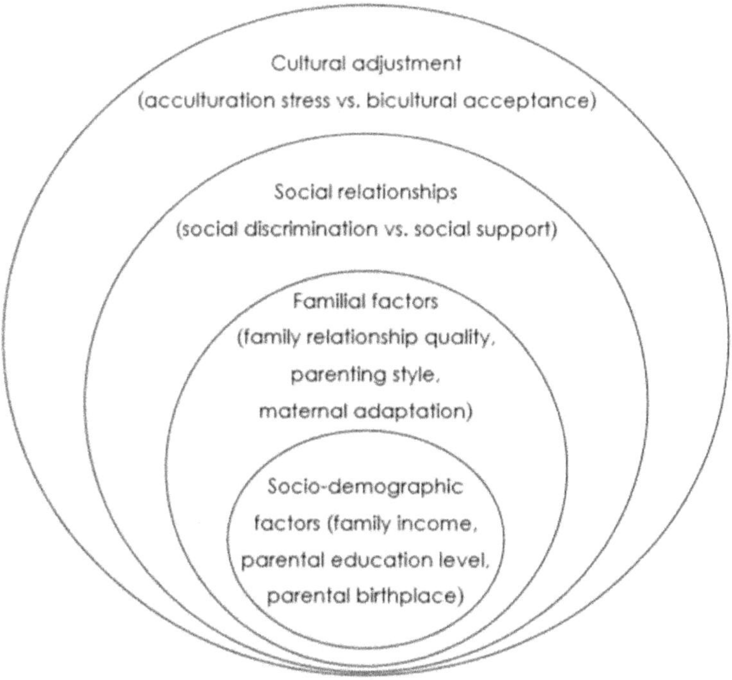

Figure 15.2 Multiple Layers of Contextual Factors Affecting Multiethnic Youths Mental Health.

Proximal family variables were the most studied environmental factors for assessing associations with psychological mental health in MY. Among family-related mental health risks, separation from parents is the most consistent predictor of mental health issues, which include depression, anxiety, and suicidal ideation and attempts [19,33]. This is especially the case for immigrant MY, who experience family separation during the immigration process, which may have adverse mental health effects on them [33]; thus, the impact of long-term mental health on future integration in South Korea should be carefully considered. Moreover, poor family relationships and domestic violence predict a high risk for mental health issues in MY [38]. Previous studies involving immigrant women who married Korean men showed higher marital distress in multicultural families than in native Korean families [66]. This marital distress often presented as a high prevalence of domestic violence. Robust social protective systems are needed for MY who do not have familial support for successful multicultural adjustment.

Limited education and income opportunities partially cause ethnic disparities in access to mental health resources [67,68]. These social disadvantages pose risks for deleterious psychosocial adaptation among children, as well [69,70]. Mental health outcomes among MY in South Korea are also influenced by the parents' ethnicity and socioeconomic status [19,27,30,31]. Moreover, maternal psychosocial problems, notably depression and cultural maladjustment, increase the mental health risks of children. This is consistent with the well-established notion of "intergenerational transmission" of maternal mental health [71,72]. Given the positive influence of helpful social support provided for foreign-born mothers and for the adjustment of MY [73], social support systems for first-generation immigrants could have many secondary effects on the mental health of their children.

Social support and belonging are important for youth who feel isolated from ethnic majority groups [74]. Social discrimination has deleterious effects on the mental health of MY. However, social support can act as a buffer against social adversity [53]. Our review particularly highlights the major role of MY relationships, including peer and teacher relationships, at school. Previous studies noted that MY experience more difficulty in overall adjustment at school compared to native-born youths. The parameters for adjustment include relationships with teachers and peers, as well as academic adaptation and rule observation [20,21]. In one case-control study, MY reported more problems with peer relationships. They feel excluded or are dissatisfied with their peer group compared to their native-born peers [22]. Furthermore, studies that used data on Korean youth showed that MY were three to five times more likely to report being victims of school violence [10,12,23], and specifically those with foreign-born mothers were 4.1

times, and those with foreign-born fathers were 17.4 times at a higher risk of victimization respectively [75]. Given the critical role of peer relationships in the psychological adjustment of youth later in life [76,77] and the adverse effect of peer bullying on future psychopathology [78], interventions to enhance school connectedness and peer relationships are necessary for healthy MY adjustment.

The integration of distinct cultures and ethnic identities is another important challenge for MY. MY experience difficulties coping with being dissimilar to the majority of their peers. In addition to cultural differences, the perceived differences in appearance between MY and their peers contribute to poor school adaptation [79], which can adversely affect psychological well-being [29]. Psychological interventions could help foster more effective coping strategies. For instance, a social-belonging intervention in the United States yielded long-term positive effects on the health and academic achievement of minority students. This was accomplished by monitoring the changes in the perception of youths regarding the social consequences of one's minority status [80]. Given the effect of such societal perceptions on adaptation [61], educating native-born youths to accept ethnic and cultural differences is necessary.

Limitations

Our systematic review had a few notable limitations. First, a meta-analysis could not be conducted given the extensive heterogeneity in sample demographics (e.g., age, parental origin), outcome variables, and measurements. Second, as this review only included published articles, a publication bias could be present. Thus, conclusions regarding the true nature of MY maladjustment should take these limitations into consideration.

Suggestions for Future Research

Future studies should investigate how multiple risk and protective factors work together to impact outcomes. Although several studies have identified simple and correlational relationships between each factor and MY mental health outcomes, the effect of any individual factor cannot be fully understood without examining the complex interactions between variables [81]. Furthermore, a prospective study to investigate long-term mental health outcomes and causal relationships between variables over time is required. Lastly, given the disparities in the use of services among MY in other countries [82], the utilization of mental health services by MY must be explored. Future work is needed to address the gap between service needs and service utilization in order to tackle relevant psychosocial barriers.

CONCLUSIONS

We reviewed fifty-four studies to compare MY's mental health outcomes with those of NKRY's and to identify multiple layers of relevant environmental factors. In conclusion, empirical evidence indicated that MY has relatively heightened risks for emotional and behavioral problems. The multiple layers of contextual factors including sociodemographic factors, familial factors, social relationships, and cultural adjustment were identified and noted. Future studies must elucidate the complex interplay between multiple risk and protective factors and the long-term adaptation and mental health service utilization of MY.

NOTE

1. This chapter was previously published as Lee, Yeeun, Minji Lee, and Subin Park. "The Mental Health of Ethnic Minority Youths in South Korea and Its Related Environmental Factors: A Literature Review." *Journal of the Korean Academy of Child and Adolescent Psychiatry* 30, no. 3 (2019): 88–99.

REFERENCES

1. Castles S, De Haas H, Miller MJ. *The Age of Migration: International Population Movements in the Modern World.* 5th ed. Basingstoke: Palgrave Macmillan, 2013.
2. Ministry of Gender Equality and Family. *An Analysis on the National Survey of Multicultural Families 2015* (Original Data in Korean). Seoul: Ministry of Gender Equality and Family, 2016.
3. Ministry of Gender Equality and Family. *2018 National Survey on the Multicultural Families.* Seoul: Ministry of Gender Equality and Family, 2019.
4. Phinney JS. "Ethnic identity in adolescents and adults: review of research." *Psychol Bull* 1990;108:499–514.
5. Okazaki S. "Impact of racism on ethnic minority mental health." *Perspect Psychol Sci* 2009;4:103–107.
6. Smedley BD, Myers HF, Harrell SP. "Minority-status stresses and the college adjustment of ethnic minority freshmen." *J High Educ* 1993;64:434–452.
7. Berry JW, Kim U. "Acculturation and mental health." In: Dasen PR, Berry JW, Sartorius N, editors. *Health and Cross-Cultural Psychology: Towards Applications.* Newbury Park, CA: Sage, 1988. pp. 207–236.
8. Bronfenbrenner U. *The Ecology of Human Development.* Cambridge, MA: Harvard University Press, 1979.
9. Yi Y, Kim JS. "Korean adolescents' health behavior and psychological status according to their mother's nationality." *Osong Public Health Res Perspect* 2017;8:377–383.

10. Ahn IY, Seo J, Lee D, Lee SJ, Cha B, Lee CS, et al. "Emotional characteristics of adolescents in monocultural and multicultural families in Korea." *J Korean Acad Child Adolesc Psychiatry* 2016;27:306–312.
11. Kang JH, Yeo TC, Kim JC, Kim JH, Im JY. "Comparison of sociality between children from multi-cultural families and children from non-multi-cultural families: latent mean analysis in behavioral problems and social abilities." *J Educ Cult* 2013;19:31–62.
12. Kim JM, Kong BG, Kang JW, Moon JJ, Jeon DW, Kang EC, et al. "Comparative study of adolescents' mental health between multi- cultural family and monocultural family in Korea." *J Korean Acad Child Adolesc Psychiatry* 2015;26:279–287.
13. Ju HO, Park SY, Lee J. "Mental health and health risk behaviors of multicultural adolescents according to their mothers' native country: using data from the 11th (2015) Korea youth risk behavior web-based survey 2015." *Child Health Nurs Res* 2017;23:101–110.
14. Bahk J, Kim AM, Khang YH. "Associations of multicultural status with depressive mood and suicidality among Korean adolescents: the roles of parental country of birth and socioeconomic position." *BMC Publ Health* 2017;17:116.
15. Park JH, Nam JS. "The language development and psychosocial adjustment of multicultural children." *Stud Korean Youth* 2010;21:129–152.
16. Jang J, Park EC, Lee SA, Choi Y, Choy YS, Kim W, et al. "Association between parents' country of birth and adolescent depressive symptoms: the early stages of multicultural society." *J Korean Med Sci* 2018;33:e116.
17. Yim SY, Park MH. "Behaviors and mental health of adolescents in multicultural families compared to general families." *J Korean Data Anal Soc* 2014;16:1641–1651.
18. Park S, Lee M, Park SJ, Lee MG. "Health risk behaviors and psychological problems among South Korean, North Korean, and other multicultural family adolescents (2011–2016)." *Psychiatry Res* 2018;268:373–380.
19. Park S, Lee Y. "Factors that affect suicide attempts of adolescents in multicultural families in Korea." *Int J Environ Res Public Health* 2016;13:E1184.
20. Hwang SY, Rho BI. "A study on the factors that influence satisfaction with school life of children from multicultural families." *Korea Acad Care Manage* 2015;15:51–76.
21. Kim AY, Kim SI. "Comparisons of psychological factors related to school adjustment between children from international marriage families and from general families." *Korean J Educ Psychol* 2011;25:853–873.
22. Park E, Nahm E. "Comparative research with general family: relation between accommodation attitude of emotional expression by multi culture family mother, children's peer relation and self-esteem." *J Korean Assoc Psychother* 2011;3:53–68.
23. Lee E. "Effects of school violence on depression and suicidal ideation in multicultural adolescents." *Iran J Publ Health* 2019;48:262–269.
24. Lee JS, Kim JM, Ju AR. "A structural analysis on the effects of children's parentification in multicultural families on their psychological maladjustment comparison with children in monocultural families." *J Korea Inst Youth Facil Environ* 2018;16:117–130.

25. Park S. “Substance use and sexual behaviors of adolescents in multicultural families in Korea.” *Psychiatry Invest* 2015;12:466–473.
26. Choi C, Hums MA, Bum CH. “Impact of the family environment on juvenile mental health: eSports online game addiction and delinquency.” *Int J Environ Res Publ Health* 2018;15:E2850.
27. Yang SY, Park SK, Kim MS. “Effects of bicultural characteristics and social capital on psychological adaptation.” *J Korea Cont Assoc* 2013;13:270–282.
28. Paik JG, Yeum DM. “A latent profile analysis on depression and ego-resiliency of adolescents in multi-cultural families.” *J Multicult Soc* 2018;11:295–319.
29. Moon SH, Lee MK, Lee MJ, Shim HJ, Cho HH. “Factors influencing the experience of depression among school-aged children from multicultural families.” *Child Health Nurs Res* 2018;24:434–442.
30. Baik J, Kim J, Yu Y. “A study on affecting factors on school resilience of adolescent from multicultural families.” *Youth Facil Environ* 2013;11:157–170.
31. Cho R. “Exploring the acculturation profiles and adaptation of children in multiethnic families in South Korea.” *Asian Pacif Migrat J* 2016;25:245–274.
32. Oh S, Jwa H. “The factors affecting on depression of multi-cultural families adolescents and immigrant adolescents.” *J School Soc Work* 2015;32:385–412.
33. Ryou B, Choi J, Sohn Y, Kim K. “Understanding of migration experiences and mental health among Korean immigrant youth.” *J Korean Soc Child Welfare* 2017;58:231–262.
34. Hwang M, Heo G. “The effect of parents’ attachment on social anxiety to multi-culture children link to the northeast Asian.” *J North-East Asian Cult* 2010;23:277–287.
35. Kim SJ, Hong CH. “The effect of discrimination experience and language problems on psychosocial adjustment in children with multi-cultural family: the moderating effect of ego-resilience and family strengths.” *Korean J Youth Stud* 2017;24:195–211.
36. Oh S. “The study on the eco-systemic variables affecting multicultural family adolescents’ depression.” *J Commun Welfare* 2016;56:1–27.
37. Kim MY, Lim JY, Chung GH. “Effects of Korean proficiency and parent-child cohesion on self-esteem and acculturation among children from multicultural families.” *J Korean Acad Nurs* 2012;42:879–888.
38. Lee HB. “The influence of domestic violence and child abuse internalization and externalization in multicultural families child.” *J Welf Couns Educ* 2014;3:55–79.
39. Kim MK, Kim HY. “The effects of psychological characteristics, parent-child relationship, and coping strategies on school adjustment of multicultural family adolescents.” *Korean J Family Welfare* 2015;20:367–385.
40. Park JW, Jang JH. “The environmental and psychological factors influencing the ego identity of teenagers from multicultural families.” *Korean J Youth Stud* 2014;21:133–154.
41. Kang Y, Kim B. “The relationships between the attachment of multicultural family children to mothers and theirs psychosocial adjustments: the intervening effects of acculturation stresses and negative coping mechanisms.” *Korea J Youth Counsel* 2013;21:19–42.

42. Yeom M, Yang S. "A Study on the maternal cultural and emotional factors influencing the children's mental health in multicultural families." *J Korean Acad Psychiatr Ment Health Nurs* 2014;23:1–11.
43. Park M. "Mothers' Korean proficiency and children's self-esteem in multi-cultural families." *Health Soc Welfare Rev* 2010;30:193–218.
44. Rhee JY, Lee JY. "The influence of stress for cultural adaptation of mothers of multicultural families on children's emotional and behavioral problems." *Counsel Psychol Educ Welfare* 2016;3:19–27.
45. Park HS. "Mediated effects of acculturative stress and maternal parenting stress on internalized problems of children in multicultural families: focused on the mediating role of mothers' depression." *J School Soc Work* 2014;27:353–376.
46. Lee S. "A study of longitudinal changes and relevant factors of multicultural acceptability attitudes amongst multiethnic adolescents." *Stud Korean Youth* 2018;29:179–208.
47. Chung GH, Lim JY. "Marriage immigrant mothers' experience of perceived discrimination, maternal depression, parenting behaviors, and adolescent psychological adjustment among multicultural families in South Korea." *J Child Family Stud* 2016;25:2894–2903.
48. Jin EY. "Mediating effect of bicultural competence in the relationship between acculturative stress of children in multi-cultural families and psychosocial adjustment: focusing on gender difference." *J School Soc Work* 2015;32:303–326.
49. Lee J, Cheon YM, Wei X, Chung GH. "The role of ethnic socialization, ethnic identity and self-esteem: implications for FBI-ethnic adolescents' school adjustment." *J Child Family Stud* 2018;27:3831–3841.
50. Choi WS. "Personal characteristics, ethnic identity, experience of discrimination, self-esteem, and problem behavior of Korean-Japanese multicultural adolescents." *Korean J Family Welfare* 2012;17:49–71.
51. Jiang H, Bae EK. "The relationship between acculturation stress of adolescents in multicultural families and their psychological maladjustment: focus on the moderating effects of resilience." *J Korean Soc Child Welfare* 2018;62:131–164.
52. Park GR, Son I, Kim SS. "Perceived ethnic discrimination and depressive symptoms among biethnic adolescents in South Korea." *J Prev Med Publ Health* 2016;49:301–307.
53. Kim SG. "The psycho-social adaptation among children of multi-cultural families." *Korean J Youth Stud* 2011;18:247–272.
54. Song SR, Park M. "Social rejection and withdrawal behaviors experienced by children in multicultural families: the mediating role of dual identity." *J Future Soc Work Res* 2018;9:65–96.
55. Kim SG. "A study on influencing factors on self-esteem of multi-cultural families children in Korea." *Korean J Youth Stud* 2012;19:109–128.
56. Seol KO, Hwang D, Sim J. "Multicultural children's perceived discrimination, internalized stigma and self-esteem: a moderated mediating effect of ethnic identity." *Korean J Develop Psychol* 2018;31:71–90.
57. Yun G, Yang M. "A study on influencing to prediction risk factors of the delinquency experience on juvenile of multicultural." *Korean Police Stud Rev* 2015;14:313–338.

58. Kim EG, Kim JN. "The relationships between multi-cultural adolescents' acculturation stress and psycho-social adjustment: the mediating effect of ego-identity and the moderating effect of perceived social support." *Multicult Educ Stud* 2016;9:21–43.
59. Cho Y. "Externalizing behaviors in multicultural children of immigrant mothers: a mediation model." *J Family Issues* 2017;38:904–920.
60. Lee Y, Park R, Lee S. "A study about bicultural acceptance attitude and psychological adaption, school adaption of adolescents in multi-cultural family." *J Educ Cult* 2017;23:347–372.
61. Lee YJ. "A study on the risk factors influencing psychosocial adjustment of a multicultural family adolescent." *Korean J Family Welfare* 2009;14:103–119.
62. Alegria M, Vallas M, Pumariega AJ. "Racial and ethnic disparities in pediatric mental health." *Child Adolesc Psychiatr Clin N Am* 2010;19:759–774.
63. Alegría M, Green JG, McLaughlin K, Loder S. *Disparities in Child and Adolescent Mental Health and Mental Health Services in the U.S.* New York, NY: William T. Grant Foundation, 2015.
64. Anderson ER, Mayes LC. "Race/ethnicity and internalizing disorders in youth: a review." *Clin Psychol Rev* 2010;30:338–348.
65. Brown JS, Meadows SO, Elder GH. "Race-ethnic inequality and psychological distress: depressive symptoms from adolescence to young adulthood." *Dev Psychol* 2007;43:1295–1311.
66. Choi GY, Byoun SJ. "Domestic violence against migrant women in South Korea: addressing the needs of a uniquely situated victim population in domestic violence policy." *Int Soc Work* 2014;57:645–660.
67. Karlsen S, Nazroo JY. "Relation between racial discrimination, social class, and health among ethnic minority groups." *Am J Publ Health* 2002;92:624–631.
68. Williams DR, Yan Yu, Jackson JS, Anderson NB. "Racial differences in physical and mental health." *J Health Psychol* 1997;2:335–351.
69. Portes A, MacLeod D. "Educational progress of children of immigrants: the roles of class, ethnicity, and school context." *Sociol Educ* 1996;69:255–275.
70. Bøe T, Øverland S, Lundervold AJ, Hysing M. "Socioeconomic status and children's mental health: results from the Bergen Child Study." *Soc Psychiatry Psychiatr Epidemiol* 2012;47:1557–1566.
71. Hammen C, Shih JH, Brennan PA. "Intergenerational transmission of depression: test of an interpersonal stress model in a community sample." *J Consult Clin Psychol* 2004;72:511–522.
72. Beardslee WR, Versage EM, Gladstone TR. "Children of affectively ill parents: a review of the past 10 years." *J Am Acad Child Adolesc Psychiatry* 1998;37:1134–1141.
73. Han S, Xue Y, Cheng C, Park Y. "Relationships among immigrant women's perceived social support, acculturation stress, and their children's school adjustment." *Korean J Educ Methodol Stud* 2017;29:1–23.
74. Kia-Keating M, Dowdy E, Morgan ML, Noam GG. "Protecting and promoting: an integrative conceptual model for healthy development of adolescents." *J Adolesc Health* 2011;48:220–228.

75. Park S, Lee Y, Jang H, Jo M. "Violence victimization in Korean adolescents: risk factors and psychological problems." *Int J Environ Res Publ Health* 2017;14:E541.
76. Parker JG, Asher SR. "Peer relations and later personal adjustment: are low-accepted children at risk?" *Psychol Bull* 1987;102:357–389.
77. Hymel S, Rubin KH, Rowden L, LeMare L. "Children's peer relationships: longitudinal prediction of internalizing and externalizing problems from middle to late childhood." *Child Develop* 1990;61:2004–2021.
78. Arseneault L, Bowes L, Shakoor S. "Bullying victimization in youths and mental health problems: 'much ado about nothing'?" *Psychol Med* 2010;40:717–729.
79. Kim S, Jeon S. "School adaptation according to multicultural characteristics of children from multicultural families." *Study Child-Family Ther* 2012;10:53–67.
80. Walton GM, Cohen GL. "A brief social-belonging intervention improves academic and health outcomes of minority students." *Science* 2011;331:1447–1451.
81. Kraemer HC, Stice E, Kazdin A, Offord D, Kupfer D. "How do risk factors work together? Mediators, moderators, and independent, overlapping, and proxy risk factors." *Am J Psychiatry* 2001;158:848–856.
82. Garland AF, Lau AS, Yeh M, McCabe KM, Hough RL, Landsverk JA. "Racial and ethnic differences in utilization of mental health services among high-risk youths." *Am J Psychiatry* 2005;162:1336–1343.
83. Jeong M. "The effect of multicultural adolescent's self-resilience on mental health." *Korean J Youth Stud* 2015;22:137–162.
84. Jwa DH. "A research on the psycho-social adaptation characteristics of immigrant youths based on nationality and acculturation types." *Korean J Youth Stud* 2014;21:97–126.
85. Kim HM, Won SJ, Choi SH. "Experiences of discrimination and psychological distress of children from multicultural families: examining the mediating effect of social support." *Korean J Soc Welfare Stud* 2011;42:117–149.
86. Moon SH, An HJ. "Anger, anger expression, mental health and psychosomatic symptoms of children in multi-cultural families." *J Korean Acad Psychiatr Ment Health Nurs* 2011;20:325–333.
87. Lemmens JS, Valkenburg PM, Peter J. "Development and validation of a game addiction scale for adolescents." *Media Psychol* 2009;12:77–95.

Index

About the Editors and Contributors

Sou Hyun Jang is an assistant professor in the Department of Sociology at Sungkyunkwan University (SKKU), Seoul, South Korea. She received her PhD in Sociology from the Graduate Center of the City University of New York (CUNY). Before joining SKKU, she worked as a postdoctoral fellow in the Department of Health Services at the University of Washington and the Fred Hutchinson Cancer Research Center. Her research interests include transnational healthcare behaviors and social determinants of health disparities. She is the author of *Medical Transnationalism: Korean Immigrants' Medical Tourism to South Korea* (Lexington Books, 2018), which examines how Korean immigrants' medical transnationalism is related to their barriers to health care in the United States and other fields of transnationalism. Her previous works focusing on medical transnationalism appeared in *Social Science and Medicine, American Journal of Health Behavior, Journal of Immigrant and Minority Health,* and *International Journal of Health Services.*

Joong-Hwan Oh is a professor of sociology at Hunter College of the City University of New York (CUNY). He received his BA in sociology from Pusan National University (South Korea) and his MA and PhD from the University of South Carolina in Sociology. He teaches a wide range of courses, including urban sociology, the sociology of online communities, Asians in the United States, and peopling in New York City at Hunter College. His substantive areas of expertise in sociology are immigration, urban communities, online social networks, racial and ethnic inequalities, and East Asia. He is the author of *Examining the Use of Online Social Networks by Korean Graduate Students: Navigating Intercultural Academic Experiences* (Routledge, 2019), and *Immigration and Social Capital in the Age of Social Media: Messages of the American Social Institutions on a Korean-American*

Women's Online Community (Lexington Books, 2016). In these broad fields of his academic research, his work also appeared in more than twenty peer-reviewed journals, such as *International Migration Review*, *Urban Studies*, *New Media & Society*, *Social Science & Medicine*, *Asian Women*, *American Journal of Economics and Sociology*, and *Sociological Inquiry*.

Kimin Kwon is a specialist in the Department of Occupational and Environmental Medicine at Hansin Medipia Medical Health Promotion, Seoul, South Korea. He received him MD from the University of Ajou. Before joining Hansin Medipia, he worked as a public doctor in the Uiseoung Medical Center.

Jae Bum Park is a professor in the Department of Occupational and Environmental Medicine at Ajou University, Suwon, South Korea. He received his PhD in medicine from the Graduate School of Ajou University. His research interests include occupational stress, health effect of noise, and health problems among precarious workers. His previous works focusing on occupational health appeared in Annals of Occupational and Environmental Medicine and Industrial Health.

Kyung-Jong Lee is a professor in the Department of Occupational and Environmental Medicine at Ajou University Hospital.

Yoon-Sik Cho is an occupational environmental medicine specialist and works at Ajou University Hospital. He graduated from Ajou University School of Medicine, completed his training course at Ajou University Hospital, and is currently completing his PhD at Ajou University Graduate School. He is the author of "Short rest between shifts and risk of hypertension in hospital workers" (*Journal of Hypertension*, 2019), which examines the relevance of workers' working conditions to their health. His previous studies on workers' health have been published in *Annals of Occupational and Environmental Medicine*, *Industrial Health*, and *Journal of Hypertension*.

Sehee Han holds a MA in public administration from Hanyang University.

Heaseung Kim obtained her PhD in political science from Ewha Woman's University in 1990.

Hee-Sun Lee is a professor of public administration at Hanyang University. He received his PhD in public administration from the University of Pittsburgh in 1989. His research interests include research methods and public policy analysis. He has published over eighty peer-reviewed articles.

TaeJin Lee is a professor in the Department of Health Policy and Management at Seoul National University. He received his PhD in Health Services Management from the University of Manchester in 2000. His research interests include economic evaluation of health technology and equity in healthcare financing.

Yang Heui Ahn is a professor in the Department of Nursing at Yonsei University Wonju College of Medicine. She received her PhD Nursing from Yonsei University.

Ok Kyung Ham is a professor in the Department of Nursing at Inha University. She received her PhD in Health Sciences from Texas Woman's University in 2002.

Soo Hyun Kim is a professor in the Department of Nursing at Inha University. She received her PhD in Nursing from Yonsei University in 2008.

Chang Gi Park is a research assistant professor in the Department of Health Systems Science at University of Illinois at Chicago.

Jun-Taek Song is affiliated with the Department of Occupational Environmental Medicine at Kyung Hee University Hospital.

Goeun Lee is a doctor of occupational environmental medicine. She was trained at Kyung Hee University Hospital and received her MPH from the Graduate School of Catholic University. She works in the Korea Workers' Compensation & Welfare Service Ansan Hospital, Ansan, Gyeonggi, South Korea. She is interested in occupational disease and workers' psychological health of work place and epidemiological research.

Jongho Kwon is affiliated with the Department of Occupational Environmental Medicine at Kyung Hee University Hospital.

Jung-Woo Park is affiliated with the Department of Occupational Environmental Medicine at Kyung Hee University Hospital.

Hyunrim Choi is a professor in the Department of Occupational Environmental Medicine at Kyung Hee University Hospital.

Sinye Lim is an associate professor in the Department of Occupational Environmental Medicine at Kyung Hee University Hospital. She received her MPH and PhD in Public Health from Seoul National University.

Jin-soo Park is affiliated with the Department of Occupational Environmental Medicine at Kyung Hee University Hospital.

Seyoung Kim is affiliated with the Department of Occupational Environmental Medicine at Kyung Hee University Hospital.

Chulin Baek is a chief in the Department of Occupational & Environment Medicine at Shihwa Medical Center, Siheung, South Korea. Before joining Shihwa Medical Center, he completed the residency program in the department of Occupational & Environment Medicine at Ajou University Hospital and received master's degree in Public Health from the Ajou University Graduate School of Public Health.

Kyungjong Lee is a professor in the Department of Occupational and Environmental Medicine at Ajou University, Suwon, South Korea. He received his Dr. PH from The Graduate School of Yonsei University. His research interests include occupational diseases and health care for workers. His previous works focusing on occupational health appeared in *American Journal of Public Health, and Industrial Health.*

Jaehyuk Jung is an occupational and environmental medicine physician and currently serving as a short-term medical officer in the Republic of Korea navy. He received his MD from Ajou University School of Medicine, Suwon, South Korea. He received his M.P.H. in safety promotion and occupational health from Ajou University Graduate School of Public Health, Suwon, South Korea. His research interests include effects of occupational stress on health of workers.

Sujin Hong is affiliated with the Department of Occupational Medicine at Korea University Hospital.

Harin Jeong is affiliated with the Department of Occupational Medicine at Korea University Hospital.

Yunjeong Heo is professor in the Department of Humanities and Social Medicine at Ajou University.

Hosun Chun is affiliated with the Department of Occupational Medicine at Korea University Hospital.

Jongtae Park, MD, MPH, PhD, is director of Center of Occupational and Environmental Medicine, Korea University Anan-Hospital. He graduated from college of Medicine, Korea University and trained in Preventive Medicine & Occupational and Environmental Medicine. He also obtained master's degree in Public health from Seoul National University. He has been performing health examinations for workers and evaluation of work-relatedness & fitness for work. He has built up the Workers Health Center of Gyeonggi-Seobu to provide Occupational Health Services for small-scale workplaces since 2011. His research interests include workplace health risk assessment and management of occupational health services.

Daeseong Kim is clinical professor in the Department of Occupational Medicine at Korea University Hospital.

Jungsun Park is professor in the Department of Occupational Health at Catholic University of Daegu.

Soo Geun Kim is professor in the Department of Occupational Medicine at Kangbuk Samsung Hospital and Sungkyunkwan University.

Jong-shik Park is affiliated with Yonsei University.

Boyoung Han is affiliated with Yonsei University.

Kab Bae Kim is affiliated with Occupational Safety and Health Research Institute, Korea Occupational Safety and Health Agency.

Yangho Kim is a professor in the Department of Occupational and Environmental Medicine at Ulsan University Hospital, University of Ulsan College of Medicine, Ulsan, South Korea. He received his PhD in medicine from Kumamoto University in Japan. Before joining University of Ulsan, he worked as a senior researcher in the Occupational Safety & Health Research Institute (OSHRI) at the Korea Occupational Safety and Health Agency (KOSHA). His research interests include occupational safety and health in vulnerable workers in Korea.

Seonhye Lee is a professor in the Department of Nursing at Gyeongnam National University of Science and Technology.

Chang Heon Cheong is a professor in the Department of Architectural Engineering at Gyeongnam National University of Science and Technology.

Jimee Kim is an assistant professor in the Department of Nursing at Dongnam Health University. She received her PhD in nursing from the department of nursing of Hanyang University. Her research interests include the relationship between health and environment, and the health inequality that can occur among them.

Jaeeon Yoo graduated from Iowa State University with a PhD in Human Development and Family Studies (Minor in Women's Studies and Gerontology) and served as an associate research fellow at the Korea Institute for Health and Social Affairs. He is now an assistant professor in the Department of Social Welfare at Gachon University.

Hyoung-Ryoul Kim is a professor in the Department of Occupational and Environmental Medicine, College of Medicine at the Catholic University Korea.

Kyungwon Choi is an assistant professor in the Department of Nursing at Korea National University of Transportation. She received her PhD from Seoul National University in 2010. Her research interests are in the field of gender differences in health behaviors and well-being, and frail elderly. Previous works on gender differences in health outcome appeared in the journals *Asian Pacific Psychiatry* and *International Journal of Environmental Research and Public Health.* Articles related to frailty of the elderly were published in *Journal of Aging and Health, Journal of Women and Aging, and International Journal of Environmental Research and Public Health.*

Hyekyeong Kim is an associate professor in the Department of Health Convergence at Ewha Woman's University.

Seunghyun Yoo is a professor of Cities, Communities & Health Promotion in the Graduate School of Public Health at Seoul National University, Seoul, South Korea. She received her Dr PH in Community Health Sciences from Tulane University School of Public Health & Tropical Medicine in New Orleans, Louisiana. Her research interests include urban-built environment and community health, perceived environment and community participation, partnership building, and qualitative research methods. Her current work focuses on developing qualitative multimethods to explore urban mobility of older adults, and integrating such approaches into comprehensive qualitative GIS. Dr. Yoo collaborates on public health training internationally, with the University of Tokyo Graduate School of Medicine and Nagasaki University School of Tropical Medicine & Global Health in Japan.

Seon Cho is affiliated with Health Promotion Research Institute, Korea Association of Health Promotion.

Eun-Joo Kwon is affiliated with Health Promotion Research Institute, Korea Association of Health Promotion.

Suyoung Kim is affiliated with Health Promotion Research Institute, Korea Association of Health Promotion.

Ji-Youn Park is affiliated with Health Promotion Research Institute, Korea Association of Health Promotion.

Yeeun Lee is affiliated with the Department of Psychology at Korea University.

Minji Lee is affiliated with Clinical Research Center, Mental Health Research Institute at the National Center for Mental Health.

Subin Park is affiliated with Department of Research Planning, Mental Health Research Institute at the National Center for Mental Health. She received her PhD in neuropsychiatry in 2012 and her major interests are in child and adolescent psychiatry and social psychiatry.

www.ingramcontent.com/pod-product-compliance
Ingram Content Group UK Ltd.
Pitfield, Milton Keynes, MK11 3LW, UK
UKHW020839290926
15470UKWH00004B/1441

9 781793 632104